CONTRIBUTORS

Editor-in-Chief

P.M. Kris-Etherton, PhD, RD

Associate Editors

Patricia Volz-Clarke, MS, RD, Kristine Clark, MS, RD, Anne M. Dattilo, PhD, RD

Technical Editor

Mary E. Russell, MS

Research Committee

Debra Krummel, PhD, RD, *Chair*, Kim Bibow, MS, RD, Catherine F. Flanagan, MS, RD, Cynthia Gorczyca, MA, RD, Alice Henneman, MS, RD, Janet Horowitz, MS, RD, Christopher Karam, MS, RD, Roseanne Scott Liebhart, Gail Mark, Linda McDonald, RD, Ann Mesaros, RD, Carol Forsythe Hall, MEd, RD, Margaret S. Raymond, RD, Josephine Reisman, MS, RD, Karen Reznik, MS, RD, Karen Ross, MA, RD, Karen G. Schwartz, MS, RD, Tracy Taylor-Baker, RD, Susan Weiner, MS, RD

Writing Committee

Darlene Dreon, MS, MPH, RD, *Chair*, Jane Andrews, MS, RD, Patricia Booth, MS, RD, Daniele Brauchi, RD, Susan Bryant, RD, Marilyn Buzzard, PhD, Sonja L. Connor, MS, RD, Zakera Chowdhury, MS, RD, Janice Daly, RD, Dottie Dolezal, RD, Maria Donohue, MS, RD, Bethene Ervin, MS, RD, Gail C. Frank, DPH, MPH, RD, Barbara Frey-Hewitt, MS, Joyce Ann Gilbert, MS, RD, Karen Glanz, PhD, MPH, Randall Gretebeck, PhD, RD, Lauren Hatcher, MS, RD, Lisa Hill, RD, Janine M. Hughes, MS, RD, Steve L. Ink, PhD, RD, Rita Johnson, MS, RD, James J. Kenney, PhD, RD, Bela Lauber, MS, RD, Lisa Martin, RD, Linda S. McDonald, RD, John B. McKinlay, PhD, Mary Carol McMann, MPH, Carolyn Moore, PhD, RD, Rebecca Mullis, PhD, RD, Suzanne P. Murphy, PhD, RD, Alison Murray, RD, Anne O'Donnell, MPH, RD, Sally Ortiz, RD, Donna Payne, PhD, RD, Patricia Peterson, MS, RD, Shirley K. Powell, MS, RD, Cindy Ragin, Lynne W. Scott, MA, RD, Marilyn Schorin, PhD, RD, Ann R. Semenske, MD, RD, Peg Seng, MA, RD, Raksha Shah, MS, RD, Ann Marie Sherry, RD, Kevin W. Smith, MA, Anastasia Snelling, RD, Joyce L. Sokolik, MS, RD, Anne H. Snyder, RD, Kristi Thurber, RD, Rachael Trevethan, RD, Linda V. Van Horn, PhD, RD, Laura Walsh, Sarah E. Whitis, MS, RD, RN, Monika Woolsey, RD

Editing Committee

Kathie M. Swift, MS, RD and Ellen Coleman, MA, MPH, RD, *Chairs*, Nadine Braunstein, MS, RD, Anne-Marie Davee, MS, RD, Mary A. Engelland, MEd, RD, Wanema Frye, MS, RD, Evette M. Hackman, PhD, RD, Janice Henske, MPH, RD, Jacqueline B. Marcus, MS, RD, Terry Galvin Matthews, MS, RD, Linda Zorn Newcomb, MA, RD, Diane Petruska, RD, Iris Plafker, RD, Jay Rush, Lynne W. Scott, MA, RD, Lisa E. Smith, RD, Amy Tuttle, RD, Lori Valencia, MEd, RD, LD, Linda V. Van Horn, PhD, RD, Martha Wilkins, MS, RD

Expert Review Committee

June Alberici, MS, Jane Andrews, MS, RD, Sonja Connor, MS, RD, Barbara H. Dennis, PhD, RD, Dottie Dolezal, MS, RD, Karen Donato, MS, RD, Ginny Dowd, Nancy Ernst, MS, RD, Joyce Gilbert, MS, RD, Evette M. Hackman, PhD, RD, Karen Hare, RD, Jeanette V. Harris, MS, RD, Carolyn Crimmins Hintlian, MPH, RD, Steve L. Ink, PhD, RD, Ruth Johnson, MS, RD, James J. Kenney, PhD, RD, Debra Krummel, PhD, RD, Kathy McManus, MS, RD, Joanne Milkereit, MHSA, RD, Jayne L. Newmark, MS, RD, Lorraine Partlow, RD, Karen Reznik, MS, RD, Jay Rush, Lynne Scott, MS, RD, Marilyn Schorin, PhD, RD, Lisa Stollman, MA, RD, Linda Van Horn, PhD, RD, Patricia Volz-Clarke, MS, RD

SCAN Publications Review Committee

Jackie Berning, MS, RD, Kristine Clark, MS, RD, Karen Hare, RD, Jeanette V. Harris, MS, RD, Joanne Milkereit, MHSA, RD, Lorraine Partlow, RD, Karen Reznik, MS, RD, Madelyn Wheeler, RD

Support Staff

Elaine McDonnell, Vikkie Mustad, MS, Debbie Salabsky

Typist

Nancy Hopkins

TABLE OF CONTENTS

PREFACE

This second SCAN manual, *Cardiovascular Disease: Nutrition for Prevention and Treatment,* was developed for registered dietitians whose efforts are directed toward the prevention and treatment of coronary heart disease (CHD).* We hope it will help dietitians become more effective interventionists in dealing with both individuals and groups.

The manual is divided into four parts. Part 1 (chapters 1 through 3) offers scientific background on coronary heart disease, with chapters on CHD risk factors, the relationship between diet and CHD, and lipoprotein metabolism.

Part 2, Nutrition Intervention (chapters 4 through 8), offers practical information, with chapters on nutritional assessment, the prevention and treatment of CHD by diet, the nutritional management of cardiac surgery patients, pediatric prevention and treatment, and weight management.

Part 3, Treatment Approaches for CHD (chapters 9 through 12), provides additional intervention information, with chapters on exercise intervention, behavior-modification strategies, and drug treatment. Chapter 12 offers an overview of cardiac rehabilitation that may be useful to dietitians who would like to become professionally active in their communities.

Chapter 13, Resources, lists a multitude of publications and organizations that can provide further information. Finally, the appendix (chapter 14) contains additional tables, guidelines, and recommendations.

As we health professionals embark on the major undertaking of reducing coronary heart disease in the United States, we will need information and strategies to achieve the goal. Help us with future revisions of this manual by letting us know what you found useful and what more is needed. We value your expertise and opinions.

Address your comments to: Editors, SCAN CV Manual, The American Dietetic Association, 216 W. Jackson Boulevard, Suite 800, Chicago, IL 60606-6995.

ACKNOWLEDGMENTS

We are indebted to the leadership of SCAN for providing assistance and encouragement throughout the development and preparation of this manual. We offer thanks to the four SCAN chairpersons who were involved: Janet Horowitz, Jacqueline Marcus, Jean Storlie, and Jeannette Harris. In addition, many SCAN members gave generously of their time at a moment's notice. Without their dedicated and enthusiastic participation, the production of this manual would not have been possible.

This manual has truly been a group effort. For us, in particular, it has been a professionally rewarding experience. We feel privileged to have had the opportunity to interact with so many talented professionals.

*The first SCAN manual, *Sports Nutrition: A Guide for the Professional Working With Active People,* was published in 1986.

We would like to thank Barbara Wellsteed for her fruitful comments during the manual's developmental stages. To Nancy Hopkins, words are inadequate to describe our gratitude and appreciation for her perseverance and stamina while typing the manuscript.

We would also like to thank Dr. Helen Guthrie, head of the Nutrition Department at The Pennsylvania State University, for providing an environment that enabled this manual to be written. We applaud the efforts of nutritionists at the Penn State Nutrition Center who patiently reviewed countless files to collect resources (tables, figures, and so on). We are also grateful to the Publications Department staff of The American Dietetic Association for their help.

For all of us, this project has been a family effort, as our spouses (and children) offered support and encouragement in many special ways. Terry Etherton contributed countless hours of writing, editing, and proofreading. Mark and Phillip Etherton deserve special recognition for their patience and understanding. Noel Clarke good-naturedly shared his home with piles of manuscript, while Barry Clark lost a devoted cycling companion. John Dattilo, unaware that this project would occupy part of his first year of marriage, nevertheless showed continued support.

Without the professional involvement, commitment, and enthusiasm of everyone involved, this manual would not have come to fruition. We sincerely thank you all.

Penny Kris-Etherton
Pat Volz-Clarke
Kris Clark
Anne Dattilo

INTRODUCTION*

Despite a considerable decrease in the incidence of coronary heart disease (CHD) since the late 1960s, it still remains the leading cause of death in the United States. Nearly 50% of all deaths are due to cardiovascular disease (CVD)[1]; in fact, many health professionals identify CVD as one of the major public health problems in the United States. In 1986 nearly 1 million Americans died from heart and blood-vessel diseases, while approximately the same number died from all other causes combined.[1] One fifth of deaths attributed to CVD and 45% of all heart attacks occur in people younger than 65.[1] Both the prevalence and economic cost of CVD are staggering; almost 66 million Americans are affected.[1] The American Heart Association estimates that the cost of CVD in 1989 was $88.2 billion.[1]

High blood cholesterol is a major modifiable risk factor for CHD. Clinical investigations and numerous epidemiological, animal-experimental, human-migration, and human-pathology studies have clearly established a strong positive association between elevated blood cholesterol levels and the prevalence and incidence of CHD. Until recently, the missing link in the lipid hypothesis has been conclusive evidence demonstrating that lowering cholesterol reduces the incidence of CHD. While numerous clinical trials demonstrated beneficial effects of cholesterol lowering on CHD morbidity and mortality, none provided unequivocal evidence, largely because of experimental design and methodological problems. Recently, however, results from the Lipid Research Clinics Coronary Primary Prevention Trial,[2,3] the Oslo Heart Trial,[4] the Leiden Intervention Trial,[5] the National Heart, Lung and Blood Institute's Type II Coronary Intervention Study,[6] and the Cholesterol-Lowering Atherosclerosis Study[7] have demonstrated the efficacy of cholesterol lowering in the primary and secondary prevention of CHD. These landmark investigations are of major importance to the practice of medicine and dietetics.

Although considerable attention has been focused on cholesterol lowering, other modifiable risk factors for CHD have also been identified. Two of these factors are linked to nutrition practices: obesity and hypertension. Other strong nonnutrition risk factors include cigarette smoking and physical inactivity.

The Lipid Research Clinics Coronary Primary Prevention Trial (LRC-CPPT)[2,3] is the first major double-blind, controlled clinical investigation to demonstrate unequivocally the benefits of cholesterol lowering on CHD morbidity and mortality. A total of 3,806 asymptomatic middle-aged men with primary hypercholesterolemia were randomly allocated to one of two groups. Both groups followed a moderate cholesterol-lowering diet (containing approximately 35% of kilocalories from fat, less than 300 mg cholesterol daily, and a polyunsaturated to saturated fatty acid ratio—P/S—of 0.7). Men in the treatment and control groups received bile acid sequestrant (cholestyramine) and a placebo, respectively, for an average of 7.4 years. Plasma total-cholesterol and LDL-cholesterol levels were reduced 13.4% and 20.3%, respectively. A 19% reduction in CHD risk ($p < 0.05$), defined by definite CHD death, definite nonfatal myocardial infarction, or both, was reported for the treatment group. Larger reductions in CHD risk were reported with a greater lowering in plasma total cholesterol and LDL cholesterol. Specifically, a 25% reduction in plasma total cholesterol and a 35% reduction in LDL cholesterol (typical responses to

*By P. M. Kris-Etherton

cholestyramine therapy) were associated with a 49% reduction in the incidence of CHD. The results of this trial have shown that even small changes in plasma total cholesterol can beneficially affect CHD incidence. A 1% reduction in plasma total cholesterol is associated with a 2% reduction in CHD risk.

The Oslo Heart Trial[4] provides further support for the benefits of cholesterol lowering in the primary prevention of CHD. In this study, dietary intervention (28% of kilocalories from fat, dietary cholesterol less than 300 mg daily, and a P/S of 1.0) was associated with a 13% reduction in plasma total cholesterol. Diet modification in conjunction with a reduction in cigarette smoking resulted in a 47% decrease in cardiovascular events. Of this, 60% was attributed to dietary-induced cholesterol lowering. Taken together, the results of the Oslo Heart Trial and the LRC-CPPT provide strong evidence for a causal role of plasma cholesterol in the pathogenesis of CHD. Moreover, the Oslo Heart Trial strongly implicates diet in the primary prevention of CHD.

Diet intervention is also efficacious in the secondary prevention of CHD. Two years of rigorous dietary intervention (vegetarian diet, less than 100 mg cholesterol daily, and a P/S of 2.0) prevented atherosclerotic lesion growth in 18 of the 39 participants of the Leiden Intervention Trial.[5] Coronary lesion growth was related to initial plasma lipids and changes in plasma lipids, apparently mediated by diet. In the National Heart, Lung and Blood Institute's Type II Coronary Intervention Study,[6] significant reductions in plasma total and LDL cholesterol mediated by drug therapy and diet modification (a P/S of 1.0, with 100 to 200 mg cholesterol daily) were associated with a decrease in atherosclerotic plaque progression in patients with hypercholesterolemia and presumptive evidence of coronary artery disease (myocardial infarction, angina, positive exercise stress test, or coronary calcification on fluoroscopy). Together these studies have shown that rigorous intervention targeted to major modifiable risk factors (ie, an elevated level of plasma total cholesterol and LDL cholesterol) is beneficial in both and primary and secondary prevention of CHD.

More recently, the Cholesterol-Lowering Atherosclerosis Study,[7] a randomized, angiographic drug trial, demonstrated the regression of atherosclerosis in approximately 17% of the subjects in the experimental group who were treated with a diet low in saturated fatty acids, cholesterol, and total fat (26% of calories) and with combined colestipol hydrochloride and niacin therapy. The participants in this study were patients who had undergone coronary artery bypass. Lowering plasma total cholesterol resulted in a significant reduction in the progression of atherosclerosis in the native coronary arteries and new lesion formation in venous bypass grafts. Plasma cholesterol lowering was associated with fewer adverse changes in coronary atherosclerosis and a significantly improved overall coronary status.

These studies have served as an impetus for a number of recent activities and developments in the diet-heart area. In 1984, the National Heart, Lung and Blood Institute convened a Consensus Conference Panel on Lowering Blood Cholesterol to Prevent Heart Disease. A panel of experts reviewed available data on the relationship between blood cholesterol levels and CHD and identified steps that should be taken to treat people with elevated blood cholesterol levels. Recommendations were made for the treatment of elevated blood cholesterol levels.[8] These recommendations were instrumental in beginning a fundamental approach to cholesterol management; *Cholesterol Counts: Steps for Lowering Your Patient's Blood Cholesterol*[9] was published in 1985 by the US Department of Health and Human Services. In 1985 the National Cholesterol Education Program (NCEP) was begun. In October 1987 the NCEP-Adult Treatment Panel (NCEP-ATP) announced guidelines for the detection, evaluation, and treatment of high blood cholesterol.[10]

These events provide remarkable new opportunities to expand the role of the registered dietitian in the health care process. Ernst et al[11] encourage registered dietitians to update their knowledge of how diet affects blood cholesterol levels and to learn the Step One and Step Two diets that are recommended by both the NCEP-ATP and the American Heart Association. Dietitians must be ready to provide Americans with information, education, and guidance on the role of diet in the prevention and treatment of CHD. As practitioners involved in the primary and secondary prevention of CHD, we play a significant role in educating patients on risk-factor management. To achieve this objective, it is essential that dietetic practitioners keep abreast of the advances that are important to our practice.

We must be prepared to intervene aggressively with diet therapy because it costs significantly less than drug treatment.[12] Moreover, side effects associated with diet therapy are virtually nonexistent. With evidence documenting the effectiveness of blood cholesterol lowering on the primary and secondary prevention of CHD and the benefits on overall mortality,[13] we have developed this manual as a resource for dietitians working in CHD prevention and rehabilitation. Nutrition intervention can save lives, especially for people at risk of premature fatal heart attack. Preventive and therapeutic nutrition can also improve the quality of life for many others as well.

References

1. American Heart Association. *1989 Heart Facts.* Dallas, Tex: American Heart Association; 1989.
2. Lipid Research Clinics Program. The Lipid Research Clinics Coronary Primary Prevention Trial results, I: reduction in incidence of coronary heart disease. *JAMA.* 1984; 251:351.
3. Lipid Research Clinics Program. The Lipid Research Clinics Coronary Primary Prevention Trial results, II: relationship of reduction in incidence of coronary heart disease to cholesterol lowering. *JAMA.* 1984; 251:355.
4. Hjermann I, Byre KV, Holme I, et al. Effect of diet and smoking intervention on the incidence of coronary heart disease: report from the Oslo Study Group of a randomized trial in healthy men. *Lancet.* 1981; 2:1303.
5. Arntzenius AC, Kromhout D, Barth J, et al. Diet, lipoproteins, and the progression of coronary atherosclerosis: the Leiden Intervention Trial. *N Engl J Med.* 1985;312:805.
6. Brensike J, Levy R, Kelsey S, et al. Effects of therapy with cholestyramine on progression of coronary arteriosclerosis: results of the NHLBI Type II Coronary Intervention Study. *Circulation.* 1984;69:313.
7. Blankenhorn DH, Nessim SA, Johnson RL, et al. Beneficial effects of combined colestipol-niacin therapy on coronary atherosclerosis and coronary venous bypass grafts. *JAMA.* 1987;257:3233.
8. Consensus Conference. Lowering blood cholesterol to prevent heart disease. *JAMA.* 1985;253:2080.
9. *Cholesterol Counts: Steps for Lowering Your Patient's Blood Cholesterol.* US Dept of Health and Human Services; 1985.
10. National Cholesterol Education Program Expert Panel. Report on detection, evaluation, and treatment of high blood cholesterol in adults. *Arch Intern Med.* 1988;148:36.
11. Ernst ND, Mullis R, Sooter-Bochenek J, et al. The National Cholesterol Education Program: implications for dietetic practitioners from the Adult Treatment Panel Recommendations. *J Am Diet Assoc.* 1988;88:1401.
12. Kinosian B, Eisenberg J. Cutting into cholesterol: cost-effective alternatives for treating hypercholesterolemia. *JAMA.* 1988;259:2249.
13. Carlson LA, Rosenhamer G. Reduction of mortality in the Stockholm Ischaemic Heart Disease Secondary Prevention Study by combined treatment with clofibrate and nicotinic acid. *Acta Med Scand.* 1988;223:405.

Table
Heart-Disease Definitions

angina pectoris — a condition in which transient chest pains occur, especially during exertion, as a result of partial blockage of the coronary arteries and consequent deprivation of an adequate supply of blood and oxygen to a portion of the heart.

aneurysm — dilation of the aorta due to an area of weakening.

arteriosclerosis — a number of pathological conditions in which there is thickening, hardening, and loss of elasticity in the arterial wall.

atherosclerosis — a form of arteriosclerosis consisting of accumulation of lipids, complex carbohydrates, blood products, fibrous tissue, and calcium deposits, which form plaques in the artery wall.

cardiovascular disease (CVD) — any disease pertaining to the heart and blood vessels.

cerebrovascular disease — ischemic (atherothrombotic) stroke and hemorrhagic stroke.

congestive heart disease — damage to myocardium or valves that does not allow normal output of blood flow.

coronary artery disease (CAD) — narrowing of the coronary arteries, preventing adequate blood supply to the myocardium, usually due to atherosclerosis.

coronary heart disease (CHD) — myocardial damage due to insufficient blood supply, caused by pathological changes in coronary arteries.

coronary thrombosis — occlusion of one or more of the coronary arteries of the heart.

hypertensive heart disease — hypertensive cardiomegaly, hypertensive cardiopathy, hypertensive CVD, and hypertensive heart failure.

intermittent claudication — typical pain due to arterial stenosis in a limb, which, when exercised, uses more oxygen than the narrowed artery can supply.

ischemic heart disease — temporary, localized deficiency of the blood supply in the heart.

lipoproteins — particles found in plasma that transport lipids such as cholesterol, triglyceride, and phospholipids. They have a hydrophobic lipid core and a hydrophilic surface comprised of unesterified cholesterol, phospholipids, and apolipoproteins. They are categorized by chemical properties and density.

1. **high-density lipoproteins (HDL)** — a family of protein-rich lipoprotein particles found in the plasma that are involved in reverse cholesterol transport (a process by which cholesterol in peripheral tissues is excreted). HDL comprises two fractions: HDL_3 and HDL_2. HDL_3 is the precursor of HDL_2. HDL_2 is a better predictor of CHD risk than either total HDL or HDL_3.
2. **low-density lipoproteins (LDL)** — cholesterol-rich lipoproteins found in the plasma that account for about 70% of plasma total cholesterol.
3. **intermediate-density lipoproteins (IDL)** — an intermediary lipoprotein that is formed in the catabolism of VLDL to LDL.
4. **very-low-density lipoproteins (VLDL)** — triglyceride-rich lipoproteins found in the plasma that transport triglycerides derived from hepatic synthesis.
5. **chylomicrons** — triglyceride-rich lipoproteins found in the plasma that transport triglycerides of dietary origin.

myocardial infarction (MI) — irreversible myocardial damage resulting from prolonged hypoxia.

plasma — the fluid portion of blood, containing electrolytes, sugars, proteins, lipids, bilirubin, and dissolved gases.

serum — the plasma portion minus factors such as fibrinogen; the clear liquid that separates from blood on clotting.

sudden death — massive MI or ischemia-related electrical instability and fatal arrhythmia; death within 1, 2, or 24 hours of onset of symptoms.

PART 1
SCIENTIFIC BACKGROUND

1. RISK FACTORS FOR CORONARY HEART DISEASE

A risk factor for coronary heart disease (CHD) has been defined as a trait that increases the probability that some manifestation of cardiovascular disease (CVD) will develop.[1] Coronary risk factors are both statistically and causally related to CHD. Thus, identified CHD risk factors are: (1) statistical correlates of CHD, (2) factors that cause CHD, and/or (3) personal characteristics that predispose a person to CHD.

Coronary risk factors have been identified through evidence derived from an enormous number of studies that used many different scientific approaches. The research conducted involved studies of animal models, epidemiological and observational studies, and clinical investigations. Coronary risk factors are frequently classified into two groups: well-established risk factors and "other" risk factors.[2] Well-established risk factors are cigarette smoking, high blood cholesterol, high blood pressure, and diabetes mellitus.[2] Other factors that may affect CHD risk include physical inactivity, obesity, stress, and certain drugs.[2]

Coronary risk factors can be classified as either unmodifiable or modifiable. Unmodifiable risk factors include genetic predisposition (family history), gender, hormonal factors, and age. Modifiable risk factors include plasma lipids, blood pressure, weight, diabetes, cigarette smoking, physical activity, stress, personality type, and oral contraceptive use. Risk factors often cluster and the effect is usually synergistic rather than additive. A brief discussion of the major coronary risk factors follows. In addition, the risk of CHD when more than one risk factor is present is addressed.

UNMODIFIABLE RISK FACTORS*

Family History and Genetic Predisposition

The risk of CVD is two to five times higher in people with familial hyperlipidemia and a family history of premature CHD than in people without such family histories.[3,4] It is not known whether the clustering of CHD within families is simply due to higher levels of known risk factors in these families.[1] For example, an elevated plasma total-cholesterol or LDL-cholesterol level may be a genetic condition that affects the pathophysiology of atherosclerosis or other related diseases. Behavioral factors that affect coronary risk factors (eg, weight, physical activity, diet) can also contribute to the familial aggregation of coronary events.

Data from the Framingham Study demonstrated that CHD clustered in families.[1] In men, a significant sibling association for CHD was reported after taking other risk factors into account.[1] Coronary mortality in grandparents was related to the serum and lipoprotein cholesterol levels of their grandchildren.[4] Specifically, the presence of CHD in grandfathers was correlated to the grandchildren's plasma total-cholesterol, LDL-cholesterol, and HDL-cholesterol levels.[4]

The genetic link to CHD has been most clearly demonstrated in children who have homozygous familial hypercholesterolemia, a rare disorder afflicting fewer than 250 children in America.[5] This disease is characterized by a markedly elevated LDL-cholesterol level, which may be as high as

*By Kristi Thurber

1,000 mg/dL. CHD frequently develops in these children and adolescents during the first two decades of life. Prevalence of the heterozygous form of familial hypercholesterolemia is about 1 in 500 people.[5] Premature CHD usually develops in those with heterozygous familial hypercholesterolemia in the middle decades of life.[6] LDL cholesterol is usually above the 90th percentile in affected people.

Table 1.1
Types of Primary Hyperlipoproteinemia

Type	Lipid Abnormalities	Lipoprotein Abnormalities*	Usual Age of Expression	Familial Forms	Some Clinical Features
I: Familial hyperchylomicronemia	Cholesterol: normal or elevated Triglyceride: elevated (>1000 mg/100 mL)	Severe chylomicronemia	Infancy and childhood	Rare and usually familial (recessive)	Bouts of abdominal pain, pancreatitis, eruptive xanthomas, hepatosplenomegaly.
IIa: Familial hypercholesterolemia	Cholesterol: elevated (300–600 mg/100mL) Triglyceride: normal	LDL increased	At birth, if genetic	Most obvious genetic form is expressed in heterozygote, more severe in homozygote; many mild examples are not obviously familial	Premature vascular disease; in familial forms, tendon and tuberous xanthomas
IIb or III: Familial combined hyperlipidemia	Cholesterol: elevated (300–600 mg/100 mL) Triglyceride: elevated (150–1000 mg/100 mL)	IIb—LDL increased, plus excess VLDL III—increased ILDL	Adulthood (over age 20)	Frequently familial and if so appears recessive, sporadic	Glucose intolerance, tuberoeruptive or planar xanthomas, premature vascular disease (especially peripheral vascular disease); worsened by alcohol excess
IV: Familial endogenous hypertriglyceridemia	Cholesterol: normal or elevated Triglyceride: elevated (400–1000 mg/100 mL)	VLDL increased	Usually third decade or later; can occur in children	When genetic, is dominant; sporadic	Glucose intolerance in about 50%, excess caloric intake common; occasionally eruptive xanthomas, hyperuricemia; worsened by alcohol excess; accelerated by coronary vessel disease
V: Mixed hyperlipemia	Cholesterol: elevated Triglyceride: elevated (>1000 mg/100 mL)	VLDL increased, chylomicrons present	Adulthood, very rare in children	When familial, more than half of close relatives have either type IV or type V	Bouts of abdominal pain and pancreatitis, eruptive xanthomas, hepatosplenomegaly, excess caloric intake common, hyperuricemia; most patients have glucose intolerance; worsened by alcohol excess

*LDL = low-density lipoproteins; VLDL = very-low-density lipoproteins; ILDL = intermediate-low-density lipoproteins.

Adapted with permission from Levy RI, Fredrickson DS, Shulman R, et al. Dietary and drug treatment of primary hyperlipoproteinemia. *Ann Intern Med.* 1972;77:287; and Havel RJ. Approach to the patient with hyperlipidemia. *Med Clin North Am.* 1982;66:319.

Table 1.2
Types and Causes of Primary Hypertriglyceridemia

Type	Lipid Abnormalities	Lipoprotein Abnormalities	Usual Age of Expression	Familial Forms	Clinical Features
I: Familial hyperchylomicronemia (deficiency of lipoprotein lipase or its cofactor, apo C-II)	Cholesterol: normal Triglyceride: elevated (>1000 mg/100 mL) On a typical American diet, lipemia is usually severe (2000–25,000 mg/dL)	Severe chylomicronemia	Infancy and childhood; may go unnoticed until an attack of pancreatitis occurs or lipemic serum is noted; thus, diagnosis may be delayed until as late as middle age	Rare and usually familial (recessive)	Patients are classically not obese and have normal carbohydrate metabolism. Bouts of abdominal pain, pancreatitis, eruptive xanthomas, hepatosplenomegaly. Estrogens intensify the lipemia by stimulating production of VLDL by liver. No apparent increase in the risk of atherosclerosis.
IV: Familial endogenous hypertriglyceridemia	Cholesterol: normal or elevated Triglyceride: elevated (400–1000 mg/dL)	VLDL increased	Third decade or later; can occur in children	When genetic, is dominant; sporadic	Glucose intolerance in about 50%, excess caloric intake common; occasional eruptive xanthomas, hyperuricemia; worsened by alcohol excess; accelerated by coronary vessel disease
V: Mixed hyperlipemia	Cholesterol: elevated Triglyceride: elevated (>1000 mg/dL)	VLDL increased, chylomicrons present	Adulthood, very rare in children	When familial, more than half of close relatives have either type IV or type V	Bouts of abdominal pain and pancreatitis, eruptive xanthomas, hepatosplenomegaly, excess caloric intake common, hyperuricemia; most patients have glucose intolerance; worsened by alcohol excess

Adapted with permission from Levy RI, Fredrickson DS, Shulman R, et al. Dietary and drug treatment of primary hyperlipoproteinemia. *Ann Intern Med.* 1972;77:287; Havel RJ. Approach to the patient with hyperlipidemia. *Med Clin North Am.* 1982;66:319.

The categorization of lipoprotein abnormalities by Fredrickson and Levy[7] contributed to our understanding of the relationship between high plasma lipid levels and atherosclerosis, the underlying disease process in CHD. The phenotypic classification of hyperlipoproteinemias defined initially by Fredrickson and Levy appears in *Table 1.1.* The table has been modified to summarize the types and causes of primary hypertriglyceridemia (*Table 1.2*).

Gender and Hormonal Factors

From the Framingham Study, it has been established that CHD develops in men 60 years of age or younger at approximately twice the rate as that of women (*Table 1.3*). Postmenopausal women have a higher incidence of CHD than premenopausal women of the same age. Both natural and surgical menopause are associated with an increased risk of CHD.[8]

Table 1.3
Incidence of Cardiovascular Disease by Age and Sex—Framingham Study: 20-Year Follow-up

Age at Examination (yr)	Rate per 1,000 per Year	
	Men	**Women**
29 to 34	3.4	0.8
35 to 39	2.9	0.7
40 to 44	5.7	1.3
45 to 49	9.1	3.1
50 to 54	16.5	6.1
55 to 59	25.1	10.2
60 to 64	27.6	18.1
65 to 69	26.7	22.1
70 to 74	37.8	26.2
75 to 79	53.0	50.4

Reproduced with permission from Kannel WB, Hjortland MC, McNamara PM, et al. Menopause and risk of cardiovascular disease. *Ann Intern Med.* 1976;85:447.

Women in their childbearing years are at lower risk for CHD.[9] This could be related to the influence of female hormones on lipoprotein levels. Levels of HDL cholesterol, which is protective against CHD, and LDL cholesterol, which is associated with increased CHD risk, differ between men and women.[10] Data from the Lipid Research Clinics (LRC) Prevalence Study show that, between the ages of 20 and 59, HDL-cholesterol levels in women are higher than in men[10] (*Figure 1.1*).[11] Furthermore, until approximately age 50, LDL-cholesterol levels in women who are not undergoing hormone therapy are lower than levels in men of the same age.[10] However, after menopause, the LDL-cholesterol levels of women are higher than those of men, although the ratio of LDL cholesterol to HDL cholesterol in women never exceeds that in men (Tables 14.1, 14.2, 14.3, 14.4, and 14.5 in the appendix.)[9] It should be noted, however, that most data indicate that LDL cholesterol is a weaker predictor of CHD risk in women than HDL cholesterol.[12]

Age

Atherosclerosis is thought to begin in childhood. Fatty streaks are present during childhood (frequently between 10 and 20 years of age) and are thought to be a precursor of atherosclerosis. Autopsies of young men who were killed at war established the presence of atherosclerosis in early adulthood. In about 40% of children, childhood blood cholesterol levels are significant predictors of cholesterol levels in adulthood. For both men and women, the incidence of CVD increases with advancing age. In men, the highest incidence of clinical manifestations of CVD occurs between the ages of 50 and 60. In women, the highest incidence of CVD is between 60 and 70.[13] Correspondingly, rates of death due to atherosclerosis increase with age[14] (*Figure 1.2*). Approximately 75% of coronary-related deaths are due to atherosclerosis.

Fig. 1.1
Regression estimates of mean plasma lipoprotein-cholesterol values by age for males, females not taking sex hormones, and females on sex-hormone preparations. Lipid Research Clinics Prevalence Study, visit 2, random sample. Adapted from Heiss G, Tamir I, Davis CE, et al. Lipoprotein-cholesterol distributions in selected North American populations: the Lipid Research Clinics Program Prevalence Study. **Circulation.** ***1980;61:302.***

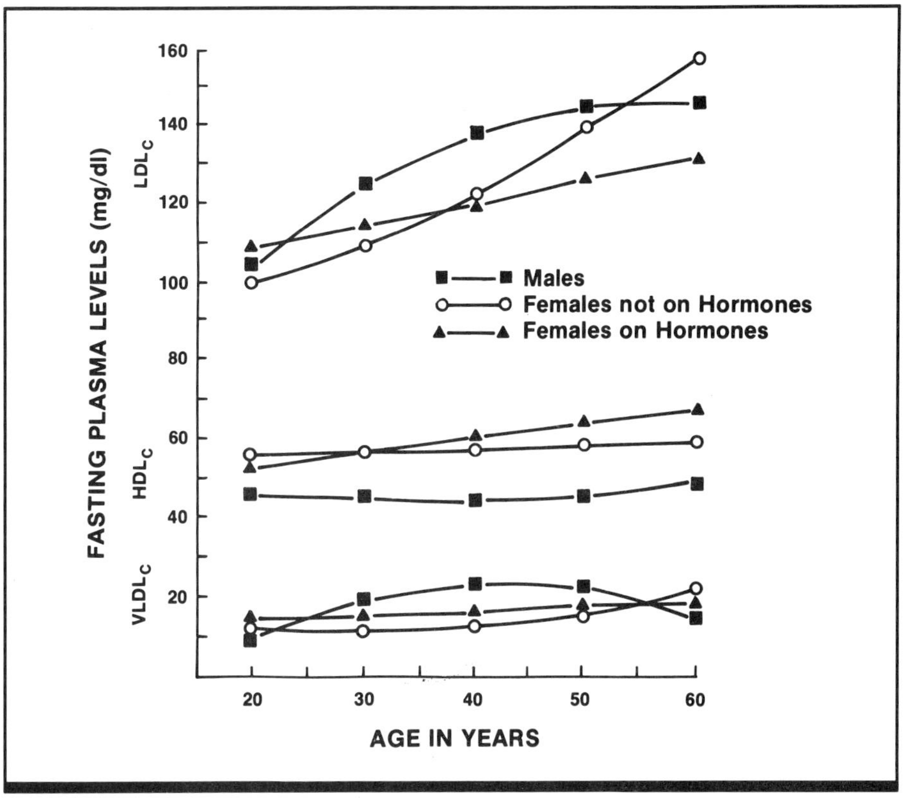

Fig. 1.2
Estimated prevalence of coronary heart disease in people age 20 and over in a US population. Adapted from American Heart Association. Reproduced with permission. **1989 Heart Facts,** ***1988. American Heart Association.***

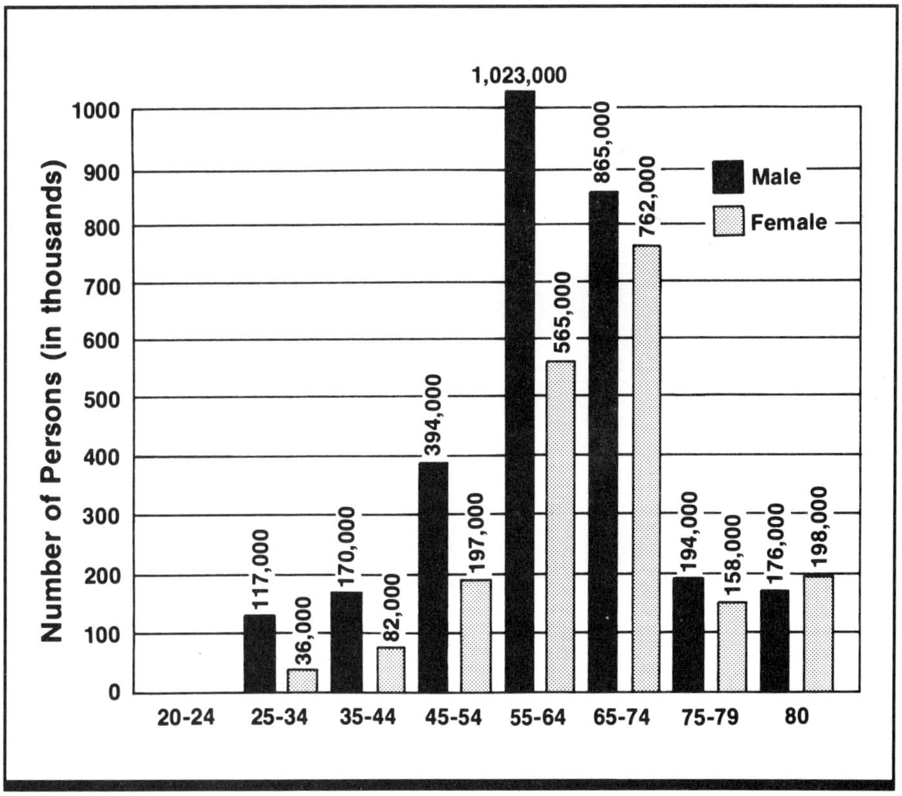

MODIFIABLE RISK FACTORS

Plasma Lipids*

Epidemiological evidence has demonstrated that total serum cholesterol and triglycerides, as well as their lipoprotein fractions, including VLDL cholesterol, LDL cholesterol, and HDL cholesterol, have both positive and negative associations with the development of CVD, especially atherosclerosis.[3,4,14–32] Clinical trials such as the Stockholm Ischemic Heart Disease study and the 102-month follow-up of the Oslo Diet/Smoking study have found that decreasing plasma cholesterol levels lead to reductions in total mortality.[33,34]

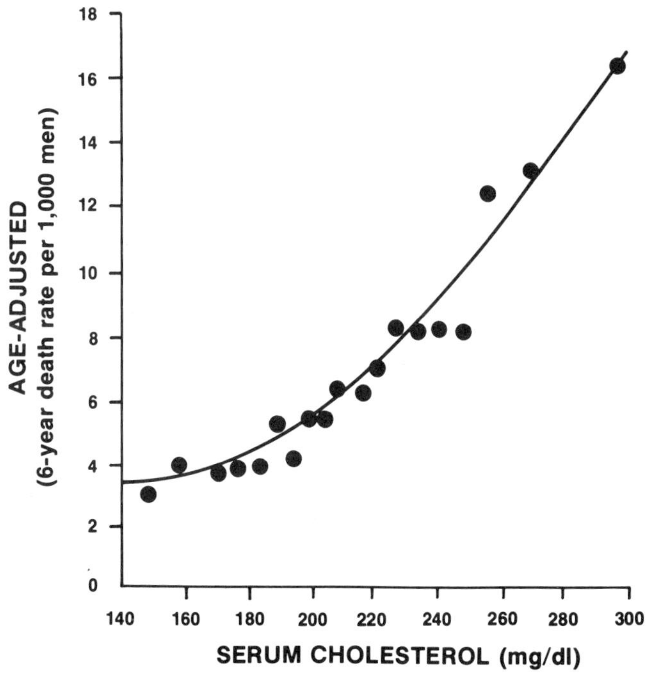

Key points:
(1) The risk increases steadily, and particularly above 200 mg/dl.
(2) The magnitude of the increased risk is large - fourfold in the top 10% as compared to the bottom 10%.

Fig. 1.3
Relationship of serum cholesterol to CHD death in 361,662 men aged 35 to 57 during an average follow-up of six years in the Multiple Risk Factor Intervention Trial. Each point represents the median value for 5% of the population. Reproduced from National Cholesterol Education Program Expert Panel. Report on detection, evaluation, and treatment of high blood cholesterol in adults. **Arch Intern Med.** ***1988;148:36.***

An elevated serum cholesterol is a major independent risk factor for CHD[15-17] (*Figure 1.3*).[6] Some, in fact, believe that serum cholesterol is the single most important risk factor in the development of CHD.[35] Risk of CHD increases steadily, particularly for plasma total-cholesterol levels greater than 200 mg/dL. At the upper part of the curve (see Figure 1.3), small changes in the serum cholesterol level result in large changes in CHD risk. In the Pooling Project (US population), serum cholesterol levels were categorized into five quintiles: I (<194 mg/dL); II (195 to 218 mg/dL); III (219 to 240 mg/dL); IV (241 to 268 mg/dL); and V (>268 mg/dL). Relative CHD risk increased from quintile I to quintile V (risk ratio per quintile = 1.0 for I; 1.0 for II; 1.50 for III; 1.64 for IV; and 1.99 for V). A greater risk ratio (V/II + I) was observed for ages 45 to 49 than for ages 60 to 64 (risk ratio 3.6 versus 1.5).[18,19] In the Framingham Study, the risk of CHD's developing in people with plasma total-cholesterol levels less than 200 mg/dL was less than half that of the total population, whereas CHD was twice as likely to develop in those with plasma total-cholesterol levels greater than 260 mg/dL.[17] People with a serum cholesterol level below 150 mg/dL were free of CHD,[35] while those with a serum cholesterol level below

*By Shirley K. Powell

180 mg/dL had the highest survival rate.[6] The average adult plasma total-cholesterol level that consistently has been associated with a low risk of CHD is 140 to 180 mg/dL.[15] It is of interest that CHD risk increases—albeit to a small degree—with increasing serum cholesterol levels even below 200 mg/dL (see Figure 1.3). Nonetheless, many Americans with a serum cholesterol level below 200 mg/dL suffer ischemic events due to atherosclerosis.[36]

Desirable plasma cholesterol levels have been defined by various groups. According to the American Heart Association in 1982, the ideal adult plasma total-cholesterol level is 130 to 190 mg/dL.[18] The National Cholesterol Education Program (NCEP) defines a desirable blood cholesterol level as less than 200 mg/dL. A borderline-high blood cholesterol is 200 to 240 mg/dL and a high blood cholesterol level is greater than 240 mg/dL.[37] The Lipid Research Clinics' established reference values for the serum cholesterol level indicate that moderate hypercholesterolemia occurs in the 75th to 90th percentile, and severe hypercholesterolemia exists when the value exceeds the 90th percentile. The National Institutes of Health (NIH) Consensus Report recommended aggressive treatment of serum cholesterol levels above the 75th percentile.[21]

The level of LDL cholesterol is positively correlated with the serum total-cholesterol level and CHD, and LDL is considered to be the most atherogenic lipoprotein. In the Bogalusa Heart Study the relationship of CVD risk to early atherosclerotic lesions was assessed in 35 subjects (average age at death, 18 years).[21] The percentage of aortic fatty streaks was positively correlated with both plasma total-cholesterol and LDL-cholesterol levels. As the extent of aortic involvement increased, the level of LDL cholesterol increased.

HDL cholesterol appears to be protective against CHD, and evidence has shown that for every 10 mg/dL increase in the HDL-cholesterol level there is a 50% difference in CHD.[15–17,20–23] HDL cholesterol is inversely associated with CHD incidence and mortality. The degree to which HDL-cholesterol levels predicted fatal and nonfatal CHD outcomes in initially asymptomatic 35- to 59-year-old hypercholesterolemic men who participated in the Lipid Research Clinics Coronary Primary Prevention Trial (LRC-CPPT) was studied by Gordon et al.[36] Plasma HDL cholesterol was a strong predictor of CHD incidence in men in both the treatment and control groups. In the Framingham Study,[38] the incidence and mortality rates from CHD were approximately twice as great in men with baseline HDL-cholesterol levels under 40 mg/dL than in men with baseline HDL-cholesterol levels of 50 mg/dL or higher (*Figure 1.4*).[39] Men with HDL-cholesterol levels between 40 and 49 mg/dL had an intermediate incidence of CHD. In the Framingham Study, HDL cholesterol was the most powerful single lipid indicator of risk for CHD, at least in people older than 50. In support of this finding, the Helsinki Heart Study [40] reported that hypercholesterolemic men treated with gemfibrozil had a reduction in plasma total-cholesterol and LDL-cholesterol levels and an increase in HDL-cholesterol levels. CHD was reduced by 34% in the treatment group. Of particular interest was the finding that the decrease in LDL cholesterol accounted for only about one half of the reduction in new coronary events. Thus, the remainder of the reduction in CHD was the result of either the decrease in plasma triglycerides or the increase in HDL-cholesterol levels or both.

The protective effect of an elevated HDL-cholesterol level in people with both very high LDL cholesterol and systolic blood pressure is striking (*Figure 1.5*). The less dense HDL subfraction, HDL_2 ($d = 1.063$ to 1.125 g/dL, versus HDL_3, for which $d = 1.125$ to 1.21 g/dL) appears to be the protective subfraction.[41] More recently, the Coordinating Committee of the NCEP, recognizing that HDL cholesterol is an independent risk factor for CHD, identified

Fig. 1.4
HDL cholesterol and CHD risk in the Framingham population. Reproduced with permission. Physicians Cholesterol Education Speaker Support Slide Set, 1987. American Heart Association.

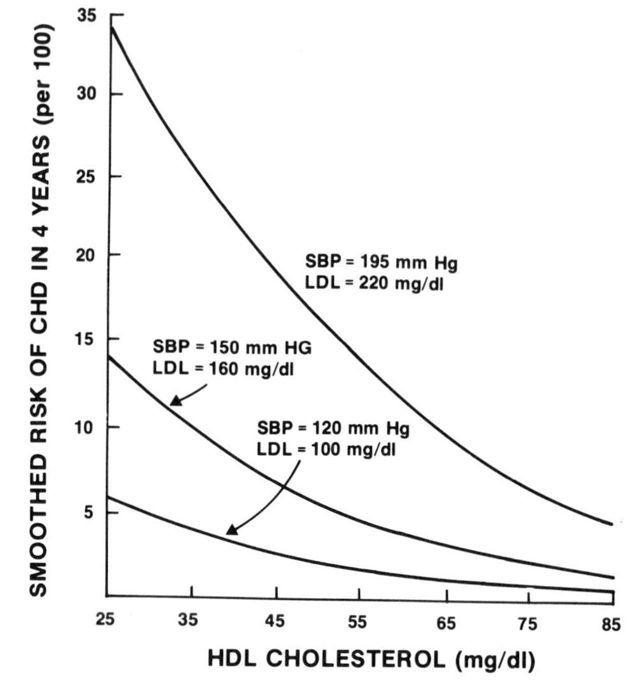

Fig. 1.5
Risk of coronary heart disease according to levels of high-density-lipoprotein cholesterol; men aged 55, Framingham Study, 24-year follow-up. CHD indicates coronary heart disease; SBP, systolic blood pressure; and LDL, low-density lipoprotein. Reproduced with permission from Kannel WB, Castelli WP, Gordon T. Cholesterol in the prediction of atherosclerotic disease: new perspectives based on the Framingham Study. Ann Intern Med. ***1979;90:85.***

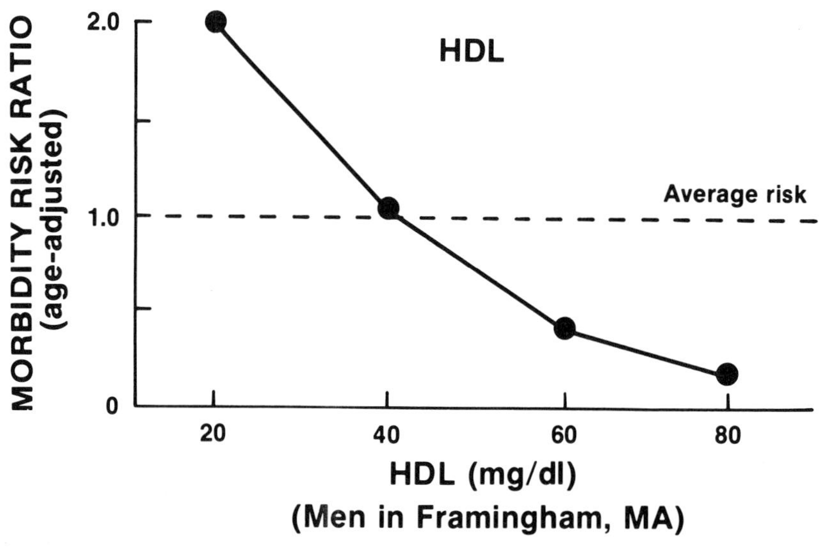

standards for risk.[42] With 45 mg/dL as a baseline level, the following HDL-cholesterol values present associated increases in CHD risk: 40 mg/dL (increase 10% to 15%), 35 mg/dL (increase 20% to 30%), 25 mg/dL (increase 40% to 60%). Thus, hypo-HDL increases the risk of CHD even when the blood cholesterol level is desirable.

People with a desirable blood cholesterol level are also at risk for CHD if they have a recently defined condition, hyperapo B. Hyperapo B is a condition in which LDL particles are smaller, cholesterol-depleted, and contain more apolipoprotein B than normal LDL particles. This smaller LDL is more dense and possibly more atherogenic.[43] Recently another lipoprotein, lipoprotein(a) [Lp(a)], has been recognized as a strong risk factor for CHD.[44] Lp(a) is a better predictor of the severity of atherosclerosis than either LDL-cholesterol or HDL-cholesterol levels.[44] Of particular concern is the accumulating evidence that suggests Lp(a) levels are not effectively modified by diet nor drug therapy. Presently, this lipoprotein fraction is not quantified in clinical practice.

The ratios of LDL cholesterol to HDL cholesterol and total cholesterol to HDL cholesterol are used as predictors of CHD risk. Ratios of total cholesterol to HDL cholesterol greater than 4.5 are considered to place a person at high risk for CVD. An optimal total-cholesterol/HDL-cholesterol ratio for low CVD risk is less than 3.5.[15,22,23] Gordon and associates[45] advise against using these ratios because some people may have similar ratios yet large differences in the concentration of plasma total-cholesterol, LDL-cholesterol, and HDL-cholesterol levels. The ratios, presented alone, do not provide information on the LDL-cholesterol level, a significant risk factor for CHD.[24]

The role of plasma triglycerides as a risk factor for CHD is controversial. In an extensive review of the literature, Hully et al[46] found a significant association between triglyceride levels and CHD; however, plasma triglycerides were not predictive of CHD whan other risk factors were accounted for.[46] A recent study[47] with 38,000 Norwegian men (ages 40 to 49) showed that plasma triglyceride levels were a weak predictor of CHD. In this study, plasma triglyceride levels were a stronger predictor of CHD as plasma total-cholesterol levels increased. In the Framingham Study,[48] plasma triglyceride levels had little effect on CHD risk in men and women who had average or high HDL-cholesterol levels. An increase in CHD rate was observed in subjects with elevated plasma triglycerides only when HDL cholesterol was less than 40 mg/dL. In middle-aged women, the available evidence suggests that plasma triglyceride levels are a significant risk factor for CHD. Based on the Framingham Study,[48] it appears that elevations in plasma triglyceride levels in the presence of a high total-cholesterol to HDL-cholesterol ratio (>3.5) increases CHD risk. Recent evidence suggests an inverse relationship between plasma triglyceride levels and HDL-cholesterol levels; hence, people with low plasma triglyceride levels and high HDL-cholesterol levels are at lower risk of CHD.[49]

Abnormalities in serum lipid values and lipoprotein fractions are due to familial factors (as noted previously) or acquired factors.[3,15,18,19,22,24-27] Acquired factors that influence plasma total- and lipoprotein-cholesterol levels include: (1) diet, (2) smoking and exercise, (3) hypertension, (4) obesity, and (5) diabetes.[15,22,24,25]

Diet*

Diet is included in the category of modifiable risk factors because of its effects on primary CHD risk factors. Many epidemiological, animal,

*By Shirley K.Powell

human-migration, clinical, and human-pathology studies consistently demonstrate a relationship between diet, plasma cholesterol, and CHD. In this section, the epidemiological evidence that links diet and individual dietary constitutents to CHD will be discussed. Additional information can be found in Chapters 2 and 5.

The positive relationships of saturated-fat intake and dietary cholesterol to CHD and mortality have been well documented. The Seven Countries Study, a cross-population study that included men from Finland, the United States, the Netherlands, Italy, Japan, Yugoslavia, and Greece, showed a positive association between saturated-fat intake (expressed as a percentage of calories) and CHD.[50,51] Men from Zutphen, Netherlands, United States, and East Finland had the highest intake of saturated fatty acids (18% to 20% of total calories) and the highest death rate due to CHD. Japanese men had the lowest intake of saturated fatty acids (3% of total calories) and the lowest death rate due to CHD.[50,51]

The Ni-Hon-San Study examined the effects of dietary intake, migration, and serum lipids of Japanese men living in Japan, Hawaii, and San Francisco, California.[52,53] The intake of saturated fats (as a percentage of total calories) was estimated to be 7%, 12%, and 14% for Japanese men living in Japan, Hawaii, and California, respectively. The serum cholesterol level was higher for those who consumed more saturated fat. Serum cholesterol was 12% higher for men in Hawaii and 21% higher for men in California than for men living in Japan. As a result, the death rate due to CHD was 1.7 times greater in Hawaii and 2.8 times greater in California.[52,53]

The Western Electric Study found a positive relationship between serum cholesterol levels and CHD deaths and the intake of both saturated fat and cholesterol.[54] In this study diet and serum cholesterol were evaluated in 1,900 middle-aged men on two occasions 1 year apart and then vital status was determined at the 20th anniversary of the first examination. Baseline serum cholesterol levels and risk of death from CHD were correlated with baseline dietary intake, eg, positively with saturated fatty acid and dietary cholesterol intakes and inversely with omega-6 fatty-acid consumption.[54] Recently, Stamler and Shekelle[55] reviewed clinical and epidemiological data relating dietary cholesterol to its effects on serum cholesterol level. The authors concluded that dietary cholesterol is an independent risk factor for CHD. Dietary cholesterol and saturated fat are hypercholesterolemic in humans.

Recent studies suggest an inverse association between the consumption of both fish and omega-3 fatty acids and CHD. In the Greenland Eskimo Study, only two cases of atherosclerotic heart disease were reported in 1,300 Eskimos from 1963 to 1967. This study concluded that the high levels of omega-3 fatty acids in the diets (5.8 g per day) of Eskimos accounted for their lower serum cholesterol compared with the Danes, who consumed a diet lower in omega-3 fatty acids (0.8 g omega-3 fatty acids per day).[56] Data on the incidence of atherosclerosis in Eskimos are not available at present, although a study is underway (J. Strong, personal communication). Kromhout[57] also found an inverse relationship between fish consumption and risk of CHD in the Zutphen, Netherlands Study of 852 middle-aged men participating in the Seven Countries Study. The men were divided into five groups based on the quantity of fish consumed per day: 0 g; 1 to 14 g; 15 to 29 g; 30 to 44 g; and more than 45 g. Dietary intake was evaluated in relation to CHD from 1960 to 1980. Fish consumption was inversely related to 20-year mortality for CHD and, as the consumption of fish increased, risk ratios of death from CHD decreased. Men who consumed more than 30 g of fish per day had a risk ratio 2.5 times lower than those who did not consume fish.[57]

Calorie intake (both total and expressed per kilogram of body weight) is another variable shown to be inversely related to CHD (perhaps because of its obvious association with physical activity level).[45,58] In the Three Population Study, dietary intake was assessed and related to the development of CHD in 16,349 men, aged 45 to 64, who were from the Framingham Study (859 men), Honolulu Heart Study (7,272 men), and the Puerto Rico Health Program (8,218 men). All men were initially free of CHD and were followed for up to 6 years for the initial manifestation of CHD. Based on one 24-hour dietary recall, a greater mean caloric intake was found in men free of CHD, whereas lower mean caloric intakes were found in men in whom CHD developed.[45] The Lipid Research Clinics (LRC) Program Prevalence Study determined nutrient intake by a 24-hour recall in 8,250 free-living, white men and women. Classified by dyslipoproteinemia phenotypes, participants were aged 20 to 49 and 50 and older. This study found an inverse relationship between calorie intake and the risk of CHD.[58] Those with a high calorie intake had a lower risk of CHD. For example, both high HDL-cholesterol levels and low LDL-cholesterol levels were associated with a greater calorie intake, while low HDL-cholesterol and high LDL-cholesterol levels were associated with lower calorie intakes.[58] These studies suggest that the difference in calorie intake may be the result of greater physical activity and leaner body mass in people with a reduced CHD risk.[45,58]

Other dietary constituents (ie, total fat, animal products, sources of protein, alcohol, starch, coffee, and others) have been related to CHD. Stamler reviewed the results of data from the United Nations Food and Agriculture Organization (FAO) and the World Health Organization and found that lipid-rich diets derived largely from animal products were associated with high CHD mortality.[25] The United States, Finland, Australia, and New Zealand had the highest incidence of mortality from CHD and the highest percentage of calories from animal sources, while Japan had the lowest of both.[25] Epidemiological studies have shown that animal protein is positively ($r = 0.78$) and vegetable protein negatively ($r = -0.40$) correlated with CHD mortality.[14] The LRC Program Prevalence Study showed an association between dyslipoprotein phenotypes and percentage of calories from alcohol and carbohydrates; subjects with high HDL-cholesterol levels ingested less refined carbohydrates and more alcohol, while subjects with low HDL-cholesterol levels ingested less alcohol.[58] In a recent statistical exploration, Hegsted and Ausman[59] found a strong negative correlation between alcohol consumption and CHD. The Three Population Study showed an association between starch and alcohol consumption with CHD incidence, but the evidence was neither consistent nor strong between populations. Men who consumed more starch were at lower risk of CHD in the Honolulu and Puerto Rico studies. The Honolulu and Framingham Studies showed that men who consumed more alcohol had a lower incidence of CHD.

Numerous studies have focused on the effects of coffee consumption on CHD. One of the best controlled is the Tromso Heart Study, in which coffee consumption was a major determinant of the serum total-cholesterol level in a group of 14,667 Norwegian subjects.[60] Serum total cholesterol was 31 mg/dL higher in men who drank more than nine cups of coffee per day than in men who drank less than one cup. The magnitude of the serum total-cholesterol-raising effect of coffee was that it increased CHD risk twofold. Coffee, in this study, was one of the strongest determinants of the serum total-cholesterol level. Other studies, however, have not supported a relationship between CHD and coffee consumption.[61] An evaluation of the Framingham Study data revealed no association between coffee consumption and CVD.[62] Similarly, a recent review[63] reported no relationship between coffee consumption and CHD risk. The role of coffee in the development of CHD is at present equivocal. Tea drinking appears to have no association with serum cholesterol or CHD.

Epidemiological studies have continually shown associations between dietary intake and risk for CHD. Intervention and experimental studies have confirmed many of these observations, which are discussed in other sections.

Diabetes Mellitus*

Diabetes mellitus (DM) is a strong CVD risk factor. Both CVD morbidity and mortality are increased in people with both type I and type II DM. In fact, CVD is the leading cause of death in persons with type I diabetes. The impact is greater for women with diabetes than for men with diabetes, and it varies with coexisting risk factors. Lipid abnormalities are present and more pronounced in people with diabetes. Hyperinsulinemia is an independent risk factor for CVD.[15,22,64–67]

Diabetes mellitus doubles CVD mortality[1]; CVD is two times more prevalent in men with diabetes and three times more prevalent in women with diabetes.[15,64] However, in areas with a lower incidence of CHD (Japan, Africa), people with diabetes also have a lower risk of CVD than those who live in countries in which CHD mortality is high.[64] Clinical manifestation of CVD is greater for people with diabetes than people without it; occlusive peripheral arterial disease is a common complication of DM.[22,64,68,69] Warren and LeCompte found evidence of myocardial infarction and thrombosis in 25.4% (193/761) of persons with diabetes at time of autopsy.[70] In the Framingham Study, subjects with diabetes, especially females, had a greater incidence of coronary insufficiency, sudden death, angina pectoris, and myocardial infarction compared with subjects without diabetes.[22] At follow-up (year 26), the percentage of deaths due to myocardial infarction was 91% for women with diabetes compared with 56% for men with diabetes, 30% for men without diabetes, and 55% for women without diabetes.[22] Obese women with both diabetes and low HDL-cholesterol levels are at high risk for CHD; their risk is higher than that of men without diabetes.[15,22,71]

Diabetic cardiovascular complications are seen at both the microvascular and macrovascular levels, with type II (non–insulin-dependent) DM having greater macrovascular complications and type I (insulin-dependent) DM having greater microvascular complications.[15,22,65] Serum lipid abnormalities increase CHD risk in people with diabetes. Elevated plasma total and VLDL triglycerides in people with diabetes is related to an impaired glucose tolerance.[15,22] People with diabetes have elevated plasma total-cholesterol and LDL-cholesterol levels and low HDL-cholesterol levels, both of which are major risk factors for CHD.[15,22] People with diabetes, especially women, have higher serum total-cholesterol levels than people without diabetes. With increasing serum total-cholesterol levels, cardiac failure also increases[14,21] (*Figure 1.6*).

Psychological Factors†

Numerous social and psychological factors, such as socioeconomic status, social mobility, anxiety, and neuroticism, and their relationship to CHD risk have been studied. The most promising psychosocial risk factors for CHD are psychological stress and the type A "coronary-prone" behavior pattern. Psychological stress, as used in this section, refers to an internal state resulting from the perception of threat, physical harm, or both.[72]

*By Shirley K. Powell
†By Jane Andrews

Fig. 1.6
Risk of cardiac failure by diabetic status in the Framingham population. Reproduced with permission from Kannel WB. Lipids, diabetes, and coronary heart disease: insights from the Framingham Study. **Am Heart J.** ***1985;110:1100.***

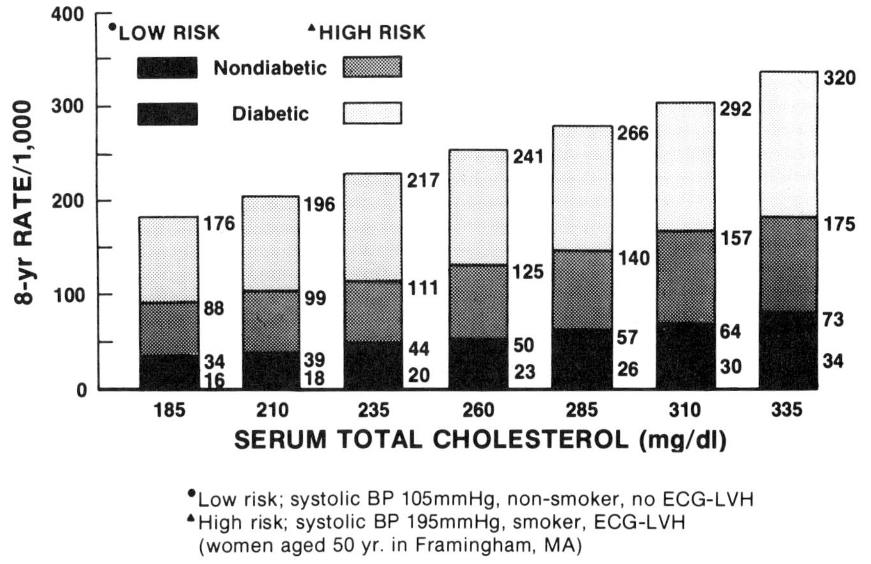

Several measures of psychological stress have been studied in relation to the development of CHD. Some research indicates that suppressed hostility, excessive workload, job responsibility, and job dissatisfaction may increase CHD risk.[73,74] Crisp, Queenan, and D'Souza prospectively studied 225 men in a general medical practice.[75] Those who suffered a myocardial infarction were more obsessive and were greater worriers than others. Moreover, in the year before their infarction they displayed high levels of sadness and anxiety-related symptoms unrelated to angina and other physical discomforts.

Another psychological factor that has important implications for CHD is the type A or coronary-prone behavior pattern.[76] Perhaps the most widely researched psychosocial risk factor for CHD, the type A pattern is characterized by excessive competitive drive, impatience, hostility, and accelerated speech and motor movements. The contrasting type B pattern displays less of these characteristics. No significant division exists between the two behavior patterns. The type B person is generally a more relaxed and easy-going person who is rarely aggressive and who is relatively devoid of time-urgent characteristics.

Twenty-five years ago epidemiological studies suggested that CHD risk was associated with the type A behavior pattern. Recent prospective research, however, has not consistently shown a relationship between type A behavior and CHD risk.[77] More recent evidence, however, has shown that those who react quickly to various situations with anger and frustration are more prone to CHD.[43]

Beyond its relevance to the primary prevention of CHD, the type A behavior pattern and its recurrence in the postmyocardial infarction patient has also been studied. Some research has indicated no relationship between a type A score and coronary mortality within a three-year follow-up after a myocardial infarction.[78] One study showed that type A subjects had a significantly lower mortality than type B subjects.[79] However, there was no difference in mortality between type A and type B patients who died within 24 hours of the coronary event. This suggests that people with the type A behavior pattern are not at increased risk for CHD mortality, and it raises the question of whether their behavior should be modified before or after a coronary event.[80] (See chapter 10 for a discussion of this topic.)

Hormones, Oral Contraceptives*

Oral contraceptive agents (OCAs) are thought to contribute to death from such CVD events as myocardial infarction, brain infarction, pulmonary embolism, subarachanoid hemorrhage, and hypertension.[81] Risk of myocardial infarction is estimated to increase by fourfold in OCA users.[82] Coronary risk in OCA users increases with age and with the presence of other risk factors, cigarette smoking and hypertension in particular. Although the relative risk is substantial, the absolute risk of 13/100,000 (average annual risk) is small, but rises to 170/100,000 for women aged 38 to 45 who smoke.[82] Some research has indicated a residual effect after discontinuation of oral contraceptives.[83]

Wahl et al[84] conducted an elaborate study to examine the effect of hormone use on lipoprotein lipid levels in premenopausal and postmenopausal women. The investigators examined the relationship of plasma lipids and lipoprotein-cholesterol concentrations to various types of estrogen-progestin formulations. LDL-cholesterol levels were 24% higher in premenopausal women using OCAs containing relatively low doses of estrogen combined with medium or high doses of progestin than in women not using hormones. HDL-cholesterol levels were significantly higher in women using OCAs high in estrogen and low in progestin. Those using a low-estrogen and high-progestin formulation had lower HDL-cholesterol levels than nonusers. LDL-cholesterol levels were 11% to 19% lower in postmenopausal women using estrogen than in nonusers. The investigators suggested that the ratios of estrogen to progestin affect LDL-cholesterol and HDL-cholesterol differently. Moreover, prolonged use of progestin-dominant OCAs may be undesirable, especially for women with known risk factors for CVD. Therefore, to reduce the risk of CVD, selecting OCAs that have a minimal effect on lipid metabolism is recommended.

There is some evidence of a beneficial association between estrogen-replacement therapy and death from ischemic heart disease in postmenopausal women.[85] Other evidence, however,[86] provides little support for a preventive effect of estrogen use against nonfatal myocardial infarction. Clearly, more work is needed in this area. A large, three-year, multicenter study is now in progress (PEPI—Postmenopausal Estrogen, Progestin Intervention—sponsored by the National Institutes of Health and the National Heart, Lung and Blood Institute) to assess the effects of estrogen-replacement therapy with and without progestin on coronary risk factors in postmenopausal women. In men, paradoxically, hyperestrogenemia may be an important CHD risk factor. Of 15 men who suffered a myocardial infarction, 7 were found to have significantly elevated levels of estradiol and estrone.[87] Others have found that male plasma estradiol levels were correlated with body weight and were also significantly higher in smokers than in nonsmokers.[88] In the Coronary Drug Project,[89] a study conducted on a large sample of men with a previous history of myocardial infarction, men receiving estrogen (5 mg/day) had a greater number of nonfatal myocardial infarcts, pulmonary embolisms, and thrombophlebitis than control subjects. Unlike the beneficial effect of estrogen on CHD risk in women, estrogen appears to raise CHD risk in men.

*By Jane Andrews

Smoking*

Cigarette smoking is a major risk factor for CHD.[90] In the United States, approximately 33% of adult men and 28% of adult women smoke cigarettes. The relative risk for CHD based on cigarette smoking alone and in combination with other risk factors from a study summarized by Paffenbarger et al is shown in *Table 1.4*. Smoking more than ten cigarettes per day alone increased coronary mortality by 1.6-fold. Coronary mortality doubled when systolic blood pressure was more than 130 mm Hg in smokers. These findings are from the entrance examinations of students at Harvard University and the University of Pennsylvania several decades ago. Smoking history was predictive of CHD risk 20, 30, and 40 years later.[91] Data from several large-scale prospective studies shown in *Table 1.5* indicate that cigarette smoking remains an important risk factor up to the seventh decade of life. The mortality ratio ranged from 1.0 for men and women who never smoked regularly to a 5.5 increase for 40- to 49-year-old men who smoked more than 40 cigarettes daily.[92]

Table 1.4
Overweight, Systolic Blood Pressure (SBP) Elevation, Cigarette Smoking, and Coronary Heart Disease Mortality Ratios in College Entrants

Group	Percentage of Entrants	Mortality Ratio
Overweight	25	1.4
SBP $\geq$ 130 mm Hg	27	1.6
Smoking $\geq$ 10 cigarettes per day	15	1.6
Overweight and SBP $\geq$ 130 mm Hg	7	2.3
Overweight and smoking	4	1.9
SBP $\geq$ 130 mm Hg and smoking	4	2.1

Adapted with permission from Paffenbarger RS, Notkin J, Kreuger DE, et al. Chronic disease in former college students, II: methods of study and observations on mortality from coronary heart disease. *Am J Public Health.* 1966;56:962.

Cigarette smoking increases the risk of nonfatal myocardial infarction in young men.[93] Age-adjusted relative risk for nonfatal myocardial infarction in men was 2.1 for light smokers (<25 cigarettes per day) and 4.0 for heavy smokers ($\geq$45 cigarettes per day) compared with nonsmokers. The relative risk for ex-smokers was similar to that of nonsmokers. Relative risk was not related to the nicotine or carbon monoxide content of the cigarette.[93]

HDL cholesterol is lower in smokers than in nonsmokers (43.5 versus 46.8 mg/dL, respectively). Smokers had a higher plasma total-cholesterol level than nonsmokers (227 versus 217 mg/dL or approximately 5% difference). LDL cholesterol is also higher in smokers than in nonsmokers (153 versus 140 mg/dL, respectively).[94]

Recent studies have examined the effect of decreasing cigarette smoking on CHD risk. The 22 Multiple Risk Factor Intervention Trial centers showed that it is possible to effect and sustain cessation of cigarette smoking in a group of high-risk middle-aged men, although mortality was not affected during the study.[29] In the Oslo Study there was a 31% reduction in cigarette smoking in the intervention group, compared with an 18% reduction in the nonintervention

*By Lisa Hill

Table 1.5
Mortality Ratios for CHD by Number of Cigarettes Smoked Daily, Men and Women by Age at Entry—Six-Year Follow-up, 1,000,000-Person Study, American Cancer Society

	Mortality Ratio for Men				
Age (yr)	**Never Smoked Regularly**	**1–9 a day**	**10–19 a day**	**20–39 a day**	**40+ a day**
40–49	1.00	1.60	2.59	3.76	5.51
50–59	1.00	1.59	2.13	2.40	2.79
60–69	1.00	1.48	1.82	1.91	1.79
70–79	1.00	1.14	1.41	1.49	1.47

	Mortality Ratio for Women				
Age (yr)	**Never Smoked Regularly**	**1–9 a day**	**10–19 a day**	**20–39 a day**	**40+ a day**
40–49	1.00	1.31	2.08	3.62	3.31*
50–59	1.00	1.15	2.37	2.68	3.73
60–69	1.00	1.04	1.79	2.08	2.02*
70–79	1.00	0.76	0.08	1.27	—

*Rates based on only five to nine deaths.

Adapted with permission from Katz LN, Stamler J, Pick R. *Nutrition and Atherosclerosis.* Philadelphia, PA: Lea & Febiger; 1958.

control group. Coronary mortality was not examined in this study.[95] The Coronary Drug Project reported that after one or more myocardial infarctions, cessation of cigarette smoking improved long-term prognosis.[96]

Recent studies indicate that passive smoke is a potential risk factor for CHD as well.[97] This has important implications for setting public health policy in designating a smoke-free environment at work, at play, and in the family.

The US has the highest average per capita consumption of cigarettes in the world; however, cigarette smoking is at its lowest point in recorded history. The prevalence of smoking has decreased by 34% for men and 17% for women since 1965.[98] Despite this, 47 million adults still smoke.

Physical Activity*

Epidemiological studies during the past 30 years have provided strong evidence that physical activity plays a protective role in the etiology of CHD. In 1953 Morris and coworkers[99] reported that London bus conductors, who actively collected tickets, had a much lower risk of CHD than the drivers, who sat for most of the day. Similarly, the London Civil Service study demonstrated that men engaged in vigorous leisure-time activities had less than half the incidence of CHD than their sedentary colleagues.[100]

A study of San Francisco longshoremen compared fatal CHD between cargoholders (who loaded and unloaded the ships and had a high level of job-related physical activity) and foremen and clerks (who had a low level of job-related physical activity) between 1951 and 1973. Men who expended 8,500 or more calories per week at work had about half the incidence of CHD mortality than their sedentary counterparts. In addition, when the data were examined

*By Lisa Hill

according to year of birth, an increase in physical activity at work was significantly associated with a lower incidence of fatal CHD in the 35- to 44-year-old and 45- to 54-year-old groups. Perhaps one reason why this was not observed in the older groups is that the younger cohorts may have included high-risk subjects who had already disappeared from the older cohorts.[101,102]

The Harvard alumni study evaluated past and present leisure-time and other lifestyle patterns in 16,936 male alumni. An important finding of this study was that current levels of physical activity, rather than history of athleticism in youth, were inversely associated with risk of CHD in all age brackets. Sedentary alumni, even ex-varsity athletes, had a high risk of CHD, while sedentary students who became physically active alumni had a low risk. Also, the rate of CHD declined consistently with increased physical activity in all age groups.[103-105] Recently, Leon et al[106] reported a modest inverse relationship between leisure-time physical activity and CHD and overall mortality in participants of the Multiple Risk Factor Intervention Trial. The authors concluded the leisure-time physical activity had a modest inverse relationship to CHD and overall mortality in middle-aged men at high risk for CHD.

Investigators from the Framingham Study found in a population of 1,909 men and 2,311 women that risk associated with a sedentary life style was modest compared with other, more powerful, risk factors studied (such as cigarette smoking, blood pressure, and serum cholesterol). However, physical inactivity in combination with these risk factors led to an overall greater CHD risk.[107]

Due to the interrelatedness of CHD risk factors, it has been difficult to ascertain whether the role of physical activity is "protective" (a cause of reduced CHD) or "selective" (an effect of CHD symptomology or other elective practices).[104] Understandably, the limitations of earlier studies have been in quantifying and characterizing a variety of work-related and/or leisure-time activities. Earlier studies were able to demonstrate a relationship between the level of physical activity and decreased mortality with as little as two multiple-choice questions. Now that the relationship has been established, more detailed information is needed. Investigators are now asking, "What kind of physical activity—with what frequency, intensity, and duration—is protective?" Several ongoing studies using more refined instruments (the Johnson and Johnson Live for Life Study, the Stanford Five-City Project)[108,109] will clarify the questions now being asked.

The positive effects of physical activity on CHD risk have raised numerous questions about how exercise protects against CHD. Since there is strong evidence to support a causal relationship between plasma lipids, lipoproteins, and apolipoproteins and the development of atherosclerosis,[104,107] numerous investigators have examined relationships between exercise and lipoprotein metabolism. The studies are both cross-sectional and longitudinal.

Observational studies have consistently shown differences in the plasma lipid profile of trained versus sedentary people.[110-114] In general, HDL cholesterol is higher[107] and plasma total triglycerides and VLDL triglycerides are lower in endurance-trained than in sedentary control subjects. LDL cholesterol is frequently lower and plasma total cholesterol is inconsistently lower in trained subjects[107]: Typically, HDL cholesterol is 20% to 35% higher in endurance-trained athletes.[115] Active people have higher levels of HDL_2 cholesterol,[110] the HDL subfraction that is negatively associated with CHD risk. HDL_3 cholesterol, which does not appear to affect CHD risk, is similar in active and sedentary people.[110]

Longitudinal studies provide important evidence of a direct causal relationship between aerobic exercise and changes in plasma lipids. Since the pioneering studies of Carlson and Mossfeldt in 1964[116] and Hoffman et al[117] in 1967 first showed a relationship between exercise and HDL-cholesterol levels, numerous longitudinal studies have been done.

Tran and coworkers[118] integrated and analyzed data collected between 1955 and 1983 and quantitatively defined the relationship between exercise and lipids and lipoproteins. Their data base represented 2,925 subjects

Table 1.6
Overall Changes in Plasma Lipids and Lipoproteins Following an Exercise Program

Total cholesterol	< 10 mg/dL*	$p < 0.01$
Total triglycerides	< 15.8 mg/dL	$p < 0.01$
HDL cholesterol	> 1.2 mg/dL	NS†
LDL cholesterol	< 5.1 mg/dL	$p < 0.05$
Total cholesterol / HDL cholesterol	< 0.48	$p < 0.01$

Note: There were no changes in the controls.
* < indicates decreased; >, increased.
† NS indicates not significant.

Adapted with permission from Tran ZV, Weltman A, Glass GV, et al. The effects of exercise on blood lipids and lipoproteins: a meta-analysis of studies. *Med Sci Sports Exer.* 1983;15:393. © by American College of Sports Medicine.

Table 1.7
Impact of Factors Affecting Plasma Lipids and Lipoproteins with Exercise

Plasma Lipid/ Lipoprotein	Factor	Change in Lipid/Lipoprotein
Total cholesterol / HDL cholesterol; Total triglycerides	Age	Larger decreases in older subjects
HDL cholesterol; LDL cholesterol	Age and sex	Larger changes in older males
All lipids and lipoproteins	Intensity	More beneficial changes at an exercise program of lower intensity (must be at least 60% of maximum heart rate) of longer duration
Total cholesterol	Vo_2max*	Larger decreases with larger increases in Vo_2max
HDL cholesterol	Vo_2	Larger increases with larger increases in Vo_2 max
Total triglycerides; Total cholesterol; LDL cholesterol	Body weight	Those with higher initial body weights and the greatest decrease in body weight had the greatest decreases
Total cholesterol / HDL cholesterol; LDL cholesterol	Percentage body fat	Greater decreases with greater decreases in percentage body fat

*Defined in chapter 9.

Adapted with permission from Tran ZV, Weltman A, Glass GV, et al. The effects of exercise on blood lipids and lipoproteins: a meta-analysis of studies. *Med Sci Sports Exer.* 1983;15:393. © by American College of Sports Medicine.

(2,086 experimental subjects and 839 controls) from 66 studies. They found that plasma total cholesterol and LDL cholesterol, total triglycerides, and the ratio of total cholesterol to HDL cholesterol were significantly decreased, and HDL cholesterol was insignificantly increased by exercise (*Table 1.6*).[118] They also found strong correlations among initial total cholesterol, total triglycerides, HDL cholesterol, and the total-cholesterol to HDL-cholesterol ratio, and their respective changes as a result of exercise (*Table 1.7*).[118] Typically, subjects with higher initial levels of total cholesterol, triglycerides, and total cholesterol to HDL cholesterol responded most (ie, had the greatest decreases) to exercise. Lower initial levels of HDL cholesterol resulted in higher levels following the exercise program. Thus, those with more "fit" plasma lipid profiles responded less to an exercise program than those with "sedentary" lipid profiles.

Exercise is associated with both a reduction in the incidence of CHD and favorable changes in plasma lipids and lipoproteins. In addition, exercise has been shown to affect favorably other cardiovascular risk factors such as blood pressure, weight, and cigarette-smoking habit.

Body Weight and Fat Distribution*

According to the National Institutes of Health Consensus Development Conference,[119] obesity has been defined as "an excess of body fat frequently resulting in a significant impairment of health." The most widely used definition of obesity is body weight greater than 120% of desirable weight for height. According to the definition using percentage of body fat as a measure, obesity is a condition in which body fat exceeds 20% of body weight in men and 28% to 30% in women. Overweight is a condition in which body weight is greater than 110% of desirable weight for height.

Historically, body weight has been assessed using "recommended" height-weight tables, the most common one developed by the Metropolitan Life Insurance Company. The 1959 standards (see Table 14.6 in the appendix) are based on the Build and Blood Pressure Study conducted by the Society of Actuaries in which the experiences of several million insured people in the United States and Canada were examined between 1935 and 1953. "Desirable" weights are those that were found to be associated with the lowest mortality. Frame sizes were indicated, but no specific guidelines were given on how they were assessed. *Relative weight* is a term commonly used; it is calculated by dividing the actual weight by the standard or desired weight for age, sex, and height and multiplying the sum by 100 (see chapter 4). In 1983 the Metropolitan Life Insurance Company issued new weight tables based on the 1979 updated Build and Blood Pressure Study (see Table 14.7 in the appendix). The new tables provide guidelines using elbow breadth to determine frame size (see chapter 4), and overall weights are controversially higher than previously published tables.[120] At this time the 1959 standards are recommended until the controversy is resolved. Unfortunately, weight tables are limited in their use, especially with nonwhite and low-income groups; they do not consider other risk factors, such as smoking; they do not measure degree of fatness or regional distribution of fat; and they rely on an ill-defined concept of frame size.[120]

Obesity is an independent risk factor for CHD. When death from CHD was used as an endpoint, obesity has been reported to be predictive when relative weight was greater than 140% or body mass index was greater than 30 kg/m^2 body surface area.[121] In a 26-year follow-up of participants in the Framingham Study, weight was a significant independent predictor of CHD

*By Shirley K. Powell

morbidity and mortality, especially in women. In the Multiple Risk Factor Intervention Trial, weight loss was associated with a reduction in plasma cholesterol. Participants who followed a fat-modified diet and lost more than 10 lb lowered their blood cholesterol level by 22 mg/dL[122]; participants who lost 5 to 9 lb lowered their blood cholesterol by 14 mg/dL. Thus, results of this study are supportive of a relationship between body weight and plasma cholesterol. According to some investigators, "If everyone were at optimal weight, there would be 25% less CHD, and 35% less congestive heart failure and brain infarction."[123,124] Design flaws in studies that have failed to observe a relationship between obesity and CHD mortality may explain the disparate findings that have been reported.

Recently, body fat and its distribution are considered to be risk factors for CHD. Measurement of body fat by skinfold thickness has been used as an index of obesity and has been shown to correlate to CHD risk.[124,125] Both increased risk of myocardial infarction and an elevated serum cholesterol level were associated with increased skinfold thickness and other measures of obesity. An elevated LDL-cholesterol and VLDL-cholesterol level were associated with a high triceps-skinfold thickness.[119]

Numerous cross-sectional investigations have examined obesity and plasma lipid relationships. In general, obesity is associated with a more atherogenic lipoprotein profile. Assessed by relative weight or body mass index, obesity was positively correlated with plasma total-cholesterol, LDL-cholesterol, and triglyceride levels and negatively correlated with HDL-cholesterol levels.[24,126,127] These associations have been reported for both adults and children.[126,128,129] Obesity has also been negatively related to HDL_2 cholesterol and HDL_3 cholesterol.[130] In the Framingham Study, Kannel and coworkers[24] showed that for each percentage increase in relative weight among males, a 1.1 mg/dL increase in serum cholesterol was predicted.[24] Approximately 0.6 mg/dL increase in serum cholesterol was found for women gaining the same amount of weight.

There is recent interest in the distribution of fat deposits versus the degree of adiposity as a predictor of CVD. Vague[131] was the first to report carbohydrate and lipid abnormalities in people with android obesity (excess fat deposits located predominately in the upper body) as opposed to gynoid (lower body) obesity. In 1965 Albrink et al[132] noted that upper body fat was more frequently associated with hypertriglyceridemia. More recently, Foster et al[133] reported that the relative contribution of body fatness to serum triglyceride, LDL-cholesterol, and HDL-cholesterol levels was insignificant compared with the effects of a central or upper fat pattern. Men and women with an elevated waist-to-hip ratio reflective of a high level of abdominal fat were more likely to have elevated plasma total-cholesterol, triglyceride, and apolipoprotein-B levels and lower HDL-cholesterol levels.[134] A recent study has shown that HDL_2-cholesterol levels are inversely correlated with truncal fat.[135] Results of the Gothenburg, Sweden, population study[136] have recently shown that the anthropometric indicator of ratio of waist-to-hip circumference was associated most strongly with the incidence of ischemic heart disease. Moreover, waist-to-hip circumference was also independently associated with the incidence of myocardial infarction. In the Honolulu Heart Program, the risk of incidence of coronary events was directly related to subscapular skinfold thickness independent of body mass index in a cohort of 7,692 men.[137] Men in the highest tertile with respect to subscapular skinfold thickness experienced more than twice the incidence of CHD in a 12-year period than men in the lowest tertile. In a recent study reported by Despres et al,[138] abdominal skinfold thickness was significantly and negatively correlated ($r = -0.16$) with the serum HDL-cholesterol concentration in 421 healthy men older than 18. Upper body fat has been shown to be metabolically different than lower body fat.

Obesity, an independent risk factor for CHD, also exacerbates other coronary risk factors in some people, placing them at higher risk for CHD. For example, not only does obesity unfavorably affect the plasma lipid and lipoprotein profile, but it also raises blood pressure and can induce diabetes and hyperuricemia.[139] Weight management is important in controlling CHD risk.

Hypertension*

With normal blood pressure currently defined as <140/<85 mm Hg,[140] hypertension is a significant independent risk factor for CHD.[141,142] From the 1960s to the 1980s, patient awareness of hypertension increased 24.5%; however, 26.6% of the US population is still unaware that they have the condition.

The Veterans Administration Cooperative Study demonstrated the effectiveness of drugs in controlling morbidity and mortality due to hypertension in men.[143–145] The Hypertension Detection and Follow-up Program further demonstrated that it is possible to screen communities throughout the country and implement a "stepped-care" drug regimen to control blood pressure. Stepped care (SC) participants were treated with antihypertensive therapy in specially set-up centers; referred care (RC) participants were referred for treatment to their usual sources of care. Results indicated a high level of long-term cooperation leading to normalization of blood pressure in the SC group compared with the RC group. A strength of this study is that it included black and white men and women from upper and lower income levels.[146] Mortality from all CVD (adjusted rate per 1,000) was significantly lower in the SC than in the RC group.

There was an overall downward trend in blood pressure in both the control and treatment groups in the Multiple Risk Factor Intervention Trial participants[29] at the end of six years of intervention. The use of antihypertensive medications by both the control and treatment group over the six years made it difficult to evaluate blood pressure changes related to weight reduction and sodium restriction. In this study, since both the treatment and intervention groups lowered their blood pressure, it was not possible to determine the blood pressure–lowering effects on coronary mortality.

Several studies have shown trends in blood pressure within families.[147–149] This clustering indicates the need to develop detection and treatment programs aimed at families rather than individuals. In the Bogalusa Heart Study, associations were found between blood pressure and the clinically measurable risk factors; however, these were not statistically significant. The findings of this study concurred with earlier findings that CHD begins early in life.[21]

INTERACTIONS OF THE MAJOR RISK FACTORS FOR CHD†

The presence of more than one risk factor increases the risk of CHD (*Figure 1.7*).[151,152] Risk increases by 30% with the presence of any one of the three major controllable risk factors (high blood pressure, high blood cholesterol, and smoking). With any two of these risk factors, the risk of CHD increases threefold. With all three of these risk factors, CHD risk increases sevenfold. Data from the Framingham Study clearly show CHD risk is strongly related to

*By Lisa Hill
†By the Editors

the serum cholesterol level; however, risk varies widely for any given plasma LDL-cholesterol concentration (see Figure 1.5).[41] The variation seems to depend on the presence of other CHD risk factors.

Fig. 1.7
Risk of coronary heart disease (CHD) by number of risk factors at initial exam in the Framingham population. From National Heart, Lung and Blood Institute.* Facts at Your Fingertips: National Heart, Lung and Blood Institute Kit '89. *Washington, DC: US Dept of Health and Human Services; 1989.

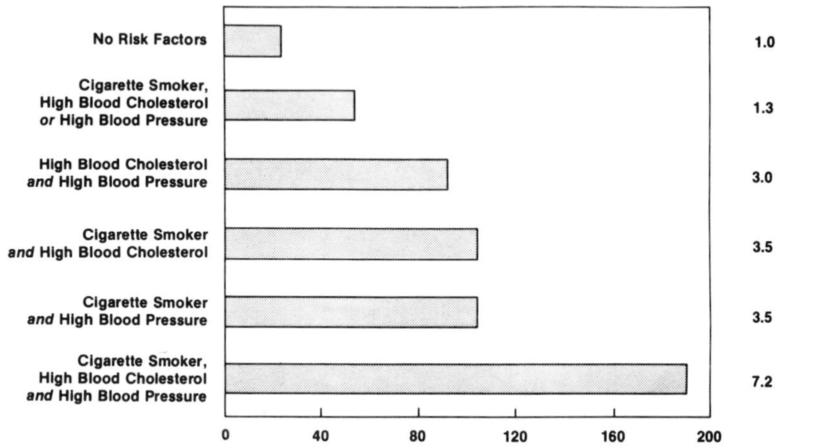

Source: Pooling Project Research Group.

The presence of any one of the three major controllable risk factors for coronary heart disease (high blood pressure, high blood cholesterol, and smoking) increases the risk by about 30 percent.

If a person has any two of these risk factors, the risk of coronary heart disease is at least three times as great as a person with no risk factors.

If a person has all three risk factors, the risk of coronary heart disease is more than seven times that of a person with no risk factors.

RISK FACTORS FOR HYPERTENSION*

Obesity. Essentially all epidemiological studies have found that obesity is among the strongest risk factors for hypertension.[152-154] In the Hypertension Detection and Follow-up Program, 60% of the hypertensive participants were more than 20% overweight. Weight loss alone without sodium restriction has been shown to reduce blood pressure significantly in hypertensive persons. Centrally distributed body fat is a stronger risk factor for hypertension than peripherally distributed body fat.

Sodium. Many epidemiological studies have demonstrated a significant, positive relationship between salt intake and systolic and diastolic blood pressures in men and women.[154,155] However, some studies have not shown such a relationship.

Long-term clinical trials have shown that approximately 40% of hypertensive patients can control blood pressure by reducing sodium intake to less than 50 mEq/day.[154] Furthermore, about one third of patients with mild hypertension can control their blood pressure by reducing sodium intake to less than 75 mEq/day. A number of studies have also shown that even a modest reduction in sodium intake sustained for a prolonged period may reduce—but not normalize—blood pressure.

*By Patricia Volz-Clarke

A reduced sodium diet seems to be most effective for controlling systolic pressures in older hypertensive patients and patients with initially high blood pressure. It is unclear whether sodium restriction attenuates the age-related increase in blood pressure; the long-term effectiveness of sodium restriction in people with hypertension also remains to be clarified.

Exercise. Physical inactivity is a risk factor for hypertension; the relative risk is 1.5 times higher in sedentary people than in physically active people. To date, five out of six studies have reported a modest, but significant, blood pressure–lowering effect of aerobic exercise.

Fiber. High-fiber diets may be mildly hypotensive.

Chloride, phosphorus, and magnesium. The dietary intake of these nutrients may be important in the pathogenesis of hypertension. High intakes of chloride do not appear to contribute to hypertension, but chloride appears to play a role in salt-induced increases in blood pressure. A low intake of dietary phosphorus increases blood pressure in rats and in humans with and without hypertension, and the addition of phosphorus to the diet attenuates hypertension in the spontaneously hypertensive rat. In humans, these relationships remain to be established. Preliminary data suggest that a low intake of magnesium is associated with an increased risk for hypertension.

Fat. The role of fat quality and quantity in the etiology and treatment of hypertension remains to be clarified. Some evidence suggests that low-fat diets with a relatively high P/S ratio reduce both systolic and diastolic blood pressures (approximately 9 and 8 mm Hg, respectively).[154] There is also evidence that increasing dietary polyunsaturated fatty acids and lowering saturated fatty acids lower blood pressure. Some information indicates that diets high in either monounsaturated fatty acids or omega-3 fatty acids lower blood pressure.

Stress. Chronic resting blood pressure is, for the most part, not influenced by stressful events, even in people with hypertension.

Cigarettes. There is no evidence that cigarette smoking contributes to the development of hypertension.

Alcohol. Population studies have shown a positive relationship between blood pressure and alcohol consumption. Evidence from clinical studies supports this relationship. Alcohol may also interfere with the efficacy of antihypertensive agents.

Calcium. Analyses of the National Health and Nutrition Examination Surveys (I and II) have not shown any relationship between dietary calcium and blood pressure.[154] Some evidence from clinical trials indicates that supplemental calcium (1,000 mg/day) has a modest (6% to 9%) blood pressure-lowering effect in hypertensive persons. Other clinical studies have not found any hypotensive effects of calcium supplements. Thus, the role of calcium in regulating blood pressure remains to be clarified.

Potassium. Population studies have shown an inverse relationship between potassium intake and blood pressure.[154] A high potassium intake reportedly does not affect blood pressure in normotensive people. In hypertensive patients, however, a high potassium intake (170 to 175 mEq/day) reduces blood pressure by 3% to 10%. Longer-term studies are needed to establish the blood pressure-lowering effects of potassium.

ADVERSE EFFECTS OF TREATMENT FOR ONE CHD RISK FACTOR ON OTHER CHD RISK FACTORS*

In general, risk-factor intervention is beneficial, and it favorably affects CHD risk. In certain instances, however, the treatment of one risk factor can adversely affect others. Gotto[156] recently reviewed some common examples to alert health professionals of potentially adverse consequences of the pharmacological modification of CHD risk factors. The examples stress the importance of monitoring patients closely during risk-factor intervention.

Fibric acid drugs (such as clofibrate) used to treat hypercholesterolemia or hypertriglyceridemia may increase the concentration of LDL cholesterol. As noted earlier, beta-blockers, which are used to treat hypertension, increase plasma total-cholesterol and triglyceride levels and decrease HDL-cholesterol levels. Some diuretics may increase the concentration of plasma total-cholesterol, triglyceride, and LDL-cholesterol levels. Thiazide diuretics and chlorthalidone increase plasma total-cholesterol and triglyceride levels and decrease HDL-cholesterol levels. Propranolol has been associated with a 15% reduction in HDL-cholesterol levels in females. As noted previously, exogenous sex hormones modify plasma lipid concentrations. Overall, estrogens increase plasma triglycerides and HDL-cholesterol levels and decrease LDL-cholesterol and total-cholesterol levels; progesterones increase LDL cholesterol and decrease triglycerides and HDL cholesterol; and androgens increase total-cholesterol and LDL-cholesterol levels and decrease HDL-cholesterol levels.

Some drugs either favorably affect plasma lipids or have no known adverse effects. The alpha-blocker prazosin has been shown to decrease LDL-cholesterol levels and increase HDL-cholesterol levels. Clonidine, hydralazine, and reserpine appear to have no adverse effects on plasma lipid levels.

CORONARY RISK-FACTOR MODIFICATION*

Evidence from numerous randomized clinical trials has shown that cholesterol lowering, especially in men at high risk for CHD, reduces the incidence of CHD. In the studies reported, cholesterol lowering has been achieved by either diet or drug therapy (see chapters 2 and 11).

The Lipid Research Clinics Coronary Primary Prevention Trial (LRC-CPPT) showed a 19% lower incidence of CHD in cholestyramine/diet-treated men versus placebo/diet-treated group. Total plasma cholesterol and LDL cholesterol were 8% and 12% lower in the cholestyramine/diet-treated group compared with the placebo/diet-treated group.[31,32] In the Multiple Risk Factor Intervention Trial, the effect of multifactor intervention for seven years on mortality from CHD was studied in 12,866 high-risk men, aged 35 to 57, who were randomized into two groups: (1) special intervention, including stepped-care hypertension reduction, nutrition modification to reduce serum total cholesterol, and smoking cessation; and (2) the usual-care group (subjects were referred to their own physicians for care). Although not statistically significant, a 7.1% decrease in mortality was observed in the special-intervention group versus the usual-care group. CHD mortality was 17.9 per 1,000 in the special-intervention group and 19.3 per 1,000 in the usual-care group.[29]

The Cholesterol-Lowering Atherosclerosis Study (CLAS) was an angiographic trial designed to assess the effects of lowering LDL cholesterol and raising HDL cholesterol on the growth of atherosclerotic lesions. One hundred sixty-two eligible men who had had coronary bypass surgery were randomized into a treatment or control group. The treatment group ($n = 80$) received colestipol-niacin and was instructed to follow a low-fat (22% calories from fat; 10% as polyunsaturated, 4% as saturated), low-cholesterol (125 mg/day) diet. The

*By the Editors

control group ($n = 82$) received placebo pills and instruction on a low-fat diet (26% calories from fat; 10% as polyunsaturated, 5% as saturated) and 250 mg of cholesterol per day. After two years, plasma total cholesterol and LDL cholesterol were lowered 26% amd 43%, respectively, and HDL cholesterol was increased 37% in the treatment group. In the placebo (diet) group, total cholesterol and LDL cholesterol were lowered by 4% and 5%, respectively. All reductions were statistically significant. The treatment group had less lesion progression and new atheroma formation in the native coronary arteries. Of major significance was that atherosclerotic regression was noted in 16.2% of the subjects in the treatment group versus 2.4% in the placebo-treated group.[154]

In the clinical trials conducted to date, the incidence of CHD morbidity and mortality can be reduced in people at high risk for CHD. In addition to the primary prevention of CHD, intervention efforts aimed at the secondary prevention of CHD are effective in reducing CHD mortality. The incidence of recurrent myocardial infarction and death due to CHD can be reduced. Lowering plasma total-cholesterol and LDL-cholesterol levels has been shown to lower the incidence of CHD consistently in both previously unaffected and affected persons.

The magnitude of the reduction in CHD has been defined for people with initial serum cholesterol levels in the 250 to 300 mg/dL range. For each 1% reduction in the serum cholesterol level, a 2% reduction in the incidence of CHD is expected.[31,32] Therefore, a 10% to 15% reduction in the serum cholesterol level (a reduction that could be reasonably achieved by the American population) should reduce CHD risk by 20% to 30%. Persons with other risk factors (such as cigarette smoking and hypertension) will probably benefit the most from cholesterol lowering. Both intervention and longitudinal studies have shown beneficial effects of both raising HDL-cholesterol levels and even small elevations in HDL-cholesterol levels. For every 1 mg/dL increment in baseline HDL cholesterol, a 3.5% to 5.5% decrease in CHD was reported in the LRC-CPPT, LRC Prevalence Study, and Framingham Study.[36] Each 1 mg/dL increase in HDL cholesterol from baseline was associated with a 4.4% reduction in CHD risk.[36]

The Veterans Administration Cooperative Study Group on Antihypertensive Agents[143–145] clearly demonstrated the positive benefits of controlling blood pressure. In middle-aged men with mean diastolic levels of 115 to 129 mm Hg, there was a 93% reduction in the rate of nonfatal plus fatal complications of CHD. For those with a diastolic blood pressure of 105 to 114 mm Hg, the reduction was 69%. Castelli[158] has noted that in most of the antihypertensive trials, the treated group, in the short term, has had a significant reduction in the incidence of stroke. In many trials there was a reduction in the incidence of a number of CHD endpoints, even though the comparisons failed to reach statistical significance.

As noted, cigarette-smoking cessation improves CHD risk status.[159] Even after one or more myocardial infarctions, cessation of cigarette smoking improves the long-term prognosis of fatal and nonfatal CHD.[160]

In summary, elevated plasma total-cholesterol and LDL-cholesterol levels are major CHD risk factors. An elevated level of HDL cholesterol is protective against atherosclerosis. Modification of abnormal serum lipids due to genetic or acquired factors can reduce the risk of CHD,[3,4,15–32] as can the management of hypertension.

References

1. Kannel WB, Shatzkin A. Risk factor analysis. *Prog Cardiovasc Dis.* 1984;26:309.
2. American Heart Association. *Dietary Treatment of Hypercholesterolemia: A Handbook for Counselors.* Dallas, Tex: American Heart Association; 1988.
3. Morrison JA, Nambodiri K, Green P, et al. Familial aggregation of lipids and lipoproteins and early identification of dyslipoproteinemia: the Collaborative Lipid Research Clinics Family Study. *JAMA.* 1983;250:1860.
4. Moll PP, Sing CF, Weidman WH, et al. Total cholesterol and lipoproteins in school children: prediction of coronary heart disease in adult relatives. *Circulation.* 1983;67:127.
5. Brown MS, Goldstein JL. A receptor-mediated pathway for cholesterol homeostasis. *Science.* 1986;232:34.
6. National Cholesterol Education Program Expert Panel. Report on detection, evaluation, and treatment of high blood cholesterol in adults. *Arch Intern Med.* 1988;148:36.
7. Fredrickson DS, Levy RI, Lees RS. Fat transport in lipoproteins—an integrated approach to mechanisms and disorders. *N Engl J Med.* 1967;276:34, 94, 148, 215, 273.
8. Kannel WB, Hjortland MC, McNamara PM, et al. Menopause and risk of cardiovascular disease. *Ann Intern Med.* 1976;85:447.
9. Hazzard WR. Atherogenesis: why women live longer than men. *Geriatrics.* 1985;40:42.
10. Kannel WB. High density lipoproteins: epidemiological profile and risks of coronary artery disease. *Am J Cardiol.* 1983; 52:9B.
11. Heiss G, Tamir I, Davis CE, et al. Lipoprotein-cholesterol distributions in selected North American populations: the Lipid Research Clinics Program Prevalence Study. *Circulation.* 1980;61:302.
12. Crouse JR. Gender, lipoproteins, diet and cardiovascular risk. *Lancet.* 1989;1:318.
13. Knipp M, Chattion M. *Current Medical Diagnosis and Treatment.* Los Altos, Calif: Lange Medical Publications;1980:195.
14. American Heart Association. *1989 Heart Facts.* Dallas, Tex: American Heart Association; 1989.
15. Kannel WB, Doyle JT, Ostfeld AM, et al. *Optimal Resources for Primary Prevention of Atherosclerotic Disease.* Dallas, Tex: American Heart Association; 1984.
16. National Institute of Health Consensus Development Conference Statement, 1985: lowering blood cholesterol to prevent heart disease. *JAMA.* 1985;253:2080.
17. Dawber TR, Kannel WB. Susceptibility to coronary disease. *Mod Concepts Cardio Dis.* 1961;30:671.
18. Grundy SM, Bilheimer D, Blackburn H, et al. Rationale of the diet-heart statement of the American Heart Association. *Circulation.* 1982;65:839A.
19. Pooling Project Research Group. Relationship of blood pressure, serum cholesterol, smoking habits, relative weight, and ECG abnormalities to incidence of major coronary events: final report. *J Chronic Dis.* 1978;31:201.
20. Rifkind BM, Segal P. Lipid Research Clinics program reference values for hyperlipidemia and hypolipidemia. *JAMA.* 1983;250:1869.
21. Newman WP, Freedman DS, Voors AW. Relation of serum lipoprotein levels and systolic blood pressure to early atherosclerosis: the Bogalusa Heart Study. *N Engl J Med.* 1986;314:138.
22. Kannel WB. Lipids, diabetes, and coronary heart disease: insights from the Framingham Study. *Am Heart J.* 1985;110:1100.
23. Reaven GM. Looking at the world through LDL-cholesterol glasses. *J Nutr.* 1986;116:1143.
24. Kannel WB, Gordon T, Castelli WP. Obesity, lipids, and glucose tolerance: the Framingham Study. *Am J Clin Nutr.* 1979;32:1238.
25. Stamler J. Research related to risk factors. *Circulation.* 1979;60:1575.
26. West RJ, Shaw A. Dietary management of familial hyperlipidemia. *Proc Nutr Soc.* 1979;38:325.
27. Knuiman JT, West CE, Burema J. Serum total and high density lipoprotein cholesterol concentrations and body mass index in adult men from thirteen countries. *Am J Epidemiol.* 1982;116:631.

28. Miettinen TA, Huttunen JK, Naukkarinen V, et al. Multifactorial primary prevention of cardiovascular disease in middle-aged men: risk factors, changes, incidence and mortality. *JAMA.* 1985;254:2097.
29. Multiple Risk Factor Intervention Trial Research Group. Multiple Risk Factor Trial, risk factor changes and mortality results. *JAMA.* 1982;248:1465.
30. Watkins LO, Neaton JD, Kuller LH. Racial differences in high-density lipoprotein cholesterol and coronary heart disease incidence in usual care group of multiple risk factor intervention trial. *Am J Cardiol.* 1986;57:538.
31. Lipid Research Clinics Program. The Lipid Research Clinic's Coronary Primary Prevention Trial Results, II: the relationship of reduction in incidence of coronary heart disease to cholesterol lowering. *JAMA.* 1984;251:365.
32. Lipid Research Clinics Program. The Lipid Research Clinic's Coronary Primary Prevention Trial Results, I: reduction in incidence of coronary heart disease. *JAMA.* 1984;251:351.
33. Carlson LA, Bottiger LE. Risk factors for ischaemic heart disease in men and women. *Acta Med Scand.* 1985;218:207.
34. Hjermann I, Byre KV, Holme I, et al. Effect of diet and smoking intervention on the incidence of coronary heart disease: report from the Oslo Study Group of a randomized trial in healthy men. *Lancet.* 1981;2:1303.
35. Stamler J, Wentworth D, Neaton JD. Is relationship between serum cholesterol and risk of premature death from coronary heart disease continuous or graded? Findings in 356,222 primary screenees of the MRFIT. *JAMA.* 1986;256:2823.
36. Gordon DJ, Ekelund LG, Karon JM, et al. Predictive value of the exercise tolerance test for mortality in North American men: the Lipid Research Clinics Mortality Follow-Up Study. *Circulation.* 1986;74:252.
37. National Cholesterol Education Program Expert Panel. Report on detection, evaluation, and treatment of high blood cholesterol in adults. *Arch Intern Med.* 1988;148:36.
38. Gordon T, Castelli WP, Hjortland MC, et al. High density lipoproteins as a protective factor against disease: the Framingham Study. *Ann Intern Med.* 1977;90:85.
39. American Heart Association. *Physician's Cholesterol Education Slide Set.* Dallas, Tex: American Heart Association; 1988.
40. Frick MH, Elo O, Haapa K, et al. Helsinki Heart Study primary-prevention trial with gemfibrozil in middle-aged men with dyslipidemia. *N Engl J Med.* 1987;317:1237.
41. Kannel WB, Castelli WP, Gordon T. Cholesterol in the prediction of atherosclerotic disease: new perspectives based on the Framingham Study. *Ann Intern Med.* 1979;90:85.
42. Grundy SM; Goodman DS, Rifkind BM, et al. The place of HDL in cholesterol management. A perspective from the National Cholesterol Education Program. *Arch Intern Med.* 1989;149:505.
43. Kwiterovich P. *Beyond Cholesterol.* Baltimore, Md: University Press; 1989:77;149.
44. Merz B. Lp(a) joins other serum cholesterol lipoproteins as risk determinants. *JAMA.* 1989;261:2013.
45. Gordon T, Kagan A, Garcia-Palmieri N, et al. Diet and its relation to coronary heart diseases and death in three populations. *Circulation.* 1981;63:500.
46. Hully SB, Rosenman RH, Bawol RD, et al. The association between triglyceride and coronary heart disease. *N Engl J Med.* 1980;302:1383.
47. Tverdal A, Foss OP, Leren P, et al. Serum triglycerides as an independent risk factor for death from coronary heart disease in middle-aged Norwegian men. *Am J Epidemiol.* 1989;129:458.
48. Castelli WP. The triglyceride issue: a view from Framingham. *Am Heart J.* 1986;112:432.
49. Brunzell JD, Austin MA. Plasma triglyceride levels and coronary heart disease. *N Engl J Med.* 1989;320:1273.
50. Keys A, Menotti A, Aravanis C, et al. The Seven Countries Study: 2,289 deaths in 15 years. *Prev Med.* 1984;13:141.
51. Keys A. Coronary heart disease in seven countries: American Heart Association monograph 29. *Circulation.* 1970;41(suppl):1.
52. Robertson TL, Kato H, Gordon T. Epidemiologic studies of coronary heart disease and stroke in Japanese men living in Japan, Hawaii, and California: coronary heart disease risk factors in Japan and Hawaii. *Am J Cardiol.* 1977;39:244.

53. Karo H, Tillorson J, Nichaman MZ, et al. Epidemiology of coronary heart disease and stroke in Japanese men living in Japan, Hawaii, and California: serum lipids and diet. *Am J Epidemiol.* 1973;97:32.
54. Shekelle RB, Shryock AM, Paul O, et al. Diet, serum cholesterol and death from coronary heart disease: the Western Electric Study. *N Engl J Med.* 1981;304:65.
55. Stamler J, Shekelle B. Dietary cholesterol and human coronary heart disease: the epidemiological evidence. *Arch Pathol Med.* 1988;112:1032.
56. Goodnight SH, Harris WS, Connor WE, et al. Polyunsaturated fatty acids, hyperlipidemia, and thrombosis. *Atherosclerosis.* 1982;2:87.
57. Kromhout D, Bosschieter EB, Conlander L. The inverse relation between fish consumption and 20-year mortality from coronary heart disease. *N Engl J Med.* 1985;312:1205.
58. Little A, Graves K, Suchindran CM, et al. Customary diet, anthropometry and dyslipoproteinemia in selected North American populations: the Lipid Research Clinics Program Prevalence Study. *Circulation.* 1986;73:1.
59. Hegsted DM, Ausman LM. Diet, alcohol, and coronary heart disease in men. *J Nutr.* 1988;118:1184.
60. Thelle DS, Arnesen E, Forde OH. The Tromso Heart Study. *N Engl J Med.* 1983;308:1454.
61. Kris-Etherton PM, Krummel D, Russell ME, et al. The effect of diet on plasma lipids, lipoproteins, and coronary heart disease. *J Am Diet Assoc.* 1988;88:1373.
62. Wilson PW, Garrison RJ, Kannel WB, McGee DL, Castelli WP. Is coffee consumption a contributor to cardiovascular disease? *Arch Intern Med.* 1989;149:1169.
63. Thelle DS, Heyden S, Fodor JG. Coffee and cholesterol in epidemiological and experimental studies. *Atherosclerosis.* 1987;67:97.
64. Royal College of Physicians of London and British Cardiac Society. Report of a joint working party: prevention of coronary heart disease. *J Royal Physicians.* 1976;10:213.
65. Saudek CD, Young NL. Cholesterol metabolism in diabetes mellitus: the role of diet. *Diabetes.* 1981;30(suppl 2):76.
66. Stout RW. Hyperinsulinemia as an independent risk factor for atherosclerosis. *Int J Obesity.* 1982;6(suppl):111.
67. Stern MP, Haffner SM. Body fat distribution and hyperinsulinemia as risk factors for diabetes and cardiovascular disease. *Atherosclerosis.* 1986;6:123.
68. Rubler S, Dlugash J, Yuceoglu YZ, et al. New type of cardiomyopathy associated with diabetic glomerulosclerosis. *Am J Cardiol.* 1972;30:595.
69. Lester WM, Roberts WC. Diabetes mellitus for 25 years or more: analysis of cardiovascular findings in seven patients studied at necropsy. *Am J Med.* 1986;81:275.
70. Warren S, LeCompte PM, Legg MA. *The Pathology of Diabetes.* 4th ed. Philadelphia, Pa: Lea & Febiger; 1966.
71. Marble A. Coronary artery disease in the diabetic. *Diabetes.* 1955;4:290.
72. Mason JW. A re-evaluation of the concept of "non-specificity" in stress theory. *J Psych Res.* 1971;8:323.
73. Haynes SG, Feinleib M, Kannel WB. The relationship of psychological factors to coronary heart disease. *Am J Epidemiol.* 1980;111:37.
74. Jenkins CD. Recent evidence supporting psychologic and social risk factors for coronary disease. *N Engl J Med.* 1976;294:987.
75. Crisp AH, Queenan M, D'Souza MF. Myocardial infarction and emotional climate. *Lancet.* 1984;2:616.
76. Marmot M. Type A behaviour and ischaemic heart disease. *Psychol Med.* 1980;10:603. Editorial.
77. Shekelle R, Hulley S, Neaton J. Type A behavior and risk of coronary death in MRFIT. Paper presented at the twenty-third Annual Conference on Cardiovascular Disease Epidemiology; March 1983; San Diego, Calif.
78. Case RB, Heller SS, Case NB, et al. Type A behavior and survival after acute myocardial infarction. *N Engl J Med.* 1978;240:2548.
79. Rahe R. Brief group therapy in myocardial infarction rehabilitation: three-to four-year follow-up of controlled trial. *Psychol Med.* 1979;41:229.
80. Friedman M, Thoresen CE, Gill JJ, et al. Alteration of type A behavior and reduction in cardiac recurrences in myocardial infarction. *Am Heart J.* 1984;108:237.
81. Dalen JE, Hickler RB. Oral contraceptives and cardiovascular disease. *Am Heart J.* 1981;101:626.

82. Jick H, Dinar R, Herman R, et al. Myocardial infarction and other vascular diseases in young women: role of estrogen and other factors. *JAMA.* 1978;240:2548.
83. Slone D, Shapiro S, Kaufman DW, et al. Risk of myocardial infarction in relation to current and discontinued use of oral contraceptives. *N Engl J Med.* 1981;305:420.
84. Wahl P, Walden C, Knopp R, et al. Effects of estrogen/progestin potency on lipid/lipoprotein cholesterol. *N Engl J Med.* 1983;308:862.
85. Ross RK, Paganini-Hill A, Mack TM, et al. Menopausal oestrogen therapy and protection from death from ichaemic heart disease. *Lancet.* 1981;1:858.
86. Criqui MH, Suarez L, Barrett-Connor E, et al. Postmenopausal estrogen use and mortality. *Am J Epidemiol.* 1988;128:606.
87. Phillips GB. Evidence for hyperoestrogenaemia as a risk factor for myocardial infarction in men. *Lancet.* 1976;2:14.
88. Lindholm J, Winkel P, Brodthagen U, et al. Coronary risk factors and plasma sex hormones. *Am J Med.* 1982;73:648.
89. Coronary Drug Project Research Group. The Coronary Drug Project. *JAMA.* 1970;214:1303.
90. *Arteriosclerosis 1981.* US Dept of Health and Human Services; June 1981; 1. NIH publication 81-3034.
91. Paffenbarger RS, Notkin J, Krueger DE, et al. Chronic disease in former college students, II: methods of study and observations on mortality from coronary heart disease. *Am J Public Health.* 1966;56:962.
92. Hammond EC, Garfinkle L. Coronary heart disease, stroke and aortic aneurysm—factors in etiology. *Arch Environ Health.* 1969;19:167.
93. Kaufman DW, Helmrich SP, Rosenberg L, et al. Nicotine and carbon monoxide content of cigarette smoke and the risk of myocardial infarction in young men. *N Engl J Med.* 1983;308:409.
94. Stamford BA, Matter S, Fell RD, et al. Cigarette smoking, exercise, and high density lipoprotein cholesterol. *Atherosclerosis.* 1984;52:73.
95. Hjermann I. Smoking and diet intervention in healthy coronary high risk men: methods and five-year follow up of risk factors in a randomized trial: the Oslo Study. *J Oslo City Hosp.* 1980;30:3.
96. Coronary Drug Project Research Group. Cigarette smoking as a risk factor in men with a prior history of myocardial infarction. *J Chronic Dis.* 1979;32:415.
97. Garland C, Barrett-Connor E, Suarez L, et al. Effects of passive smoking on ischemic heart disease mortality of non-smokers: a prospective study. *Am J Epidemiol.* 1985;121:645.
98. National Health Interview Survey. US Dept of Commerce; 1985. Form HIS-1(SB).
99. Morris JN, Heady JA, Raffle PAB, et al. Coronary heart disease and physical activity of work. *Lancet.* 1953;2:1053, 1110.
100. Morris JN, Chave SPW, Adam C, et al. Vigorous exercise in leisure-time and the incidence of coronary heart disease. *Lancet.* 1973;1:333.
101. Paffenbarger RS, Hale WE. Work activity and coronary heart mortality. *N Engl J Med.* 1975;292:545.
102. Paffenbarger RS, Hale WE, Brand RJ, et al. Work-energy level, personal characteristics, and fatal heart attack: a birth-cohort effect. *Am J Epidemiol.* 1977;105:200.
103. Paffenbarger RS, Wing AL, Hyde RT. Physical activity as an index of heart attack risk in college alumni. *Am J Epidemiol.* 1978;108:161.
104. Paffenbarger RS, Hyde RT, Wing AL, et al. A natural history of athleticism and cardiovascular health. *JAMA.* 1984;252:491.
105. Paffenbarger RS, Hyde RT, Wing AL, et al. Physical activity, all-cause mortality, and longevity of college alumni. *N Engl J Med.* 1986;314:605.
106. Leon AS. Age and other predictors of coronary heart disease. *Med Sci Sports Exer.* 1987;19:159.
107. Kannel WB, Sorlie P. Some health benefits of physical activity: the Framingham Study. *Arch Intern Med.* 1979;139:857.
108. Wilber CS. The Johnson and Johnson program. *Prev Med.* 1983;12:672.
109. Farquhar JW, Fortman SP, Maccoby N, et al. The Stanford Five-City Project: design and methods. *Am J Epidemiol.* 1985;122:323.
110. Sallis JF, Haskell WL, Wood PD, et al. Physical activity assessment methodology in the five-city project. *Am J Epidemiol.* 1985;121:91.
111. Blair SN, Haskell WL, Ho P, et al. Assessment of habitual physical activity by a seven-day recall in a community survey and controlled experiments. *Am J Epidemiol.* 1985;122:794.

112. Klesges RC, Klesges AM, Swenson AM, et al. A validation of two motion sensors in the prediction of child and adult physical activity levels. *Am J Epidemiol.* 1985;122:400.
113. Washburn RA, Montoye HJ. The assessment of physical activity by questionnaire. *Am J Epidemiol.* 1986;123:563.
114. Camley JA, LaPorte RE, Sandler RB, et al. Comparison of methods to measure physical activity in postmenopausal women. *Am J Clin Nutr.* 1987;45:14.
115. Kris-Etherton PM. The effect of exercise on lipid and lipoprotein metabolism. In: *Nutrition and Aerobic Exercise.* Washington, DC: American Chemical Society, 1986.
116. Carlson LA, Mossfeldt F. Acute effects of prolonged heavy exercise on the concentration of plasma lipids and lipoproteins in man. *Acta Physiol Scand.* 1964;62:51.
117. Hoffman AA, Nelson WR, Gross FA. Effects of an exercise program on plasma lipids of senior Air Force officers. *Am J Cardiol.* 1967;20:516.
118. Tran ZV, Weltman A, Glass GV, et al. The effects of exercise on blood lipids and lipoproteins: a meta-analysis of studies. *Med Sci Sports Exer.* 1983;15:393.
119. Burton BT, Foster WR. Health implications of obesity: a NIH Consensus Development Conference. *J Am Diet Assoc.* 1985;85:1117.
120. Weigly ES. Average? Ideal? Desirable? A brief overview of height-weight tables in the United States. *J Am Diet Assoc.* 1984;84:417.
121. Alexander JK. The cardiomyopathy of obesity. *Prog Cardiovasc Dis.* 1985;27:325.
122. Caggiula AW, Christakis G, Farrand M, et al. The Multiple Risk Factor Intervention Trial (MRFIT), IV: intervention on blood lipids. *Prev Med.* 1981;10:443.
123. Bray GA. Effect of obesity on health and happiness. In: Brownell KD, Foryet JP, eds. *Handbook of Eating Disorders.* New York, NY: Basic Books Inc; 1986.
124. Stern MP, Haffner SM. Body fat distribution and hyperinsulinemia as risk factors for diabetes and cardiovascular disease. *Arteriosclerosis.* 1986;6:123.
125. Simopoulos AP, VanItallie TB. Body weight, health and longevity. *Ann Intern Med.* 1984;100:285.
126. Glueck CJ, Taylor HL, Jacobs D, et al. Plasma high-density lipoprotein cholesterol: association with measurements of body mass: the Lipid Research Clinics Program Prevalence Study. *Circulation.* 1980;62(suppl 4):62.
127. Brennan PJ, Simpson JM, Blacket RB, et al. Effects of body weight on serum cholesterol, serum triglycerides, serum urate, and systolic blood pressure. *Aust NZ J Med.* 1980;10:15.
128. Aristimuno GG, Foster TA, Voors AW, et al. Influence of persistent obesity in children on cardiovascular risk factors: the Bogalusa Heart Study. *Circulation.* 1984; 69:895.
129. Freedman DS, Burke GL, Harsha DW, et al. Relationship of changes in obesity to serum-lipid and lipoprotein changes in childhood and adolescence. *JAMA.* 1985;254:515.
130. Lupien PJ, Rochon J, Dagenais GR, et al. Lipid profile of a French-Canadian population, I: association of plasma-lipid and lipoprotein levels with age, relative body weight, and education. *Can Med Assoc J.* 1985;113:1127.
131. Vague J. The degree of masculine differentiation of obesities: a factor determining predisposition to diabetes, atherosclerosis, gout, and uric calculous disease. *Am J Clin Nutr.* 1956;4:20.
132. Albrink MJ, Meigs JW. The relationship between serum triglycerides and skinfold thickness in obese subjects. *Ann NY Acad Sci.* 1965;131:673.
133. Foster CJ, Weinsein RL, Birch R, et al. Obesity and serum lipids: an evaluation of the relative contribution of body fat and fat distribution and lipid levels. *Int J Obesity.* 1987;11:151.
134. Anderson AJ, Sobocinski KA, Freedman DS, et al. Body fat distribution, plasma lipids, and lipoproteins. *Arteriosclerosis.* 1988;8:88.
135. Ostlund RE Jr, Staten M, Kohrt WM, et al. The ratio of waist-to-hip circumference, plasma insulin level, and glucose intolerance as independent predictors of the HDL_2 cholesterol level in older adults. *N Engl J Med.* 1990;322:229.
136. Lapidus L, Bengstsson C, and Larrson B. Distribution of adipose tissue and risk of cardiovascular disease and death: a twelve-year follow up of participants in the population study of women in Gothenburg, Sweden. *Br Med J.* 1984;289:1257.
137. Donahue RP, Abbott RD, Bloom E, et al. Central obesity and coronary heart disease in men. *Lancet.* 1987;1:821.
138. Despres JP, Tremblay A, Perusse L, et al. Association independent from obesity and serum triglyceride concentration. *Int J Obesity.* 1988;12:1.

139. Grundy SM, Arky R, Bray GA, et al. Coronary risk factor statement for the American public: a statement of the nutrition committee. *Circulation.* 1985;72:1135A.
140. *The 1984 Report of the Joint National Committee on Detection, Evaluation and Treatment of High Blood Pressure.* US Dept of Health and Human Services, Public Health Service, National Institutes of Health; June 1984. NIH publication 84-1088.
141. Pooling Project Research Group. Relationship of blood pressure, serum cholesterol, smoking habits, relative weight and ECG abnormalities to incidence of major coronary events: final report of the Pooling Project. *J Chron Dis.* 1978;31:201.
142. Shurtleff D. Some characteristics related to the incidence of cardiovascular disease and death: the Framingham Study, 18-year follow up. In: *An Epidemiological Investigation of Cardiovascular Disease.* US Dept of Health, Education, and Welfare; February 1984. NIH publication 74-599.
143. Veterans Administration Cooperative Study Group on Antihypertensive Agents. Effects of treatment on morbidity in hypertension: results in patients with diastolic blood pressure averaging 115 through 129 mm Hg. *JAMA.* 1967;202:1028.
144. Veterans Administration Cooperative Study Group on Antihypertensive Agents. Effects of treatment on morbidity in hypertension, II: results in patients with diastolic blood pressure averaging 90 through 114 mm Hg. *JAMA.* 1970;213:1143.
145. Veterans Administration Cooperative Study Group on Antihypertensive Agents. Effects of treatment on morbidity in hypertension, III: influence of age, diastolic blood pressure and prior cardiovascular disease; further analysis of side effects. *Circulation.* 1972;45:991.
146. Hypertension Detection and Follow-up Program Cooperative Group. Five-year findings of the Hypertension Detection and Follow-up Program, I: reduction in mortality of persons with high blood pressure, including mild hypertension. *JAMA.* 1979;242:2562.
147. Connor SL, Connor WE, Henry H, et al. The effects of familial relationships, age, body weight, and diet on blood pressure and the 24-hour urinary excretion of sodium, potassium, and creatinine in men, women, and children of randomly selected families. *Circulation.* 1984;70:76.
148. Speers MA, Kasl SV, Freeman DH, et al. Blood pressure concordance between spouses. *Am J Epidemiol.* 1986;123:818.
149. Clarke WR, Schrott HG, Burns TL, et al. Aggregation of blood pressure in the families of children with labile high systolic blood pressure: the Muscatine Study. *Am J Epidemiol.* 1986;123:67.
150. Pooling Project Research Group. Relationship of blood pressure, serum cholesterol, smoking habits, relative weight and ECG abnormalities to incidence of major coronary events: final report of the Pooling Project. *J Chron Dis.* 1978;31:201.
151. Castelli WP. Epidemiology of coronary heart disease: the Framingham Study. *Am J Med.* 1984;2:4.
152. National Kidney Foundation. *Education Program on Nonpharmacologic Management of Hypertension.* New York, NY: National Kidney Foundation Inc; 1988.
153. National Research Council, National Academy of Sciences. *Diet and Health. Implications for Reducing Chronic Disease Risk.* Washington, DC: National Academy Press; 1989.
154. *The Surgeon General's Report on Nutrition and Health.* Washington, DC: US Dept of Health and Human Services; 1988.
155. Rose G, Stamler J. The INTERSALT study: background, methods, and main results. *J Human Hypertension.* 1989;3:283.
156. Gotto AM Jr. Treatment of hyperlipidemia. *Am J Cardiol.* 1986;57:11.
157. Blankenhorn DH, Nessim SA, Johnson RL, et al. Beneficial effects of combined colestipol-niacin therapy on coronary atherosclerosis and coronary venous bypass grafts. *JAMA.* 1987;257:3233.
158. Castelli WP. Epidemiology of coronary heart disease: the Framingham Study. *Am J Med.* 1984;76:4.
159. Stamler J. Lifestyles, major risk factors, proof and public policy. *Circulation.* 1978;58:3.
160. Stamler J. Introduction to risk factors in coronary artery disease. In: McIntosh HO, ed. *Cardiology Series.* Northfield, Ill: Medical Communications Inc; 1978;1 (part 3).

161. Levy RI, Fredrickson DS, Shulman R, et al. Dietary and drug treatment of primary hyperlipoproteinemia. *Ann Intern Med.* 1972;77:287.
162. Havel RJ. Approach to the patient with hyperlipidemia. *Med Clin North Am.* 1982;66:319.
163. Paffenbarger RS, Notkin J, Kreuger DE, et al. Chronic disease in former college students, II: methods of study and observations on mortality from coronary heart disease. *Am J Public Health.* 1966;56:962.
164. Katz LN, Stamler J, Pick R. *Nutrition and Atherosclerosis.* Philadelphia, Pa: Lea & Febiger; 1958.
165. National Heart, Lung and Blood Institute. *Facts at Your Fingertips: National Heart, Lung and Blood Institute Kit '89.* Washington, DC: US Dept of Health and Human Services; 1989.

2. DIET AND CHD: SUMMARY OF THE LITERATURE

Epidemiological, clinical, and laboratory investigations have established that diet plays a critical role in the prevention and treatment of coronary heart disease (CHD). Early studies clarified the roles of dietary fat quality and cholesterol on plasma lipid and lipoprotein levels. Recently, the role of other dietary factors on CHD risk status has been addressed. Ongoing investigations are studying the effects that diet and dietary factors have on plasma lipoprotein subfractions and composition, apolipoprotein concentration, mechanistic actions, hemostasis, and thrombosis. The effects of specific fatty acids and other dietary constituents on atherosclerosis are being studied extensively. Results from these studies are advancing our understanding of how diets can be most effectively modified to prevent and treat CHD.

DIETARY FACTORS THAT AFFECT PLASMA LIPIDS

Fat Quality—Saturated Fatty Acids*

Numerous epidemiological studies demonstrated a strong relationship between saturated-fatty-acid intake and plasma total-cholesterol and LDL-cholesterol levels as well as the incidence of CHD. The study most widely acknowledged was conducted by Ancel Keys after World War II.[1] Clinical and experimental studies have repeatedly confirmed these early observations.

Certain saturated fatty acids, such as lauric ($C_{12:0}$), myristic ($C_{14:0}$), and palmitic ($C_{16:0}$), are hypercholesterolemic. A recent study by Bonanome and Grundy[2] indicates that stearic acid ($C_{18:0}$) has no effect on plasma total-cholesterol and LDL-cholesterol levels. Major sources of the hypercholesterolemic saturated fatty acids are provided in the appendix (see Table 14.18). Saturated fatty acids can also be reduced by decreasing total fat intake since most food fats in the American diet have some saturated fatty acids.

Predictive equations have been developed by Keys et al[3] and Hegsted et al[4] to determine the magnitude of change in plasma cholesterol in response to changes in the fatty-acid composition of the diet. Both equations† predict that the plasma cholesterol-raising effect of saturated fatty acids is approximately twice the cholesterol-lowering effect of polyunsaturated fatty acids (omega-6). Thus, the effect of dietary fat on serum cholesterol is a function of the expression 2S − P, where S and P represent, respectively, the quantity of saturated fatty acids and omega-6 fatty acids as percentages of total calories. Saturated fatty acids are twice as potent in raising plasma total cholesterol as polyunsaturated fatty acids are in lowering plasma total cholesterol. For every 1%

*By Rachael Trevethan

†Keys (Minnesota) equation:

$$\triangle chol = 1.35(2\triangle S - \triangle P) + 1.52\triangle Z$$

Hegsted (Harvard) equation:

$$\triangle chol = 2.16\triangle S - 1.65\triangle P + 0.0677\triangle C - 0.53$$

where $\triangle chol$ = estimated change in serum cholesterol in mg/dL
$\triangle S$ = change in percentage of daily calories from saturated fat
$\triangle P$ = change in percentage of daily calories from polyunsaturated fat
$\triangle Z$ = change in the square root of daily dietary cholesterol in mg/1,000 kcal and
$\triangle C$ = dietary cholesterol in mg/day

increase in the saturated-fatty-acid intake (on a caloric basis), plasma total cholesterol increases approximately 2.7 mg/dL. Accordingly, for every 1% increase in omega-6 fatty acids, a 1.4 mg/dL reduction in plasma total cholesterol is expected.

Saturated fatty acids raise and omega-6 fatty acids lower LDL-cholesterol levels. Most often, investigators have found that diets high in saturated fatty acids (and cholesterol) raise HDL-cholesterol levels.[5] Diets high in omega-6 fatty acids often lower HDL-cholesterol levels.[6,7]

A mechanism to describe the hypercholesterolemic effect of saturated fatty acids has been recently reported. Spady and Dietschy[8] noted a decrease in hepatic LDL-receptor activity in hamsters concomitant with an increase in plasma LDL-cholesterol levels in response to a diet high in saturated fatty acids and cholesterol. This finding is of major significance to our understanding of the role diet plays in the development of atherosclerosis.

Fat Quality—Unsaturated Fatty Acids

*Chemistry of unsaturated fatty acids.** There are four different classes of unsaturated fatty acids found in mammals: omega-3, omega-6, omega-7, and omega-9. The distinction among these classes is the position of double bonds relative to the CH_3 end group. Omega-3 fatty acids have their first double bond positioned between the third and fourth carbons from the CH_3 end group. Likewise, omega-6 fatty acids have their first double bond positioned between the sixth and seventh carbons. Thus, omega-7 and omega-9 fatty acids have their first double bond positioned between the seventh and eighth carbons and the ninth and tenth carbons, respectively.

*Omega-6 fatty acids (polyunsaturated fatty acids).** Traditionally, a diet high in polyunsaturated fatty acids, especially omega-6 fatty acids, was recommended to reduce CHD risk. Omega-6 fatty acids elicit a direct hypocholesterolemic effect.[9,10] In addition, omega-6 fatty acids replace saturated fatty acids in the diet.[6] A diet high in fatty acids has a greater lowering effect on plasma total cholesterol than does manipulation of dietary cholesterol.[11] The hypocholesterolemic effects of the omega-6 fatty acids are the result of changes in VLDL-cholesterol and LDL-cholesterol levels (and sometimes HDL-cholesterol levels).[11]

Although the P/S ratio of the diet has been widely used as an indicator of the relative polyunsaturated fatty-acid and saturated fatty-acid composition, it is of limited usefulness. For example, diets with markedly different quantities of total fat (and, therefore, polyunsaturated fatty acids and saturated fatty acids) could have identical P/S ratios. Because of this, it is preferable to use percentage of calories from saturated fatty acids, monounsaturated fatty acids, and polyunsaturated fatty acids, since this provides a more accurate description of the amounts of the respective fatty-acid classes in the diet.[12]

There is no specific P/S (omega-6 fatty acids to saturated fatty acids) ratio recommended. In following the Step One and Step Two diets, however, the P/S ratio will be approximately 1.0–1.3. A very high P/S ratio does not provide additional hypocholesterolemic benefits and may cause a decrease in HDL-cholesterol levels.[6,9,10]

*By Rachael Trevethan

It is recommended that saturated fatty acids provide not more than 10% of calories to the diet. Saturated fatty acids can be partially replaced by substituting either polyunsaturated or monounsaturated fatty acids. Examples of foods rich in polyunsaturated and monounsaturated fatty acids are provided in the appendix (see Tables 14.19, 14.20, 14.22, and 14.23). However, it is recommended that no more than 10% of total calories come from polyunsaturated fatty acids. Monounsaturated fatty acids should also provide approximately 10% of total calories if a diet provides less than 30% of calories from fat.

*Omega-3 fatty acids.** There was not a great deal of interest in the effect of fish oils on plasma lipids until the 1970s, when epidemiological studies suggested that marine lipids have a protective role against CHD. Many studies have shown that the consumption of large amounts of fish oil (approximately 90 to 120 g/day) markedly lowers plasma triglyceride levels. Much smaller quantities (approximately 8 g/day) also affect plasma triglyceride levels.[13] The fatty acids that confer the hypotriglyceridemic effect are the omega-3 fatty acids. The principal omega-3 fatty acids in fish oil are eicosapentenaenoic acid (EPA, $C_{20:5}$) and docosahexaenoic acid (DHA, $C_{22:6}$).

In a recent review, Harris[13] summarizes the effect of fish oil on plasma lipids and lipoproteins. Studies have shown little effect of fish oil on the plasma total-cholesterol level. Hypertriglyceridemic persons have even experienced increases in LDL-cholesterol levels of 10% to 20% during omega-3 fatty-acid supplementation. Some studies have also found that HDL cholesterol may increase (about 5% to 10%) when fish oil is consumed. The mechanisms responsible for the changes in LDL cholesterol and HDL cholesterol are not known. Harris[13] notes that in studies that have shown a plasma cholesterol-lowering effect of fish oil supplements, saturated-fatty-acid intake was lower during the treatment phase of the experiment compared with baseline.

The mechanism by which fish oil affects plasma triglyceride levels is primarily by inhibiting VLDL production.[14] Omega-3 fatty acids are also antithrombotic. There is some evidence that these effects are due to the changes that omega-3 fatty acids have on platelet and endothelial-cell function. It should be noted, however, that this evidence is based on in vitro studies. Future studies are necessary to resolve the effects that omega-3 fatty acids have on platelet function. Omega-3 fatty acids reduce platelet aggregation (and blood clots) and also are antiinflammatory.

The amount of omega-3 fatty acids required for effective long-term management of plasma lipid levels is not known. Eskimos consume 4 to 5 g of EPA daily,[15] an amount present in 18 oz to 3 lb of fish rich in omega-3 fatty acids. It is unrealistic to believe that many in the general US population will consume this quantity of fish each day. The use of fish-oil supplements (*Table 2.1*) to increase omega-3 fatty acid consumption is not recommended. Questions have been raised about the safety, proper dosages, duration of treatment, and side effects of long-term ingestion. Furthermore, taken in the doses recommended by the manufacturer, these supplements contribute only very small quantities of omega-3 fatty acids to the diet. Food sources of omega-3 fatty acids are listed in the appendix (see Tables 14.24 and 14.25).

At this time it is prudent to recommend that the public consume more fish, since it has been shown to beneficially affect CHD risk. In addition, substituting fish for foods high in saturated fatty acids is an effective way to reduce both saturated-fatty-acid and total fat intake. All types of fish are recommended.

*By Rachael Trevethan

Table 2.1
Selected Fish-Oil Products*

Product*	Mode	Omega-3 Fat Content	Dosage
MaxEPA (Scherer)	1000-mg capsules	180 mg EPA 120 mg DHA	1–2/day (with meals)
SuperMaxEPA (Twin Labs)	1200-mg capsules	225 mg EPA 150 mg DHA	2/day
Promega Parke-Davis	1000-mg capsules	350 mg EPA 150 mg DHA	1–2/day (with meals)
Proto-chol (Squibb)	1000-mg capsules	180 mg EPA 120 mg DHA	1–2/day (with meals)

*Recommended by manufacturer (not endorsed by SCAN).

Adapted with permission from Abramowicz M, ed. Fish oil for the heart. *Med Ltr.* 1987;29:7.

*Monounsaturated fatty acids.** The basis for the growing interest in the role of monounsaturated fatty acids in dietary treatment of hyperlipoproteinemia is based on information from some cohorts in the Seven Countries Study. In spite of the decrease in cardiovascular disease (CVD) in the United States, cardiovascular deaths are still approximately twice as high as in Mediterranean nations. Researchers found that although study subjects on the Mediterranean island of Crete ate a diet containing 40% of its calories from fat, they had a very low incidence of CHD.[16] Analysis of possible explanations for this finding led to the observation that differences lay in the high intake of olive oil in Crete. Olive oil is a good source of the most common monounsaturated fatty acid, oleic acid. When compared with the Cretan diet, the typical American diet is higher in total fat, saturated fatty acids, and polyunsaturated fatty acids, and is lower in monounsaturated acids (*Table 2.2*).

Table 2.2
Mean Percentage of Calories From Total Fat, Monounsaturated Fatty Acids, Saturated Fatty Acids, and Polyunsaturated Fatty Acids in American and Greek Diets

Country	Total Fat, %	Mono-unsaturated, %	Saturated, %	Poly-unsaturated, %
USA, typical diet	37	14	13	7
Corfu, Greece	33	18	6	4
Crete, Greece	36	26	8	3

Adapted with permission from Aravanis C, Corcondilas A, Dontas AS, et al. The Greek islands of Crete and Corfu. *Circulation.* 1970;41(suppl 1):I-88; and *Designing Foods*; ©1988 by the National Academy of Sciences, National Academy Press, Washington, D.C.

Fifteen-year data from the Seven Countries Study indicate that relationships between death rates and dietary factors were positive for saturated fatty acids and negative for monounsaturated fatty acids, and that death rates were not related to omega-6 fatty acids, protein, carbohydrate, and alcohol.[17] Death rates were negatively related to the ratio of monounsaturated fatty acids to saturated fatty acids.

Mattson and Grundy[18] examined the effects of substituting monounsaturated fatty acids for saturated fatty acids on plasma lipoproteins. Other

*By Lynne W. Scott and Mary C. McMann

studies have since investigated dietary components that can be substituted for saturated fatty acids in the American diet.[19-25] While some of these studies have substituted monounsaturated fatty acids for saturated fatty acids, others have used diets high in omega-6 fatty acids or low in total fat and high in carbohydrate. Particular emphasis has been placed on lowering LDL-cholesterol levels without lowering HDL-cholesterol levels. Some general conclusions can be drawn, based on the results of these studies[26]:

1. A diet low in saturated fatty acids is effective in lowering elevated plasma levels of total and LDL cholesterol.
2. Partially replacing the calories from saturated fatty acids with carbohydrate calories can lead to reductions in plasma total cholesterol, LDL cholesterol, and HDL cholesterol and may cause slight (not statistically significant) elevation in triglyceride levels.
3. Partially replacing the calories from saturated fatty acids with omega-6 fatty acids leads to a decrease in both LDL cholesterol and HDL cholesterol.
4. Partially replacing the calories from saturated fatty acids with monounsaturated fatty acids leads to a decrease in plasma total cholesterol and LDL cholesterol at least as great as with diets that are either low in total fat or that partially replace saturated fatty acids with omega-6 fatty acids. *Table 2.3* indicates that using monounsaturated fatty acids does not significantly change HDL-cholesterol or triglyceride levels.[18]

Table 2.3
Mean Levels of Various Plasma Lipids in Subjects Fed Diets High in Saturated Fatty Acids, Monounsaturated Fatty Acids, and Polyunsaturated Fatty Acids

Diet	Total Cholesterol, mg/dL	Triglyceride, mg/dL	LDL Cholesterol, mg/dL	VLDL Cholesterol, mg/dL	HDL Cholesterol, mg/dL
Saturated	224	259	143	42	39
Monounsaturated	197	249	119	40	38
Polyunsaturated fatty acids (omega-6)	191	231	120	36	35

Adapted with permission from Mattson FH, Grundy SM. Comparison of effects of dietary saturated, monounsaturated, and polyunsaturated fatty acids on plasma lipids and lipoproteins in man. *J Lipid Res.* 1985;26:194.

Table 2.4 summarizes lipoprotein changes from several studies, showing only the groups that received a source of monounsaturated fatty acids as their primary fat source. All of the studies were conducted with small groups over short periods of time (usually three to four weeks). With one exception,[20] these studies used high levels of fat (37% to 50% of total calories). Monounsaturated fatty acids made up more than 15% of calories and saturated fatty acids were usually lower than the maximum levels recommended by the American Heart Association (AHA) and the National Cholesterol Education Program.[27]

Table 2.4
Lipoprotein Values in Studies Using Monounsaturated Fatty Acids

Author (Year)	Fat Source	Diet: Fat % cal	Mono % cal	Sat % cal	Serum Lipoproteins: Chol mg/dL	Tg* mg/dL	HDL-C mg/dL	LDL-C mg/dL
Mattson (1985)[18]	High-oleic safflower oil	40	NA	NA	263 −31	249 −9	38 −1	150 −31
Grundy (1986)[19]	High-oleic safflower oil	40	28	4	251 −43	171 +7	43 −4	179 −43
Sirtori (1986)[20]	Olive oil 1st	30	18	7	241 −4	157 +14	38 +1	175 −4
	2nd	30	18	7	273 −19	130 +2	46 0	205 −15
Mensink (1987)[21]	Olive oil and margarine	41	24	10	197 −18	88 −11	57 +2	NA
Garg (1988)[22]	Olive oil	50	33	10	225 −29	285 −122	32 +2	135 −1
Baggio (1988)[23]	Olive oil	38	28	10	229 −25	86 −23	50 0	159 −19
Grundy (1988)[24]	High-oleic safflower oil	40	27	7	227 −19	127 −23	51 −1	143 −3
Mensink (1989)[25]	Olive oil	37	15	13	189 −28	88 −4	53 −4	127 −23

*Tg, triglyceride.

Oils high in monounsaturated fatty acids include high-oleic safflower and sunflower oil (which is used by only a few food manufacturers and is not currently available on the retail market), olive oil, and canola oil (*Table 2.5*).

Table 2.5
Percentage of Monounsaturated Fatty Acids, Polyunsaturated Fatty Acids, Saturated Fatty Acids, and P/S Ratio of Various Oils High in Monounsaturated Fatty Acids

Oils	Mono-unsaturated, %	Poly-unsaturated, %	Saturated, %	P/S
High-oleic safflower oil	75.3	14.2	6.1	2.3
Olive oil	73.7	8.4	13.5	0.6
Canola oil	62.0	32.0	6.0	5.3
Peanut oil	46.2	32.0	16.9	1.9

Adapted from Reeves JB III, Weihrauch JL. *Composition of Foods: Fats and Oils—Raw, Processed, and Prepared.* US Dept of Agriculture handbook 8-4 (revised); 1979.

Some nutritionists feel that a reduction in total fat with an increase in monounsaturated fatty acids may be an effective lipid-lowering diet. It is important to note, however, that other plasma cholesterol-lowering diets (such as the AHA Step One Diet) have been shown to be very effective despite having a relatively low level of monounsaturated fatty acids (approximately 10% of calories). In the Cholesterol-Lowering Atherosclerosis Study,[29] the regression of atherosclerotic lesions was noted in 3.6% of the subjects in the control group, which followed a diet containing 29% of calories from fat, 10% from monounsaturated fatty acids, 8% from saturated fatty acids, and 9% from polyunsaturated fatty acids. The use of monounsaturated fatty acids may provide an alternative approach to the very-low-fat diets and diets with higher levels of polyunsaturated fatty acids that are presently used to achieve a cholesterol-lowering effect. In particular, the substitution of monounsaturated fatty acids for saturated and polyunsaturated fatty acids may be used for those who have difficulty reducing dietary fat to recommended levels (less than 30% of calories). It should be noted, however, that diets with more than 15% of calories from monounsaturated fatty acids and less than 10% of calories from saturated fatty acids are difficult to plan, as both types of fatty acids are often present in the same foods. In meat, a major source of saturated fatty acids, monounsaturated fatty acids and saturated fatty acids occur in equal amounts.

Fat Quantity*

Although early epidemiological studies indicated a relationship between total fat intake and the incidence of CHD, fat quality (specifically saturated fatty acid intake) was not controlled. Nichaman and Hamm[30] recently reported that the effect of fat quality on plasma total cholesterol was independent of fat quantity. The authors noted that low-fat diets (<30% calories from fat) affect plasma lipid levels by virtue of their fatty-acid composition. A similar conclusion is supported for high-fat diets (>35% of calories from fat) by Blackburn[31] from data collected in the Seven Countries Study. Therefore, some scientists feel that fat quantity is not significant in the development of CHD.

Others believe, however, that total fat plays a more significant role in the development of CHD than previously thought. Two recent population studies[32,33] reported a significant relationship between total fat intake and the incidence of CHD morbidity and mortality. Additional studies in this area are needed. Within the next decade the relative contribution of total fat intake independent of fat quality to CHD morbidity and mortality should be resolved.

A reduction in total fat is recommended for the prevention and treatment of CHD to facilitate reducing saturated fatty acids and calories, both of which affect blood lipid levels. Diets lower in fat (and, likely, in calories) are beneficial for long-term weight control. While there is no question that reducing saturated fatty acids is effective in the prevention and treatment of CHD, there is a growing uncertainty about the best approach for reducing dietary saturated fatty acids. Should total fat and, hence, saturated fatty acids be reduced? Or should unsaturated fatty acids (monounsaturated or omega-3 fatty acids) replace saturated fatty acids in the diet, leading to the consumption of higher-fat diet (approximately 35% of calories)? The efficacy of different lipid-lowering diets with respect to weight control and adherence also needs to be clarified.

It is well accepted that fat quality has a more significant effect on the plasma lipid response than fat quantity. It will be important to resolve the usefulness and practicality of diets higher in total fat but low in saturated fatty acids in the management of plasma lipids. Should this approach prove to be effective, practitioners will have more options in counseling patients.

*By Rachael Trevethan

Vegetarianism*

It is evident that the consumption of a vegetarian diet (which is typically low in total fat, saturated fatty acids, and cholesterol) is associated with a favorable plasma lipoprotein profile.[34,35] Furthermore, population studies have shown that vegetarians have a reduced risk of CHD.[36] In addition to the reduction in plasma total-cholesterol and LDL-cholesterol levels, vegetarianism has been associated with lower concentrations of apolipoprotein A-I, B, and E.[34,37] In addition, LDL production rates have been reported to be lower in vegetarians.[38]

It is not clear what factors account for the differences in plasma lipid levels between vegetarians and omnivores that have been reported in cross-sectional studies. It is likely that differences in total fat, saturated fatty acids, cholesterol, and fiber intake contribute to the differences in plasma lipid levels. In addition, other dietary constituents may play a contributory role.

Recently it has been reported that serum from vegans (vegetarians who avoid all animal products) had a higher linoleic-acid content and a lower arachidonic-acid content than omnivores.[39] Since arachidonic acid is a precursor of thromboxane A-2, which causes vasoconstriction and platelet aggregation, fatty-acid composition may play some role in the protective effects of a vegetarian diet on CHD.

Carbohydrate†

Since fat and carbohydrate (CHO) are inversely related in the diet, recommendations to lower total fat are also recommendations to increase carbohydrate. Carbohydrate represents approximately 45% of the dietary energy intake of the American diet.[40] Approximately one third to one half of the carbohydrate in the diet is simple sugar. Many nutritionists recommend that carbohydrate comprise at least 50% of calories, with an emphasis on complex (and unrefined) carbohydrates.

Interpopulation studies have established that high-carbohydrate diets are associated with a lower risk of CHD.[41] The consumption of a diet that contains approximately 80% of calories as carbohydrate (ie, a very-high-carbohydrate and very-low-fat diet) is associated with low plasma total-cholesterol, LDL-cholesterol, and HDL-cholesterol levels.[42,43] Diets with less carbohydrate but that are, nonetheless, still high in carbohydrate (approximately 50%) are associated with a favorable plasma lipid profile. Clinical studies have supported the population data. When subjects are switched from a typical American diet to one that is lower in saturated fatty acids, cholesterol, and total fat and is higher in soluble fiber, expected changes in plasma lipids occur.[44]

Despite the beneficial effects of a habitual high-carbohydrate diet, some scientists have expressed concern over the findings that HDL-cholesterol levels are lower and plasma triglyceride levels are elevated on high-carbohydrate diets. It should be noted, however, that in populations with high carbohydrate intakes the incidence of CHD is low even though HDL-cholesterol levels are relatively

*By Rachael Trevethan
†By Anne O'Donnell

low. In populations with a habitual high-carbohydrate diet, however, new evidence suggests plasma triglycerides are higher (C. West and M. Katan, Wageningen University, the Netherlands, personal communication). In addition, there is recent information that plasma triglyceride levels begin to normalize after subjects switch to a high-carbohydrate diet and follow it for months.[45]

Carbohydrate type also plays an important role in determining the plasma triglyceride response. The issue of carbohydrate type (simple versus complex) has been reviewed recently[46] and will not be discussed further. The evidence suggests that simple carbohydrate may cause a greater plasma triglyceride response than complex carbohydrate. Implementation of the present dietary recommendations of the Surgeon General and the Committee on Diet and Health of the Food and Nutrition Board (ie, lower the total fat, saturated fatty acid, and cholesterol intake) will lead to a greater carbohydrate intake. The ideal dietary approach—how carbohydrate is increased, by what amount, with what type of carbohydrate, and with how much and what type of fiber—for increasing dietary carbohydrate to elicit the most beneficial lipid response needs to be clarified.

Protein*

Dietary protein is thought to be a minor risk factor for CHD. Residents of the United States consume about 16% of their calories from protein. Protein intake remains rather constant despite large changes in fat and carbohydrate intake. Epidemiological studies have shown that consumption of animal protein is postively correlated with CHD mortality, whereas vegetable protein is negatively correlated.[41] It is important to note, however, that increases in animal protein and saturated fatty acids parallel each other in the diet and, therefore, it is difficult to evaluate their effects independently in population studies.

Until recently, studies with rabbits, rats, and pigs have shown that consumption of animal protein caused hypercholesterolemia, whereas vegetable protein consumption caused hypocholesterolemia. With humans, however, most studies in which the effect of dietary protein source on plasma lipid response has been evaluated have not shown any clear results.[47-49] Although some studies have shown an effect of protein quality on plasma lipid levels in humans,[50] the cumulative findings to date suggest that while protein source may influence the plasma lipid status, its influence is of lesser significance than other dietary constituents (eg, saturated fatty acids and cholesterol).

Dietary Cholesterol†

Dietary cholesterol has been shown to raise plasma total-cholesterol and lipoprotein-cholesterol levels.[51-53] It is half as potent as saturated fatty acids in raising the plasma cholesterol level (S. Connor, University of Oregon, personal communication). It has been recommended that intake not exceed 300mg/day.[27]

In 1978, Connor et al[41] were the first to report a correlation between dietary cholesterol and the plasma cholesterol level in a free-living population. Recently, Stamler and Shekelle[54] reported that dietary cholesterol was an independent risk factor for CHD. A relationship between egg consumption and the

*By the Editors
†By Joyce L. Sokolik

incidence of CHD was not noted in the Framingham Study,[55] possibly because of the relatively small variation in cholesterol intake among the subjects studied.

Over the years there has been controversy over the effect of dietary cholesterol on the plasma cholesterol response. Between 1959 and 1972 many metabolic ward studies were conducted to examine the effects of dietary cholesterol on serum cholesterol levels.[56-62] In all cases, dietary cholesterol caused a significant increase in serum cholesterol levels.

From 1976 to 1981 a series of studies was conducted with normal free-living subjects,[63-65] hospitalized patients not in a metabolic ward setting,[66] and free-living subjects eating food prepared in a university metabolic kitchen[67] or at home. Dietary cholesterol fed as whole eggs reportedly had no significant effect on the plasma or serum cholesterol level. Egg intake varied from none to four per day (0 to 1,000 mg cholesterol). There are several reasons why no significant effects were observed in these studies.[51] First, experimental conditions were not tightly controlled. (In tightly controlled studies, dietary cholesterol has had a predictable response on plasma total cholesterol levels.) Subjects were often instructed to "add two eggs (or more) daily" to their habitual diet. Compliance to the recommended diet is questionable. Moreover, since diet was not controlled, subjects consumed uncontrolled amounts of cholesterol. In none of these studies were double-blind procedures used. Furthermore, in many of the studies only plasma total-cholesterol levels were measured. Unmeasured changes may have occurred in individual lipoproteins. In addition, often only one blood sample was collected for analysis. In several studies, individual plasma cholesterol responses to dietary cholesterol varied markedly.[65-67]

To investigate the influence of whole eggs on the plasma total-cholesterol level of free-living people, a well-designed study was conducted in which whole eggs (0.5 cup = 500 mg cholesterol) or a cholesterol-free egg substitute were administered (in a double-blind and random order) to 16 normal outpatients. This study confirmed the results of earlier metabolic ward studies[56,62] in which feeding high-cholesterol diets elevated the plasma total-cholesterol level. In recent years the results of this study have been further confirmed.[53,68,69]

In studies conducted to investigate the effect of egg consumption on the distribution of cholesterol among the various lipoprotein fractions, eggs were shown to increase LDL cholesterol,[53,68,70-72] IDL cholesterol,[73] and HDL_2 cholesterol.[72] An elevated cholesterol/triglyceride ratio in the LDL fraction in one study[70] suggested that the diet altered both the concentration and composition of LDL.

A review of the literature reveals variation in the plasma cholesterol response of individual subjects fed high-cholesterol diets.[67-69,72,74,75] In some, plasma total cholesterol is affected less than predicted by dietary cholesterol, whereas other subjects show a greater-than-predicted response to dietary cholesterol.[67-69,72,74,75] Most subjects, however, respond as predicted, and the incidence of hyperresponsiveness and hyporesponsiveness is small. The plasma cholesterol response to dietary cholesterol is also affected by the type of fat in the diet. The quantities of saturated fatty acids (SFAs), omega-6 fatty acids, and cholesterol are all important in determining plasma lipid response. While omega-6 fatty acids reduce the plasma response to a cholesterol challenge, they do not negate it.

Predictive mathematical models to describe the plasma total-cholesterol response to dietary cholesterol have been developed. Within the range of practical interest (0 to 400 mg/1,000 calories), a 100 mg increase in dietary cholesterol in a 2,500-calorie diet increases the plasma total-cholesterol level about 4 mg/dL.[73] Other values in the literature are a 5, 7, and 12 mg increase in the plasma total-cholesterol level for every 100 mg increase in dietary cholesterol per 1,000 calories or per total calorie intake.[76-78]

American men and women currently consume 435 and 304 mg of cholesterol per day, respectively, which is lower than the amounts reported in 1968, when the per capita cholesterol consumption was 520 mg/day.[79] Since the average large egg contains approximately 213 mg of cholesterol (rather than the previously published value of 274 mg),[80] cholesterol intake may be less than reported.

Alcohol*

Population studies have established a significant negative correlation between moderate alcohol consumption (which is defined as not exceeding two drinks per day) and CHD.[81-85] A positive association between moderate alcohol consumption and an elevated HDL-cholesterol level has also been observed in numerous population studies.[82,86-91] This association was significant even after potentially confounding factors such as sex, age, body weight, hormone use, smoking, or exercise were taken into consideration.[82,87,89-91] Controlled clinical studies support the positive relationship between alcohol consumption and HDL-cholesterol levels.[92-94] In these studies, attention has focused on identifying alcohol's effects on the HDL subfractions.

In recent studies[95,96] serum HDL_3 concentrations were observed to decrease with alcohol cessation in moderate drinkers and to increase when drinking was resumed. Serum HDL_2 was unaffected by changes in alcohol consumption. The investigators interpreted these observations to suggest that either HDL_3 is not inert in the development of CHD or the association between reduced incidence of CHD and moderate alcohol intake is due to factors unrelated to HDL_2.[95,96] Burr and associates,[97] however, reported that the increase in HDL cholesterol in response to alcohol was the result of an increase in the HDL_2, not the HDL_3, fraction. Methodological differences in the isolation of the HDL subfractions may explain discrepant findings in this area. Studies[93,95,98] have shown that serum apolipoprotein A-I or A-II, or both, decreased significantly with alcohol cessation in moderate drinkers and increased significantly when drinking was resumed. These observations suggest that the association between moderate alcohol intake and the reduced risk of CHD may be mediated in part by increased levels of serum apolipoprotein A-I or A-II, or both.[98]

Possible mechanisms by which moderate alcohol consumption relates negatively to CHD include the prevention of plaque formation, changes in the concentration of HDL and distribution of its subfractions, alterations in nutritional intake, and the reduction of stress.[84] More extensive clinical and epidemiological trials are needed to identify the mechanisms by which alcohol favorably affects CHD risk.

While moderate alcohol consumption appears to be negatively associated with CHD, it should not be recommended to reduce CHD risk. Alcohol

*By Joyce L. Sokolik

increases plasma triglyceride levels; affects hypertension, alcohol hepatitis, cirrhosis, and certain cancers; causes fetal alcohol syndrome and cardiomyopathy; and can cause social and psychological problems.

Coffee*

In 1983, the Tromso Heart Study[99] identified a positive relationship between coffee intake and elevated plasma total-cholesterol levels. Numerous epidemiological studies conducted to date have produced conflicting results.[99-110] In several population studies, coffee consumption has been shown to be associated with elevated plasma total-cholesterol levels in both sexes.[99-102] In one study,[103] coffee had a significant effect on plasma total-cholesterol levels in males only. In other studies,[104,105,110] a significant association was observed only in females. The positive association between coffee intake and CHD risk reported in one study[106] became statistically insignificant when cigarette smoking was taken into account. Other population studies[107-109] have shown no significant association between coffee consumption and plasma total-cholesterol levels in either gender. Although the emerging consensus suggests that coffee consumption elevates plasma lipids, inconsistencies exist in the literature. The variability in these findings may reflect differences among the studies with respect to methods used to measure coffee consumption, adjustment for cigarette smoking and diet, and failure to account for interpopulation differences.

In several of the above studies[100,101,103,104] investigators studied the relationship of caffeine-containing beverages other than coffee to plasma total-cholesterol levels to determine if caffeine was linked to an elevated plasma total-cholesterol level. Tea and cola beverages had no effect on plasma total-cholesterol levels[100,101,103] in either males or females; however, in one study[104] the caffeine in tea, cola, and chocolate was significantly related to the plasma total-cholesterol levels in females but not males.

In a recent controlled trial with 77 middle-aged sedentary, healthy men,[111] Stanford researchers observed a significant association between coffee intake and plasma LDL-cholesterol and apolipoprotein-B levels. These effects were observed with coffee intake exceeding two to three cups per day. The confounding factors that were considered were stress, nutrient intake (including alcohol), age, cigarette use, adiposity, and aerobic capacity. The researchers caution against extrapolating these coffee-lipoprotein associations to the general population without further research.

Researchers at The Johns Hopkins University recently published results of a prospective investigation of the effect of coffee consumption on CHD in 1,130 male medical students who were followed from 19 to 35 years.[112] Adjustments were made for age, current smoking, hypertension status, and baseline level of serum cholesterol. The researchers concluded that there was an independent dose-responsive association between coffee consumption and clinically evident CHD, which is consistent with a twofold to threefold elevation in risk among heavy coffee drinkers (five or more cups per day).

As with other coronary risk factors, research on the effects of coffee consumption is difficult because of potentially confounding factors, including: dietary habits, age, sex, body mass index, exercise, cigarette smoking, alcohol consumption, estrogen use, ethnicity, occupation, stress, drugs, and the baseline plasma total-cholesterol level. The coffee-cholesterol relationship is further confounded by the type of coffee used (origin of coffee beans) and the method

*By Joyce L. Sokolik

of preparation (instant, drip, boiled, percolated), as well as the water itself. There is some evidence to suggest that consumption of boiled—but not filtered—coffee adversely affects the plasma lipid profile. Nonetheless, it is premature at this time to implicate coffee as a coronary risk factor. Further trials are needed to establish whether there is a relationship between coffee consumption and plasma total-cholesterol and lipoprotein-cholesterol levels and to determine the responsible constituent(s). Practitioners are advised to assess the coffee consumption of their patients and to intervene when indicated. Coffee consumption may be of clinical importance for hypercholesterolemic patients. Recently, decaffeinated coffee was reported to increase LDL-cholesterol and apolipoprotein-B levels significantly in males.[113] When subjects changed from drinking caffeinated to decaffeinated coffee for four months, LDL cholesterol increased by approximately 9 mg, compared with subjects that consumed an equal amount of caffeinated coffee or no coffee. More research in this area is needed before the relationship of decaffeinated coffee to CHD risk is fully understood.

Fiber*

Dietary fiber refers to nonstarch polysaccharides and lignin in the diet that are not digested by the secretions of the human digestive tract. Fiber is composed of celluloses, hemicelluloses, mucilages, pectins, gums, waxes, and lignin. Among the isolated sources of fiber, cellulose, some hemicelluloses, and lignin are generally considered to be water-insoluble molecules, while pectins, gums, mucilages, and mixed linkage betaglucans are considered soluble sources of dietary fiber.

The hypotheses of Burkitt and Trowell[114]—that many diseases of industrialized societies are associated with diets high in fat and low in fiber—have been the impetus for many studies designed to examine the physiological effects of dietary fiber. Much of this research in the heart-disease area has focused on the effect of dietary fiber on plasma lipid levels.

It has become apparent that the different types of dietary fiber have varying physiological effects and that this is especially true with respect to their effect on plasma lipid levels. Differences in the effects of various fibers on plasma lipid levels appear to be due to physiochemical properties, such as water-holding capacity, ionic charge, gel-forming characteristics, and solubility.

Insoluble dietary fiber sources are generally considered to be ineffective in reducing serum lipid levels in humans. Cellulose has been reported to have little or no effect on serum total-cholesterol and triglyceride levels when added to the diets of normocholesterolemic subjects at a level of 15 g/day.[115,116] Wheat bran, a source of insoluble dietary fiber, has been used in many studies designed to examine the effect of fiber on various blood lipids. These studies are difficult to interpret and compare due to differences in subjects' inital serum lipid profiles and to poorly defined types and amounts of dietary fiber in the experimental diets. Nonetheless, it has been concluded that wheat fiber has little or no effect on serum total-cholesterol and triglyceride levels.[117,118]

In contrast to the results found for insoluble-dietary-fiber sources, the significant lowering of certain plasma lipids has been reported for soluble or viscous fibers. The purified water-soluble fiber sources that have been studied

*By Steve Ink

include pectin, psyllium, guar, gum arabic, and locust bean gum. Food sources of soluble fiber have also been examined for their potential as hypocholesterolemic agents and include oatmeal, oat bran, barley, and legumes.

Pectin. The effect of dietary pectin on serum lipid levels was reported as early as 1961. Since then, numerous studies have confirmed the hypocholesterolemic properties of pectin both in normocholesterolemic and hypercholesterolemic subjects.[119] The magnitude of change in plasma total cholesterol elicited by pectin ingestion has been found to be quite variable, but generally 15 g of pectin per day lowers serum total-cholesterol levels by about 5% to 10% after three to four weeks. The reduction is associated with a reduction in VLDL-cholesterol or LDL-cholesterol levels or both. Pectin apparently has little effect on plasma triglyceride levels. Apple- and citrus-derived pectins have been reported to have hypocholesterolemic properties and could be used as food sources of pectins. Oranges, grapefruit, apples, bananas, carrots, potatoes, and beans provide 1 to 2 g of pectin per 3 oz.

Guar. Guar gum is another water-soluble fiber source that has been studied quite extensively for its serum lipid-altering properties. Studies with both hypercholesterolemic and normocholesterolemic subjects suggest that consumption of 15 to 20 g of guar gum per day lowers plasma total cholesterol approximately 10%.[120-125] Guar gum tends to lower LDL cholesterol without affecting HDL-cholesterol levels. The serum triglyceride response to guar gum has been found to be quite variable. An apparent disadvantage associated with guar gum supplementation relates to gastrointestinal problems in some people, including flatulence and diarrhea.

Other soluble fibers. Psyllium, gum arabic, locust bean gum, and karaya gum are all soluble fibers that have reported hypocholesterolemic properties.[115,126-128] Although the number of studies is limited, these soluble fibers have been shown to lower serum total-cholesterol levels by about 5% to 10% when 15 to 20 g of the fiber is added to the diet.

The results of the studies discussed above for pectin, guar, and other purified fiber sources suggest that these fibers have significant potential for use as adjuncts to the nutritional management of hypercholesterolemia. Unfortunately, palatability and acceptability of these soluble fibers are somewhat limiting. In addition, the purified soluble fibers do not contribute nutrients. Several foods, however, are sources of both soluble-fiber nutrients as well as calories: oats, oat bran, barley, and legumes. New evidence suggests that rice bran is also hypocholesterolemic and corn bran may have a role in cholesterol-lowering diets as well. However, neither of these will be discussed since there is insufficient literature available.

Oat fiber. As early as 1963, DeGroot and coworkers[129] reported that rolled oats decreased the serum total-cholesterol levels in hypercholesterolemic men. Subsequent studies examined the effect of oat bran consumption on serum lipid levels in hypercholesterolemic men and again showed significant reductions in plasma total-cholesterol and triglyceride levels.[130-132] These studies with hypercholesterolemic subjects have indicated that serum total-cholesterol levels can be lowered by as much as 15% when about 3 oz of oats or oat bran is consumed each day.

A recent study has assessed whether moderate intake of either rolled oats or oat bran would enhance the serum cholesterol-lowering effect of a diet low in saturated fatty acids and cholesterol in normolipidemic, free-living subjects.[133] The results of this study confirmed the hypocholesterolemic properties of oat products and suggested that ingestion of as little as 2 oz (dry weight) of oatmeal or oat bran each day could enhance the serum cholesterol reduction induced by dietary-fat modification in the general population. The lipoprotein changes associated with oat ingestion were favorable, with reductions in LDL-cholesterol levels and small increases in HDL-cholesterol levels. Plasma triglycerides were not affected. A more recent study,[134] however, failed to observe a cholesterol-lowering effect of oat bran in normocholesterolemic women and men.

There is some question about this study, however, because it was conducted with young, normocholesterolemic subjects and—more important—fat intake varied among the treatment groups. Nonetheless, a majority of studies have shown that oats and oat bran are effective in lowering plasma cholesterol levels via undefined mechanisms. When oats or oat bran or both are added to the diet, however, saturated-fatty-acid intake may decrease.[135]

A portion of the hypocholesterolemic effects of oats is due to the high water-soluble-fiber content (betaglucans) of oats. One ounce of rolled oats or oat bran contains about 3 g and 4 g of total dietary fiber, respectively, of which 40% is associated with the water-soluble fraction. Therefore, of the commonly consumed grains, only oats and perhaps barley[136] are water-soluble fibers that can realistically affect plasma lipid levels.

Legumes. Beans, such as pinto and navy, are generally good sources of soluble fiber and provide about 5 g of soluble fiber per 100 g dry weight.[137] Ingestion of 100 g or more of dried beans (navy, pinto, and kidney) per day has been found to significantly lower serum total-cholesterol levels in hypercholesterolemic subjects.[132,138] Lipoprotein changes in these studies were favorable with significant reductions in LDL-cholesterol levels. Subject compliance was found to be quite good for the high-bean diet.[138] Soybean fiber has also been used as a potential hypocholesterolemic agent in clinical trials. The results have been inconclusive, with one study showing an increase in serum lipid levels and another a modest decrease.[139,140]

The studies discussed above generally support the hypothesis that increased consumption of water-soluble fiber will lower serum total-cholesterol levels. Although the mechanisms by which soluble fibers are hypocholesterolemic have not been clearly defined, several hypotheses have been proposed based on both human and animal studies.

An increase in consumption of water-soluble fiber typically results in a greater fecal bile salt and neutral steroid excretion.[141] Since the enterohepatic recirculation of bile acids is a very efficient process, the soluble-fiber-dependent reduction in bile-acid reabsorption may result in a diversion of cholesterol from lipoprotein synthesis in the liver to bile-acid synthesis. A related theory suggests that fiber-induced changes in the bile-acid pool size and composition may account for some of soluble fibers' effect on serum lipid levels.[142] Another hypothesis proposes that soluble fibers cause an increase in the viscosity of the contents of the small intestine, which may slow nutrient absorption. This may alter the rate and site of apolipoprotein synthesis in the intestine and, in turn, affect cholesterol metabolism.[143,144] One final mechanism by which water-soluble fiber may influence cholesterol metabolism relates to the fermentation of soluble fiber in the colon and the release of short-chain fatty acids such as propionate. Propionate can then be absorbed into the circulation and removed by the liver, resulting in inhibition of cholesterol synthesis.[145]

In summary, soluble fibers including pectin, guar, psyllium, and other gums as well as food sources of soluble fiber such as oats, oat bran, barley, and legumes offer good potential for lowering serum total-cholesterol levels in hypercholesterolemic and normocholesterolemic populations. The most effective approach in using soluble fibers in the management of hypercholesterolemia would seem to be one of including them in a total dietery plan designed to lower intake of saturated fatty acids and cholesterol while increasing consumption of complex carbohydrates. The amount of purified fibers such as pectin and guar that is required to significantly decrease serum cholesterol levels is estimated to be about 15 to 30 g/day. The most practical approach may be to add food sources of soluble fiber such as oats, oat bran, barley, and legumes to the diet at levels approaching 50 g/day (dry weight) in order to lower cholesterol levels significantly. These foods provide nutrients in addition to soluble fiber.

FAT REPLACEMENTS*

Gums. Gums are not used to replace fat in formulations, but they do perform some of the functions of oils in reduced-calorie (reduced-fat) salad dressings. Xanthan gum (a high-molecular-weight polysaccharide) is used as a suspension stabilizer in pourable salad dressings. It also functions to increase the viscosity and stability of low-calorie dressings. In these products that have less oil and more water, xanthan is important for stabilizing the oil phase.

Maltrin M-040 maltodextrin. A spray-dried carbohydrate made from corn starch, Maltrin M-040 maltodextrin is used to partially replace oil in salad dressings, margarines, and frozen desserts. The manufacturer suggests that it can be used to provide formulations with 50% of the calories and 25% of the oil of the standard product formulation. Maltodextrin is completely digested and contains 4 calories per gram.

Polydextrose. Polydextrose is a water-soluble, reduced-calorie polymer of dextrose with small amounts of sorbitol and citric acid. It provides 1 calorie per gram and is only partially metabolized. Although it is not a fat, it is used to partially replace fats to produce low-calorie and reduced-calorie foods. Polydextrose functions as a bulking agent, texturizing agent, and humectant in a variety of foods. The FDA has approved its use in several foods.

Simplesse. Simplesse is made from the protein of fresh egg whites or milk by simply changing its physical form (size, shape, and texture). These proteins are microparticulated—a cooking and blending process aggregates the protein into small, spherical particles. These particles are small enough so that the tongue perceives them as a fluid rather than a solid. This creates a sensation of smoothness, richness, and creaminess normally associated with fat. When incorporated into foods, Simplesse makes fat reduction possible with little or no change in flavor. Typically, 1 g of Simplesse (1.33 calories) replaces 1 g of fat (9 calories). Thus, Simplesse can be used to lower total fat intake. Since Simplesse turns rubbery when heated, this particular fat replacement will be used in salad dressings, cheeses, and other dairy products.

Sucrose polyester. Sucrose polyester (Olestra) is a noncaloric fat replacement that is neither digested nor absorbed. Sucrose polyester consists of six, seven or eight long-chain fatty acids esterified to a sucrose core. Procter & Gamble intends to use sucrose polyester in shortening and oils in homes, restaurants, and commercially prepared snack foods (*Figure 2.1*). The proposed levels of substitution are up to 35% of the fat used in shortenings and cooking oils for home use and up to 75% of the fat used in commercial deep-fat fryers

*By the Editors

and in fried snack foods such as potato chips. At this level of substitution in conjunction with typical food consumption patterns, the expected consumption of sucrose polyester would be approximately 5 g per day.

It has been estimated that the addition of sucrose polyester to the American food supply could reduce total fat intake from 37% to 35% of calories. Clinical studies have shown that sucrose polyester (approximately 30 g/day) decreases plasma cholesterol about 7% to 15%.[146] Other studies have shown that cholesterol absorption is also decreased.[147] Since sucrose polyester does not contribute calories to the diet, it may be useful for the promotion of weight loss and may contribute to the alterations in plasma lipid levels observed with weight loss.

Fig. 2.1
Reduction of fat and caloric content of commonly used cooking fats. Reproduced with permission of Procter & Gamble Co.

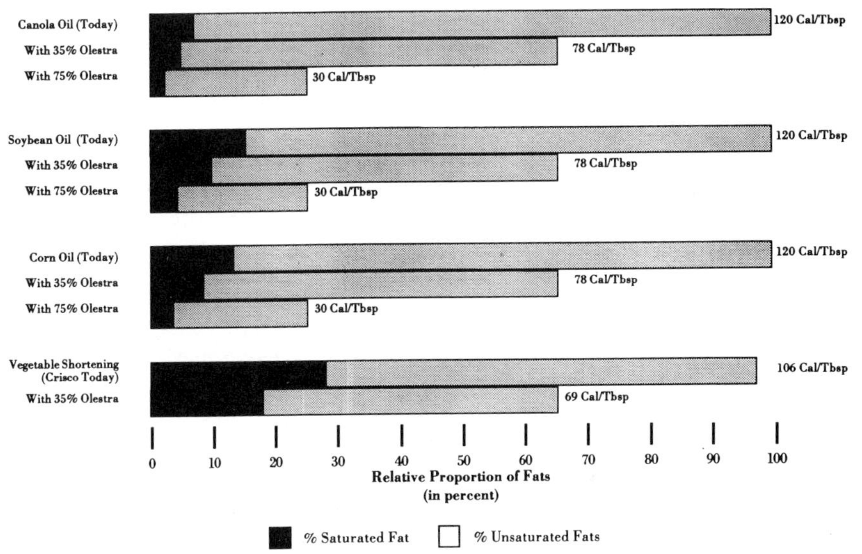

All available evidence indicates that sucrose polyester is safe. There is a need to supplement sucrose polyester with vitamin E (1 mg per gram of sucrose polyester), but no need for other fat-soluable vitamins has been identified. Some early studies indicated that sucrose polyester resulted in anal leakage. This problem has been solved by increasing the saturation of fatty acids esterified into sucrose.

Sucrose polyester is palatable and heat stable and is another tool to consider when planning cholesterol-lowering diets. There are concerns that consumers eager to eliminate calories could abuse products with sucrose polyester. It will be important for dietitians to instruct patients on how to incorporate fat replacements in their diets (and at what level) to ensure that the diet is nutritionally adequate.

Tapioca dextrin. Tapioca dextrin is used to replace fat in food products. It is used to replace 30% to 50% of the oil in salad dressings. It contains 4 calories per gram and is typically used at 25% concentration (ie, replace 4 parts of fat or oil with 1 part tapioca dextrin and 3 parts water). This product has been marketed in the United States since 1984.

Other fat substitutes. A number of fat substitutes are presently in various stages of development. Arco Chemical Company has developed a noncaloric fat substitute from propylene oxide. Possible uses for this fat-replacement product are conventional oils, salad dressings, baked goods, spreads, and ice cream. Refined jojoba oil may be a suitable fat substitute. An oil substitute has been developed from polycarboxylic acid that appears to be thermally stable. Other synthetic oils are being developed by many food companies.

References

1. Keys A. Coronary heart disease in seven countries. *Circulation.* 1970;41:1.
2. Bonanome A, Grundy SM. Effect of dietary stearic acid on plasma cholesterol and lipoprotein levels. *N Engl J Med.* 1988;318:1244.
3. Keys A, Anderson JT, Grande F. Serum cholesterol response to changes in the diet, IV: particular saturated fatty acids in the diet. *Metabolism.* 1965;14:776.
4. Hegsted DM, McGandy RB, Meyers ML, et al. Quantitative effects of dietary fat on serum cholesterol in man. *Am J Clin Nutr.* 1965;17:281.
5. Tan MH, Dickinson MA, Albers JJ, et al. The effect of a high cholesterol and saturated fat diet on serum high-density lipoprotein-cholesterol, apolipoprotein A-7 and apolipoprotein E levels in normolipemic humans. *Am J Clin Nutr.* 1980;33:2559.
6. Grundy SM, Nix D, Whelan MF, et al. Comparison of three cholesterol-lowering diets in normolipemic men. *JAMA.* 1986;256:2351.
7. Shepherd J, Packard CJ, Patsch JR, et al. Effect of dietary polyunsaturated and saturated fat on properties of high density lipoproteins and the metabolism of apoprotein A-1. *J Clin Invest.* 1978;61:1582.
8. Spady DK, Dietschy JM. Interaction of dietary cholesterol and triglycerides in the regulation of hepatic low density lipoprotein transport in the hamster. *J Clin Invest.* 1988;81:300.
9. Jackson RL, Kashyap ML, Barnhart RL, et al. Influence of polyunsaturated and saturated fats in plasma lipids and lipoproteins in man. *Am J Clin Nutr.* 1984;39:595.
10. Gustafson I, Vessby B, Karlstrom B, et al. Effects on the serum lipoprotein concentrations by lipid-lowering diets with different fatty acid compositions. *J Am Col Nutr.* 1985;4:241.
11. Oh SY, Monaco PA. Effect of dietary cholesterol and degree of fat unsaturation on plasma lipid levels, lipoprotein composition, and fecal steroid excretion in normal young adult men. *Am J Clin Nutr.* 1985;42:399.
12. Kris-Etherton PM, Krummel D, Russell ME, et al. The effect of diet on plasma lipids, lipoproteins, and coronary heart disease. *J Am Diet Assoc.* 1988;88:1373.
13. Harris WS. Fish oils and plasma lipid and lipoprotein metabolism in humans: a critical review. *J Lipid Res.* 1989;30:785.
14. Nestel PJ, Connor WE, Reardon MF, et al. Suppression by diets rich in fish oil of very low density lipoprotein production in man. *J Clin Invest.* 1984;74:82.
15. Bang HO. More on fish oil. *N Engl J Med.* 1987:316:624. Letter.
16. Aravanis C, Corcondilas A, Dontas AS, et al. The Greek islands of Crete and Corfu. *Circulation.* 1970;41(suppl I):I-88.

17. Keys A, Menotti A, Karvonen MJ, et al. The diet and 15-year death rate in the Seven Countries Study. *Am J Epidemiol.* 1986;124:903.
18. Mattson FH, Grundy SM. Comparison of effects of dietary saturated, monounsaturated, and polyunsaturated fatty acids on plasma lipids and lipoproteins in man. *J Lipid Res.* 1985;26:194.
19. Grundy SM. Comparison of monosaturated fatty acids and carbohydrates for lowering plasma cholesterol. *N Engl J Med.* 1986;314:745.
20. Sirtori CR, Tremoli E, Gatti E, et al. Controlled evaluation of fat intake in the Mediterranean diet: comparative activities of olive oil and corn oil on plasma lipids and platelets in high-risk patients. *Am J Clin Nutr.* 1986;44:635.
21. Mensink RP, Katan MB. Effect of monosaturated fatty acids versus complex carbohydrates on high-density lipoproteins in healthy men and women. *Lancet.* 1987:17:122.
22. Garg A, Bonanome A, Grundy SM, et al. Comparison of a high-carbohydrate diet with a high-monosaturated-fat diet in patients with non-insulin-dependent diabetes mellitus. *N Engl J Med.* 1988;319:829.
23. Baggio G, Pagnan A, Muraca M, et al. Olive-oil-enriched diet: effect on serum lipoprotein levels and biliary cholesterol saturation. *Am J Clin Nutr.* 1988;47:960.
24. Grundy SM, Florentin L, Nix D, et al. Comparison of monounsaturated fatty acids and carbohydrates for reducing raised levels of plasma cholesterol in man. *Am J Clin Nutr.* 1988;47:965.
25. Mensink RP, Katan MB. Effect of a diet enriched with monounsaturated or polyunsaturated fatty acids on levels of low-density and high-density lipoprotein cholesterol in healthy men and women. *N Engl J Med.* 1989;321:436.
26. Mattson FH. A changing role for dietary monounsaturated fatty acids. *J Am Diet Assoc.* 1989;89:387.
27. Ernst ND, Cleeman J, Mullis R, et al. The National Cholesterol Education Program: implications for dietetic practitioners from the Adult Treatment Panel Recommendations. *J Am Diet Assoc.* 1988;88:1401.
28. National Academy of Sciences. *Designing Foods—Animal Product Options in the Marketplace.* Washington, DC: National Academy Press; 1988.
29. Blankenhorn DH, Nessim SA, Johnson RL, et al. Beneficial effects of combined colestipol-niacin therapy on coronary atherosclerosis and coronary venous bypass grafts. *JAMA.* 1987;257:3233.
30. Nichaman MZ, Hamm P. Low-fat, high carbohydrate diets and plasma cholesterol. *Am J Clin Nutr.* 1987;45:1155.
31. Blackburn H. Diet and mass hyperlipidemia: a public health view. In: Levy RI, Rifkind BM, Dennis BH, et al, eds. *Nutrition, Lipids and Coronary Heart Disease.* New York, NY: Raven Press; 1979.
32. Gordon T, Kagan A, Garcia-Palmicri M, et al. Diet and its relation to coronary heart disease and death in three populations. *Circulation.* 1981;63:500.
33. Shekelle, RB, Shryock AM, Paul O, et al. Diet, serum cholesterol, and death from coronary heart disease: the Western Electric Study. *N Engl J Med.* 1981;304:65.
34. Burselm J, Schonfeld G, Howald MA, et al. Plasma apoprotein and lipoprotein lipid levels in vegetarians. *Metabolism.* 1978;27:711.
35. Gear JS, Mann JI, Thorogood M, et al. Biochemical and hematological variables in vegetarians. *Br Med J.* 1980;280:1415.
36. Phillips RL, Lemon FR, Beeson WL, et al. Coronary heart disease mortality among Seventh-Day Adventists with differing dietary habits: a preliminary report. *Am J Clin Nutr.* 1978;31(suppl 10):S191.
37. Lock DR, Varhol A, Grimes S, et al. Apolipoprotein E levels in vegetarians. *Metabolism.* 1982; 31:917.
38. Nestel PJ, Billington T, Smith B. Low density and high density lipoprotein kinetics and sterol balance in vegetarians. *Metabolism.* 1981;30:941.
39. Melchert HU, Limsathayourat N, Mihajlovic H, et al. Fatty acid patterns in triglycerides, diglycerides, free fatty acids, cholesteryl esters and phosphatidylcholine in serum from vegetarians and non-vegetarians. *Atherosclerosis.* 1987;65:159.
40. Nutrition Committee, American Heart Association. Dietary guidelines for healthy American adults. *Circulation.* 1988;77:721A.
41. Connor WE, Cerqueira MT, Connor R, et al. The plasma lipids, lipoproteins, and diet of the Tarahumara Indians of Mexico. *Am J Clin Nutr.* 1978;31:1131.
42. Keys A, Fidanza F, Scardi V, et al. Studies on serum cholesterol and other characteristics of clinically healthy men in Naples. *Arch Intern Med.* 1954;93:328.

43. Keys A, Kimur N, Bronte-Stewart B, et al. Lessons from serum cholesterol studies in Japan, Hawaii, and Los Angeles. *Ann Intern Med.* 1958;48:83.
44. Hallfrisch J, West S, Fisher C, et al. Modification of the United States' diet to effect changes in blood lipids and lipoprotein distribution. *Atherosclerosis.* 1985;57:179.
45. Katan MJ. Diet and HDL. In: Miller NE, Miller GJ, eds. *Metabolic Aspects of Cardiovascular Disease, vol 3: Clinical and Metabolic Aspects of HDL.* Oxford, England: Elsevier;1984:103-131.
46. Glinsmann WH, Irausquin H, Park YK. Evaluation of health aspects of sugar contained in carbohydrate sweeteners: report of Sugars Task Force, 1986. *J Nutr.* 1986;116(suppl):S5.
47. Carroll KK, Giovannetti PM, Huff MW, et al. Hypocholesterolemic effect of substituting soybean protein for animal protein in the diet of healthy young women. *Am J Clin Nutr.* 1978;31:1312.
48. VanRaaij JM, Katan MB, Hautvast JG, et al. Effects of casein versus soy protein diets on serum cholesterol and lipoproteins in young, healthy volunteers. *Am J Clin Nutr.* 1981;34:1261.
49. Sacks FM, Breslow JL, Wood PG, et al. Effect of a lack of dairy protein (casein) and soy protein on plasma cholesterol of strict vegetarians: an experiment and a critical review. *J Lipid Res.* 1983;24:1012.
50. Carroll KK. Hypercholesterolemic and atherosclerosis: effect of dietary protein. *Fed Proc.* 1982;41:2792.
51. Roberts SL, McMurray MP, Connor WE. Does egg feeding (ie, dietary cholesterol) affect plasma cholesterol levels in humans? the results of a double-blind study. *Am J Clin Nutr.* 1981;34:2092.
52. Chenoweth W, Ullmann M, Simpson R, et al. Influence of dietary cholesterol and experimental conditions on serum lipids in men. *J Nutr.* 1981;111:2069.
53. Sacks FM, Salazar J, Miller L, et al. Ingestion of egg raises plasma low density lipoproteins in free-living subjects. *Lancet.* 1984;1:647.
54. Stamler R, Shekelle J. Dietary cholesterol and risk of death in middle-aged men. *CVD Newsletter.* Abstract. 1988;43:168
55. The Framingham Study—an epidemiological investigation of cardiovascular diseases. In: *The Framingham Diet Study.* Washington, DC:US Dept of Health, Education, and Welfare; 1970: sec 24.
56. Beveridge JMR, Connell WF, Mayer GA, et al. The response of man to dietary cholesterol. *J Nutr.* 1960;71:61.
57. Connor WE, Hodges RE, Bleiler RE. The serum lipids in men receiving high cholesterol and cholesterol-free diets. *J Clin Invest.* 1961; 40:894.
58. Connor WE, Stone DB, Hodges RE. The interrelated effects of dietary cholesterol and fat upon human serum lipid levels. *J Clin Invest.* 1964;43:1691.
59. Hegsted DM, McGandy RB, Myers ML, et al. Quantitative effects of dietary fat on serum cholesterol in man. *Am J Clin Nutr.* 1965;17:281.
60. Steiner A, Howard EJ, Akgun S. Importance of dietary cholesterol in man. *JAMA.* 1962;181:186.
61. Connor WE, Hodges RE, Bleiler RE. Effect of dietary cholesterol upon serum lipids in man. *J Lab Clin Med.* 1961;57:331.
62. Mattson FH, Erickson BA, Klingman AM. Effect of dietary cholesterol on serum cholesterol in man. *Am J Clin Nutr.* 1972;25:589.
63. Porter MW, Yamanaka W, Carlson SD, et al. Effect of dietary egg on serum cholesterol and triglycerides of human males. *Am J Clin Nutr.* 1977;30:490.
64. Flynn MA, Nolph GB, Flynn TC, et al. Effect of dietary egg on human serum cholesterol and triglycerides. *Am J Clin Nutr.* 1979;32:1051.
65. Slater G, Mead J, Dhopeshwarkar G, et al. Plasma cholesterol and triglycerides in men with added eggs in the diet. *Nutr Rep Int.* 1976;14:249.
66. Kummeraw FA, Youngja K, Hull J, et al. The influence of egg consumption on the serum cholesterol level in human subjects. *Am J Clin. Nutr.* 1977;30:664.
67. Flaim E, Ferreri LF, Thye FW, et al. Plasma lipid and lipoprotein cholesterol concentrations in adult males consuming normal and high cholesterol diets under controlled conditions. *Am J Clin Nutr.* 1981;34:1103.
68. Oh SY, Miller LT. Effect of dietary egg on variability of plasma cholesterol levels and lipoprotein cholesterol. *Am J Clin Nutr.* 1985;42:421.
69. Katan MB, Benyen AC, DeVries JHM, et al. Existence of consistent hypo- and hyperresponders to dietary cholesterol in man. *Am J Epidemiol.* 1986;123:221.

70. Applebaum-Bowden D, Hazzard WR, Cain J, et al. Short-term egg yolk feeding in humans: increase in apolipoprotein B and low density lipoprotein cholesterol. *Atherosclerosis.* 1979;33:385.
71. Schonfeld G. Patsch W, Rudel LL, et al. Effects of dietary cholesterol and fatty acids on plasma lipoproteins. *J Clin Invest.* 1982;69:1072.
72. Mistry P, Miller E, Laker M, et al. Individual variation in the effects of dietary cholesterol on plasma lipoproteins and cellular cholesterol homeostasis in man. *J Clin Invest.* 1981;67:493.
73. Hegsted, DM. Serum-cholesterol response to dietary cholesterol: a re-evaluation. *Am J Clin Nutr.* 1986;44:299.
74. Packard CJ, McKinney L, Carr K, et al. Cholesterol feeding increases low density lipoprotein synthesis. *J Clin Invest.* 1983;72:45.
75. Bronsgeest-Schoute DC, Hermus RJJ, Dallinga-Thie GM et al. Dependence of the effects of dietary cholesterol and experimental conditions on serum lipids in man, III: the effect of removal of eggs from the diet of free-living habitually egg-eating people. *Am J Clin Nutr.* 1979;32:2193.
76. Malmros H. The relation of nutrition to health: a statistical study of the effect of wartime on atherosclerosis, tuberculosis, and diabetes. *Acta Med Scand.* 1950;246:137.
77. Hegsted DM, McGandy RB, Meyers ML, et al. Quantitative effects of dietary fat on serum cholesterol in man. *Am J Clin Nutr.* 1965;17:281.
78. Grundy SM, Bilheimer D, Blackburn H, et al. Rationale of the diet-heart statement of the American Heart Association. *Circulation.* 1982;65:839A.
79. Marston R, Raper, N. Nutrient content of the US food supply. *Nat Food Rev.* 1987; 36:18.
80. Egg Nutrition Center. Today's egg contains 25% less cholesterol. *Nutr Close-Up.* 1989;6:1.
81. Hennekens CH, Willett W, Rosner B, et al. Effects of beer, wine and liquor in coronary deaths. *JAMA.* 1979;242:1973.
82. Yano K, Rhoads GG, Kagan, A. Coffee, alcohol and risk of coronary heart disease among Japanese men living in Hawaii. *N Engl J Med.* 1977;297:405.
83. Klatsky AL, Friedman GD, Siegelaub AB. Alcohol consumption before myocardial infarction: results from the Kaiser-Permanente epidemiologic study of myocardial infarction. *Ann Intern Med.* 1974;81:294.
84. LaPorte RE, Cresanta JL, Kuller, LH. The relationship of alcohol consumption to atherosclerotic heart disease. *Prev Med.* 1980;9:22.
85. St Leger AS, Cochrane AL, Moore, F. Factors associated with cardiac mortality in developed countries with particular reference to the consumption of wine. *Lancet.* 1979;2:1017.
86. Heiss G, Johnson NJ, Reiland S, et al. The epidemiology of plasma high-density lipoprotein cholesterol levels: the Lipid Research Clinics program prevalence study. *Circulation.* 1980;62(suppl IV):IV-116.
87. Gordon T, Ernst N, Fisher M, Rifkind, B. Alcohol and high-density lipoprotein cholesterol. *Circulation.* 1981;64(suppl III):III-63.
88. Castelli W, Gordon T, Hjortland MC, et al. Alcohol and blood lipids: the Cooperative Lipoprotein Phenotyping Study. *Lancet.* 1977;2:153.
89. Ernst N, Fisher M, Smith W, et al. The association of plasma high-density lipoprotein cholesterol with dietary intake and alcohol consumption: the Lipid Research Clinics program prevalence study. *Circulation.* 1980;62(suppl IV):IV-41.
90. Willett W, Hennekens CH, Siegel AJ, et al. Alcohol consumption and high-density lipoprotein cholesterol in marathon runners. *N Engl J Med.* 1980;303:1159.
91. Williams P, Robinson R, Bailey A. High-density lipoprotein and coronary risk factors in normal men. *Lancet.* 1979;1:72.
92. Crouse JR, Grund SM. Effects of alcohol on plasma lipoproteins and cholesterol and triglyceride metabolism in man. *J. Lipid Res.* 1984;25:486.
93. Fraser GD, Anderson JT, Foster N, et al. The effect of alcohol on serum high density lipoprotein (HDL). *Atherosclerosis.* 1983:46:275.
94. Hulley SB, Gordon S. Alcohol and high-density lipoprotein cholesterol: causal inference from diverse study designs. *Circulation.* 1981;64(suppl III):III-57.
95. Williams PT, Krauss RM, Wood PD, et al. Associations of diet and alcohol intake with high-density lipoprotein subclasses. *Metabolism.* 1985;34:525.
96. Haskell WL, Camargo C, Williams PT, et al. The effect of cessation and resumption of moderate alcohol intake on serum high-density-lipoprotein subfractions. *N Engl J. Med.* 1984;310:805.

97. Burr ML, Fehily AM, Butland BK, et al. Alcohol and high-density-lipoprotein cholesterol: a randomized controlled trial. *Br J Nutr.* 1986;56:81.
98. Camargo CA, Williams PT, Vranizan KM, et al. The effect of moderate alcohol intake on serum apolipoproteins A-I and A-II. *JAMA.* 1985;253:2854.
99. Thelle DS, Arnesen E, Forde, OH. The Tromso Heart Study: does coffee raise serum cholesterol? *N Engl J Med.* 1983;308:1454.
100. Haffner SM, Knapp JA, Stern MP, et al. Coffee consumption, diet and lipids. *Am J Epidemiol.* 1985;122:1.
101. Klatsky AL, Petitti DB, Armstrong MA, et al. Coffee, tea and cholesterol. *Am J Cardiol.* 1985;55:577.
102. Arab L, Kohlmeier M, Schlierf G, et al. *N Engl J Med.* 1983;309:1250. Letter.
103. Kark JD, Friedlander Y, Kaufmann NA, et al. Coffee, tea, and plasma cholesterol: the Jerusalem Lipid Research Clinic prevalence study. *Br Med J.* 1985;291:699.
104. Shirlow MJ, Mathers, CD. Caffeine consumption and serum cholesterol levels. *Int J Epidemiol.* 1984;13:422.
105. Mathias S, Garland C, Barrett-Connor E, et al. Coffee, plasma cholesterol, and lipoproteins: a population study in an adult community. *Am J Epidemiol.* 1985;121:986.
106. Dawber TR, Kannel WB, Gordon T, et al. Coffee and cardiovascular disease: observations from Framingham Study. *N Engl J Med.* 1974;291:871.
107. Shekelle RB, Gale M, Stamler J, *N Engl J Med.* 1983;309:1249. Letter.
108. Hoffman A, Van Laar A, Klein F, et al. *N Engl J Med.* 1983;309:1248. Letter.
109. Kovar MG, Fulwood R, Feinleib M. *N Engl J Med.* 1983;309:1249. Letter.
110. Wilson PW, Garrison RJ, Kannel WB, McGee DL, Castelli WP. Is coffee consumption a contributor to cardiovascular disease? *Arch Intern Med.* 1989;149:1169.
111. Williams PT, Wood PD, Vranizan KM, et al. Coffee intake and elevated cholesterol and apolipoprotein B levels in men. *JAMA.* 1985;253:1407.
112. LaCroix AZ, Mead LA, Liang KY, et al. Coffee consumption and the incidence of coronary heart disease. *N Engl J Med.* 1986;315:977.
113. Superko HR, Bortz WM, Albers JL, et al. Lipoprotein and apolipoprotein changes during a controlled trial of caffeinated and decaffeinated coffee drinking in men. *Circulation.* 1989;80:II-86. Abstract.
114. Burkitt DP, Trowell, HC. *Refined Carbohydrate Foods and Disease: The Implications of Dietary Fiber.* London, England: Academic Press; 1975.
115. Behall KM, Lee KH, Moser, PB. Blood lipids and lipoproteins in adult men fed four refined fibers. *Am J Clin Nutr.* 1984;39:209.
116. Hillman LC, Peters SG, Fisher CA, et al. The effects of the fiber components pectin, cellulose and lignin on serum cholesterol levels. *Am J Clin Nutr.* 1985;42:207.
117. Anderson JW, Chen WJL. Plant fiber: carbohydrate and lipid metabolism. *Am J Clin Nutr.* 1979;32:346.
118. Kay RM, Truswell AS. Dietary fiber: effects on plasma and biliary lipids in man. In: Spiller GA, Kay RM, eds. *Medical Aspects of Dietary Fiber.* New York, NY: Plenum Press; 1980:153.
119. Reiser S. Metabolic effects of dietary pectins related to human health. *Food Tech.* 1987;215:91.
120. Jenkins DJA, Leeds AR, Slavin B, et al. Dietary fiber and blood lipids: reduction of serum cholesterol in type II hyperlipidemia by guar gum. *Am J Clin Nutr.* 1979;32:16.
121. Jenkins DJA, Reynolds D, Slavin B, et al. Dietary fiber and blood lipids: treatment of hypercholesterolemia with guar crispbread. *Am J Clin Nutr.* 1980;33:575.
122. Aro A, Uustiupa M, Voutilanen E, et al. Effects of guar gum in male subjects with hypercholesterolemia. *Am J Clin Nutr.* 1984;39:911.
123. Jenkins DJA, Leeds AR, Slavin B, et al. Reduction of serum cholesterol in type II hyperlipidaemia by guar gum. *Proc Nutr Soc.* 1977;36:94A.
124. Bosello O, Cominacini L, Zocca I, et al. Effects of guar gum on plasma lipoproteins and apolipoproteins C-II and C-III in patients affected by familial combined hyperlipoproteinemia. *Am J Clin Nutr.* 1984;40:1165.
125. Penagini R, Velio P, Vigorelli R, et al. The effect of dietary guar on serum cholesterol, intestinal transit, and fecal output in man. *Am J Gastroenterol.* 1986;81:123.
126. Zavoral JH, Hannan P, Fields DJ, et al. The hypolipidemic effect of locust bean gum food products in familial hypercholesterolemic adults and children. *Am J Clin Nutr.* 1983;38:285.

127. McLean AH, Eastwood MA, Anderson JR, et al. A study of the effects of dietary gum arabic in humans. *Am J Clin Nutr.* 1983;37:368.
128. Anderson JW, Zettwoch N, Feldman T, et al. Hypocholesterolemic effects of psyllium mucilloid for hypercholesterolemic men. *Fed Proc.* 1987;46.
129. DeGroot AP, Luyken R, Pikaar, NA. Cholesterol-lowering effect of rolled oats. *Lancet.* 1963;2:303.
130. Gould MR, Anderson JW, O'Mahoney S. Biofunctional properties of oats. In: Inglett GE, Munck L, eds. *Cereals for Food and Beverages: Recent Progress in Cereal Chemistry and Technology.* New York, NY: Academic Press; 1980:447.
131. Kirby RW, Anderson JW, Sieling B, et al. Oat-bran intake selectively lowers serum low-density lipoprotein cholesterol concentrations of hypercholesterolemic men. *Am J Clin Nutr.* 1981;34:824.
132. Anderson JW, Story L, Sieling RD, et al. Hypocholesterolemic effects of oat-bran or bean intake for hypercholesterolemic men. *Am J Clin Nutr.* 1984;40:1146.
133. Van Horn LV, Liu K, Parker D, et al. Serum lipid response to oat product intake with a fat-modified diet. *J Am Diet Assoc.* 1986;86:759.
134. Swain JF, Rouse IL, Curley CB, et al. Comparison of the effects of oat bran and low-fiber wheat on serum lipoprotein levels and blood pressure. *N Engl J Med.* 1990;322:147.
135. Demark-Wahnefried W, Bowering J, Cohen, PS. Reduced serum cholesterol with dietary change using fat-modified and oat bran supplemented diets. *J Am Diet Assoc.* 1990;90:223.
136. Chen WJL, Anderson JW, Gould MR. Effects of oat bran, oat gum, and pectin on lipid metabolism of cholesterol-fed rats. *Nutr Rep Int.* 1981;24:1093.
137. Chen WJL, Anderson JW. Soluble and insoluble plant fiber in selected cereals and vegetables. *Am J Clin Nutr.* 1981;34:1077.
138. Anderson JW, Story L, Sieling B, et al. Hypocholesterolemic effects of high-fibre diets rich in water-soluble plant fibres. *J Can Diet Assoc.* 1984;45.
139. Schweizer TF, Bekhechi AR, Koellreutter B, et al. Metabolic effects of dietary fiber from dehulled soybeans in humans. *Am J Clin Nutr.* 1983;38:1.
140. Shore RL, Day PJ, Willis RA, et al. Effects of soybean polysaccharide on plasma lipids. *J Am Diet Assoc.* 1985;85:1461.
141. Anderson JW, Chen WJL. Cholesterol-lowering properties of oat products. In: Webster F, ed. *Oat Chemistry and Technology.* Minneapolis, Minn: American Association of Cereal Chemists; 1986.
142. Story JA, Watterson JJ. Modification of bile acid pool size and composition by oat bran, corn bran and cellulose in rats. *Fed Proc.* 1987;46.
143. Schneeman BO, Cimmarusti J, Cohen W, et al. Composition of high density lipoproteins in rats. *J Nutr.* 1984;114:1320.
144. Liu GC, Coulston AM, Reaven GM. Effect of high-carbohydrate low-fat diets on plasma glucose, insulin and lipid responses in hypertriglyceridemic humans. *Metabolism.* 1983;32:750.
145. Chen WJL, Anderson JW, Jennings D. Propionate may mediate the hypocholesterolemic effects of certain soluble plant fibers in cholesterol-fed rats. *Proc Soc Exp Biol Med.* 1984;175:215.
146. Mellies MJ, Jandacek RJ, Taulbee JD, et al. A double-blind, placebo-controlled study of sucrose polyester in hypocholesterolemic outpatients. *Am J Clin Nutr.* 1983;37:339.
147. Crouse JR, Grundy SM. Effects of sucrose polyester on cholesterol metabolism in man. *Metabolism.* 1979;28:994.
148. Abramowicz M, ed. Fish oil for the heart. *Med Ltr.* 1987;29:7.
149. Reeves JB III, Weihrauch JL. *Composition of Foods: Fats and Oils—Raw, Processed and Prepared.* US Dept of Agriculture handbook 8-4 (revised); 1979.

3. LIPOPROTEIN METABOLISM*

There are five major classes of lipoproteins: chylomicrons, very-low-density lipoproteins (VLDL), intermediate-density lipoproteins (IDL), low-density lipoproteins (LDL), and high-density lipoproteins (HDL). As is LDL, HDL is further subfractionated into small and large particles, HDL_2 and HDL_3. The characteristics of the lipoproteins are summarized in *Table 3.1.*

Table 3.1
Characteristics and Functions of the Plasma Lipoproteins

	Chylomicron	VLDL	IDL	LDL	HDL
Density, g/mL	<0.95	0.95–1.006	1.006–1.019	1.019–1.063	1.063–1.210
Electrophoretic mobility	Origin	Pre-β	Pre-β to β	β	α
Origin	Intestine	Liver and intestine	In the circulation secondary to the catabolism of other lipoproteins		
			Liver	Liver	Liver and intestine
Physiological role	Transport of dietary triglyceride	Transport of endogenous triglyceride	LDL precursor	Major cholesterol transport lipoprotein	Reverse cholesterol transport
Composition, %					
Triglyceride	90	60	40	10	5
Cholesterol	5	12	30	50	20
Phospholipid	3	18	20	15	25
Protein	2	10	10	25	50
Major apolipoproteins	A-I A-IV B-48 C-I C-II C-III	B-100 C-I C-II C-III E	B-100 E	B-100	A-I A-II

Adapted with permission from Kris-Etherton PM, Krummel D, Russell ME, et al. The effect of diet on plasma lipids, lipoproteins, and coronary heart disease. *J Am Diet Assoc.* 1988;88:1373.

Lipoproteins have a hydrophobic core consisting of nonpolar lipids (triglyceride and cholesterol esters) coated with surfactants (phospholipids and unesterified or free cholesterol) and proteins that are referred to as *apolipoproteins.* The proportions of triglyceride, cholesterol, phospholipid, and protein differ among the specific lipoprotein classes. Chylomicrons and VLDL are triglyceride-rich lipoproteins, and LDL, the major cholesterol-transport particle in plasma, carries 70% of the plasma total cholesterol. HDL is a protein-rich particle; 50% of its mass is protein.

Conceptually, there are three lipoprotein metabolic systems: exogenous fat transport, endogenous fat transport, and reverse cholesterol transport (see Havel[1] and Breslow[2] for recent reviews). A brief description of each pathway follows; each is also summarized in *Figure 3.1.*

*By the Editors

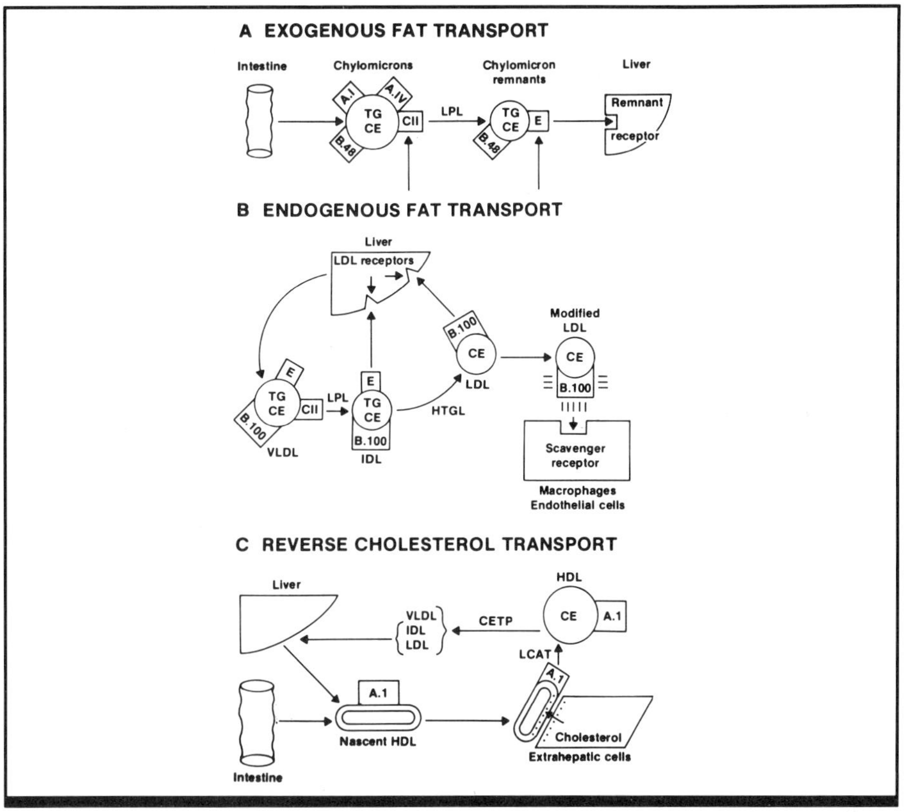

Fig. 3.1
Lipoprotein metabolic pathways. Reproduced with permission from Breslow JL. Apolipoprotein genetic variation and human disease. **Physiol Rev.** ***1988;68:85.***

Dietary triglycerides are packaged into chylomicrons in the intestine (Figure 3.1, A). They enter the circulation through the thoracic duct and acquire apolipoproteins C and E from HDL. During removal of triglyceride from the core of the chylomicron, some surface material (primarily phospholipids, cholesterol, and apolipoproteins) is transferred to HDL. Chylomicron remnants are efficiently removed by the hepatic apolipoprotein E receptor, internalized via endocytosis, and translocated to the lysosomes where the remnant lipid and protein constituents are catabolized.

Endogenous fat transport refers to the synthesis and catabolism of VLDL and LDL (Figure 3.1, B). VLDL is hydrolyzed to IDL lipoprotein lipase (LPL). Surface material from IDL is transferred to HDL. Unesterified cholesterol is esterified in HDL via the action of the enzyme lecithin-cholesterol acyltransferase (LCAT). The esterified cholesterol is transferred back to IDL leading to a cholesterol-ester enrichment of IDL. Some IDL is cleared from plasma by hepatic LDL receptors that bind apolipoprotein E. The remainder undergo rapid continued lipolysis probably by hepatic triglyceride lipase, during which time all apolipoproteins except B-100 are transferred to other lipoproteins. The result is the formation of LDL with apolipoprotein B-100 on its surface. This from of apolipoprotein B is recognized by the hepatic and extrahepatic high-affinity LDL receptors. Approximately 70% of LDL is removed from plasma via this mechanism, principally by the liver. The remaining LDL is modified in plasma and removed by scavenger receptors on macrophages and endothelial cells. Plasma LDL levels are influenced by LDL receptor number, which, in turn, is regulated by the cell's need for cholesterol. When the need is low, cells make fewer receptors and remove LDL at a reduced rate. As a result of these cellular events, the rate with which LDL is removed from the plasma decreases and there is a corresponding rise in plasma LDL.[3] In summary, the steady-state plasma LDL-cholesterol concentrations are determined by four factors: (1) the rate of LDL production, (2) the rate of receptor-dependent LDL clearance, (3) LDL receptor affinity, and (4) the rate of receptor-independent LDL clearance. When LDL-cholesterol levels increase because of some perturbation in the above scenario, there occurs a series of events that lead to and cause atherosclerosis.

Arterial uptake of LDL appears to be mediated by a receptor-independent mechanism. It has been proposed that in response to oxidative modification, LDL are removed by macrophages via the acetyl-LDL or scavenger-receptor pathway.[4] Other modifications in LDL (eg, chemical alteration, such as acetoacetyl LDL and malondialdehyde-conjugated LDL) are recognized, and the modified LDL are removed by the acetyl-LDL receptor or the scavenger receptor. A biological modification, cell-induced oxidation of LDL, may be similar to chemically modified LDL.[4]

Oxidized LDL are highly cytotoxic.[4] It has been postulated that oxidized LDL could cause functional changes in endothelial cells that favor fatty-streak formation (by causing penetration of circulating monocytes into endothelial cells or movement of LDL into the subendothelial space). Steinberg and colleagues[4] speculate that the loss of endothelial cells may not be an initiating factor in the development of atherosclerosis. Rather, injury to the arterial wall may occur after the lipid-laden macrophages become nonfunctional or die, and release cytotoxic, oxidized LDL, which could cause the loss of endothelial cells overlying the fatty streak. After injury to the endothelium a cascade of events that lead to lesion growth follows (*Figure 3.2*). The proposed relationship between the lipid-infiltration hypothesis and the endothelial-injury hypothesis is depicted in Figure 3.2.

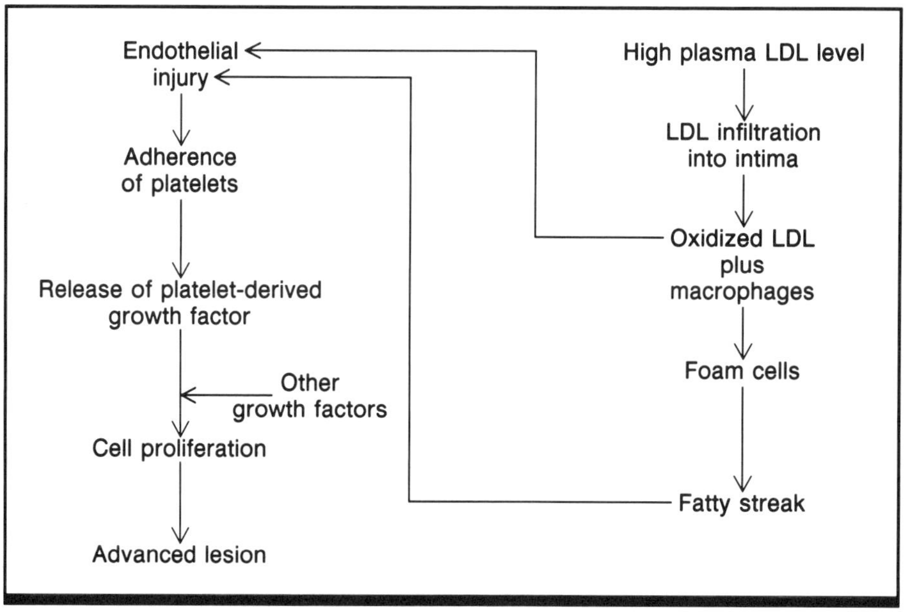

Fig. 3.2
Postulated linkage between the lipid-infiltration hypothesis and the endothelial-injury hypothesis. The lipid-infiltration hypothesis (right column) may be sufficient to account for fatty streaks, and the endothelial-injury hypothesis (left column) may account for progression of the fatty streak to more-advanced lesions. Reprinted by permission of the* New England Journal of Medicine, *1989;320:915.

HDL transports approximately 25% of circulating cholesterol. HDL functions in reverse cholesterol transport (Figure 3.1, C). This system provides a mechanism by which cholesterol in peripheral tissues can be excreted. Nascent HDL, produced in the liver and intestine, accepts unesterified cholesterol from extrahepatic cells (*Figure 3.3*). The free cholesterol is esterified via the enzyme LCAT, using apolipoprotein A-I as a cofactor, and moves to the core of HDL. The accumulation of cholesterol esters by nascent HDL leads to the formation of HDL_3, the predominant form of circulating HDL. Continued uptake of free cholesterol by HDL_3 leads to the production of HDL_{2a}. Through a series of exchange reactions, VLDL triglycerides are transferred to HDL_{2a} and, concurrently, HDL_{2a} cholesterol esters are translocated to VLDL. The resultant triglyceride-rich cholesterol-depleted HDL_{2b} is further catabolized back to HDL_3 by hepatic triglyceride lipase. HDL_2 is negatively associated with CHD risk, whereas HDL_3 seems to be unrelated.

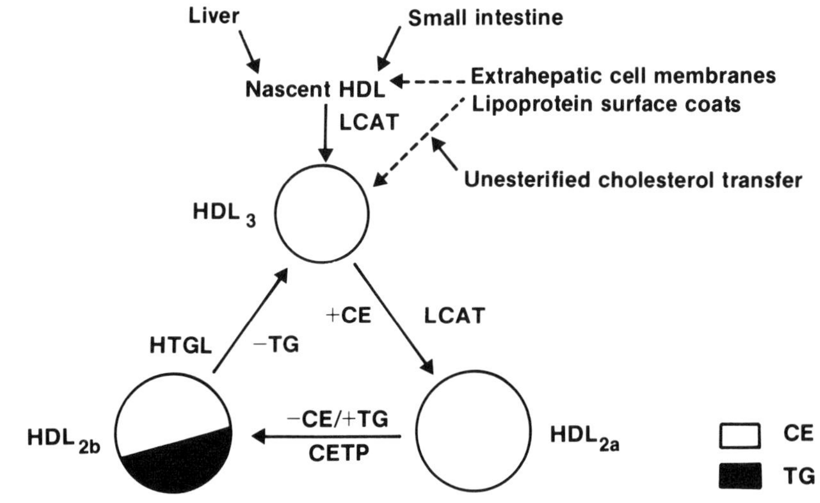

Fig. 3.3
***Metabolism of high-density lipoprotein (HDL). CE indicates cholesterol ester; CETP, cholesterol ester transfer protein; HTGL, hepatic triglyceride lipase; LCAT, lecithin-cholesterol acyltransferase; TG, triglyceride. Reproduced with permission from Grundy SM. Lessons from the Helsinki Heart Study.* **Postgrad Med.** *1988;84:217.*

Recently, an LDL-like particle first discovered 25 years ago has become the focus of considerable interest. Lp(a) is an LDL-like particle that contains both apolipoprotein B and the disulphide-linked apolipoprotein(a). Current belief is that Lp(a) is involved in the formation of atheromatous plaques.[6]

Some scientists believe that cholesterol-rich chylomicron remnants may be atherogenic, perhaps by contributing cholesterol ultimately to the arterial endothelium.[7] Cholesterol feeding leads to the appearance of HDL_c in the plasma. HDL_c is rich in cholesterol esters and floats at lower densities (d = 1.03–1.10 g/mL) than HDL. HDL_c binds to the LDL receptor and leads to an increase in the cholesterol content of fibroblasts and smooth-muscle arterial cells in culture.[8] HDL_c is thought to be an atherogenic lipoprotein particle.

The apolipoproteins play an important role in lipoprotein metabolism. The plasma transport lipoprotein for each apolipoprotein is identified in Table 3.1 and the major characteristics and functions of the apolipoproteins are summarized in *Table 3.2*.

Table 3.2
Apolipoproteins and Their Association With Human Diseases

Apolipoprotein	Plasma Concentration, mg/mL	Molecular Weight, kDa*	Function	Association with Clinical Disorders
A-I	1.0–1.2	28	Tissue cholesterol efflux LCAT activation	Apo A-I/apo C-III deficiency coronary heart disease
A-II	0.3–0.5	17		Coronary heart disease
A-III	0.06–0.07	33	Cholesterol transport	
A-IV	0.16	46		
B-100	0.7–1.0	550	VLDL production ligand for LDL receptor	Abetalipoproteinemia hypobetalipoproteinemia B-100 deficiency coronary heart disease
B-48	0.03–0.05	275	Chylomicron production	B-48 deficiency
C-I	0.04–0.06	7	LCAT activation moderate	
C-II	0.03–0.05	9	Lipoprotein lipase activation	Familial hyperchylomicronemia (type I)
C-III	0.12–0.14	9	Lipase inhibition	Apo A-I/apo C-III deficiency
E	0.03–0.05	38	Ligand for LDL and chylomicron remnant receptors	Familial dysbetalipoproteinemia (type III)

*kDa, kilodaltons.

Adapted with permission from Breslow JL. Apolipoprotein genetic variation and human disease. *Physiol Rev.* 1988;68:85.

Numerous factors affect the concentration of lipids and lipoproteins in the plasma. These are discussed in chapters 1, 2, and 9 in this manual. The major factors that affect plasma lipid and lipoprotein levels are identified in *Table 3.3.* A brief summary of their specific effects is included.

PART 2
NUTRITION INTERVENTION

4. NUTRITION ASSESSMENT

The assessment of nutritional status provides important baseline information that is used in making a diagnosis, prioritizing problems, developing a nutrition care plan, monitoring the client's progress, and evaluating treatment. Components of the process include family history, psychosocial, anthropometric, dietary, clinical, and biochemical assessment. In this chapter each area of the nutrition-assessment process is discussed, including important information for monitoring patients or for diagnosing or ruling out as well as preventing coronary heart disease (CHD).

FAMILY HISTORY*

Obtaining a detailed family history is useful in assessing the potential for genetic risk of CHD. Since CHD is so prevalent in the United States, most interviewees report some family history of it. However, a strong family history of early CHD (such as death of a sibling or parent before age 50) should prompt practitioners to evaluate existing risk factors and encourage more aggressive treatment and, preferably, encourage aggressive preventive measures. Furthermore, all family members should be assessed similarly for risk status before CHD is clinically manifested.

At minimum, a thorough family history should include specific information on the patient's first-degree relatives—ie, parents, siblings, and any offspring. Data on second-degree relatives—ie, grandparents, uncles, aunts, nephews, and nieces—may also be helpful. Age and time of onset or diagnosis of each of the major risk factors should be recorded for each family member. The age at death and cause of death for all deceased family members should be noted.

PSYCHOSOCIAL ASSESSMENT*

A comprehensive psychosocial assessment is essential to effectively evaluate and accurately identify patients' problems and needs. Together with data collected in other areas of nutrition assessment, a complete patient profile should be developed. This information is very important in establishing an effective counseling relationship and is also valuable in ensuring the success of the nutrition care plan.

Practitioners must obtain information about a client's life style; cooking, shopping, and eating habits; family structure; and other factors that affect eating behavior. Essential information is listed in *Table 4.1.*

ANTHROPOMETRIC ASSESSMENT†

When taking anthropometric measurements of healthy people, patients with hyperlipidemia, and ambulatory and bedridden coronary patients, the following considerations are important:

Appropriateness—While a broad spectrum of measurements can be made, key questions should be asked when selecting anthropometric measures: Why is the information needed? How will it be used?

Patient cooperation and general health status—An anthropometric assessment may not be appropriate for seriously ill, terminally ill, or comatose patients.[1]

*By Dottie Dolezal
†By Joyce Ann Gilbert

Table 4.1
Psychosocial Areas of Inquiry

1. Home life and meal patterns
   a. number in household (eat together?)
   b. person who does shopping
   c. person who does cooking
   d. food-storage and cooking facilities (stove, refrigerator)
   e. type of housing (home, apartment, room, etc)
   f. ability to shop and prepare food
2. Ethnic or cultural background
   a. influence on eating habits
   b. religion
   c. education
3. Economics
   a. income—frequency and steadiness of employment
   b. amount of money for food each week or month and individual's perception of its adequacy for meeting food needs
   c. eligibility for food stamps and cost of stamps
   d. public-aid recipient?
4. Appetite
   a. good, poor, any changes
   b. factors that affect appetite
   c. taste and smell perception and any changes
5. Lifestyle
   a. schedule
   b. eating out
6. Attitudes
   a. food- and diet-related
   b. health-related
7. Allergies, intolerances, or food avoidances
   a. food avoided and reason
   b. length of time of avoidance
   c. description of problems caused by foods
8. Dental and oral health
   a. problems with eating
   b. foods that cannot be eaten
   c. problems with swallowing, salivation, food sticking

Reprinted with permission from Krause MV, Mahan LK. *Food, Nutrition and Diet Therapy.* 7th ed. Philadelphia, Pa: WB Saunders Co; 1984:197.

History—An assessment of the patient's weight history, in particular, and desired weight are important in developing a realistic and attainable nutrition care plan.

Reassessment and monitoring—Three to four weeks may be required to document changes in many anthropometric measurements.

STANDARD ANTHROPOMETRIC MEASUREMENTS*

Anthropometric measurements are useful in estimating body composition, monitoring growth and development, and assessing malnutrition, obesity, and risk of CHD among others. Since overweight and obesity are risk factors for CHD, and since body weight affects plasma lipid levels, assessing and monitoring anthropometric status are very important in the prevention and treatment of CHD.

*By Joyce Ann Gilbert

Anthropometric measurements are indices of body stature, weight, and fatness. Measurements taken on an individual patient are compared to gender- and age-specific standards. Anthropometrics are particularly useful when measured at intervals over time. Measurements include height, weight, skinfold measurements, and the circumference of certain body parts.

Height and weight measurements should be taken on all persons, if possible. With this information, body mass index and percentage of ideal body weight can be determined. Percentage of body fat is also a useful measurement in assessing CHD risk.

An upright beam balance should be used to weigh an ambulatory patient. Spring-type bathroom scales are not accurate and should be avoided unless they are used at home to monitor patients' weight. Patients should be weighed with minimal clothing and after they have voided. Stature measurements require a measuring stick or nonstretchable tape attached to a flat vertical surface as well as some form of right-angle headboard.[2] The movable measuring rod attached to platform scales does not measure stature accurately.

Frame Size

Frame size can be estimated from: (1) elbow breadth (bicondylar breadth of the humerus) and (2) wrist circumference. (Other body breadths that have been used to estimate frame size include: shoulder, hip, knee, and ankle.) Elbow breadth is measured most accurately with special calipers.* The two prongs of the calipers are placed on either side of the elbow and the millimeter reading is noted. Elbow breadth for men and women with a medium frame appears in *Table 4.2* and *Table 4.3*. To determine wrist circumference, the right

Table 4.2
Elbow Breadth for Men With Medium Frame Size

Height, ft and in.*	Height, cm*	Elbow Breadth, in.	Elbow Breadth, mm
5′1″–5′2″	155.0–157.5	2½–2⅞	63.5–73.0
5′3″–5′6″	160.0–167.6	2⅝–2⅞	66.7–73.0
5′7″–5′10″	170.2–177.8	2¾–3	69.8–76.2
5′11″–6′2″	180.3–188.0	2¾–3⅛	69.8–79.4
6′3″	190.5	2⅞–3¼	73.0–82.5

*Without shoe heels.

Adaptation courtesy Statistical Bulletin, Metropolitan Life Insurance Co.

Table 4.3
Elbow Breadth for Women With Medium Frame Size

Height, ft and in.*	Height, cm*	Elbow Breadth, in.	Elbow Breadth, mm
4′9″–4′10″	144.8–147.3	2¼–1½	57.1–63.5
4′11″–5′2″	150.0–157.0	2¼–2½	57.1–63.5
5′3″–5′6″	160.0–167.6	2⅜–2⅝	60.3–66.7
5′7″–5′10″	170.1–177.8	2⅜–2⅝	60.3–66.7
5′11″	180.3	2½–2¾	63.5–69.8

*Without shoe heels.

Adaptation courtesy Statistical Bulletin, Metropolitan Life Insurance Co.

*Available from Metropolitan Life Insurance Co, Health and Safety Education Division, 1 Madison Ave, New York, NY 10160.

wrist is measured distal to the styloid process of radius and ulna at the smallest circumference. From wrist circumference and height an *r* value is calculated as follows:

$$r = \frac{\text{Height in Centimeters}}{\text{Wrist Circumference in Centimeters}}$$

A smaller *r* value is indicative of a large frame and a larger value is indicative of a small frame (*Table 4.4*).

Table 4.4
Body Frame Sizes for Men and Women Based on* r *Values

Men		Women	
***r* Value**	**Frame Size**	***r* Value**	**Frame Size**
≥10.4	Small	≥11.0	Small
9.6–10.4	Medium	10.1–11.0	Medium
≤9.6	Large	≤10.1	Large

Adaptation courtesy Statistical Bulletin, Metropolitan Life Insurance Co.

It is important to note that there are some limitations with both methods of estimating frame size. For example, elbow breadth has been shown to be correlated with percentage of body fat[4]; hence, frame size will be overestimated in relatively obese persons. Frame size is of limited usefulness in anthropometric assessment.

Body Weight

Desirable (or ideal) body weight is the weight for given gender height and frame size that is associated with health and longevity. In clinical practice, the NIH Office of Disease Prevention and Technology Transfer[5,6] recommends using the 1959 Metropolitan Life Insurance Co tables (instead of the 1983 tables) for patients with a family history or current indications of diseases or with risk factors complicated by obesity such as hypertension, hypertriglyceridemia, hypercholesterolemia, and glucose intolerance or diabetes. While some scientists recommend using the 1959 tables for everyone, others[6] note that the more liberal 1983 tables may be used for patients without complicating risk factors. The principal differences between the two tables are for men and women of shorter stature. Ideal weights are heavier in the more recent version of the table. (See Tables 14.6 and 14.7 in the appendix.)

Percentage overweight is often expressed relative to desirable or ideal body weight:

$$\text{Percentage Overweight} = \frac{\text{Observed Body Weight}}{\text{Desired Body Weight}} \times 100$$

People who are 110% above desirable body weight are overweight. Obesity is defined as being greater than 120% of desirable weight for height.

The body mass index,

$$\frac{\text{W kg}}{\text{H}^2\ \text{cm}}$$

(weight in kilograms divided by height in centimeters squared), can be determined simply from height and weight measurements. A nomogram for determining body mass index (BMI) appears in *Figure 4.1*. The ideal BMI goal for women is 21.5 to 22.4 and for men is 22.0 to 22.7.[7] A BMI that warrants intervention is 25.8 to 26.9 for women and 26.4 to 27.2 for men.

Fig. 4.1
Nomogram to determine body mass index, weight divided by stature squared

$\frac{W}{S^2}$

Directions

1. **Locate the person's stature on the left column. Numbers in this column *increase* going down the scale.**
2. **Locate the person's weight on the right column. Numbers in this column *decrease* going down the scale.**
3. **Lay a ruler or straightedge so that it touches these two points—stature and weight.**
4. **Note where the straightedge crosses the slanted line between these two columns. This is the person's W/S^2 value.**
5. **Enter the W/S^2 value in the person's record.**

Used with permission of Ross Laboratories, Columbus, OH 43216, from* Nutritional Assessment of the Elderly Through Anthropometry. *© 1984 Ross Laboratories. (Adapted from* Am J Clin Nutr. *1981;34:2831.)

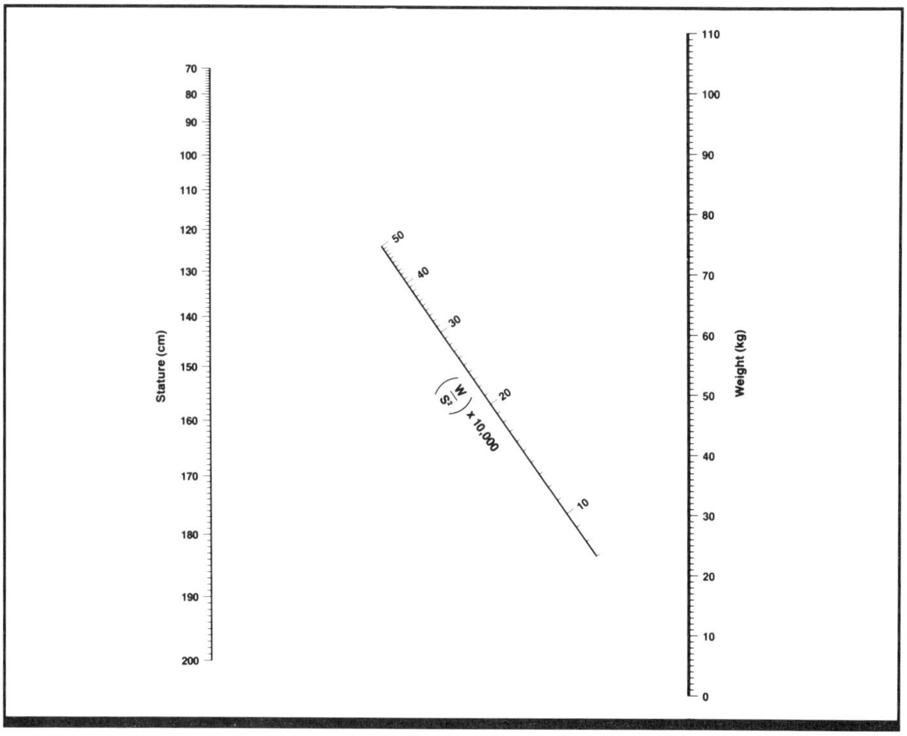

Body Compositional Analysis

There are numerous traditional and new methods for determining body composition.[8] Assessing body fatness is useful in diagnosing and treating obesity. The average adult male has 12% to 15% body fat, whereas average adult females have between 22% and 25%. Men are considered obese if body fat exceeds 25% of body weight. Women are considered obese when body fat is greater than 28% to 30% of body weight.

Skinfold measurements are frequently used to indirectly estimate body fatness. The technique assumes that the thickness of the subcutaneous adipose tissue reflects a constant proportion of the total body fat and that the sites measured represent the average thickness of the subcutaneous adipose tissue.[8] There are more than 100 prediction equations that are age-, race-, and gender-specific.

Triceps and subscapular skinfold thickness measurements are taken most frequently. Some of the equations that estimate the percentage of body fat use only triceps-skinfold measurements or measurements from sites on the upper body. If body fat is unevenly distributed between the upper and lower body, the limitations of the equation and the method are obvious.

Successive skinfold measurements should be made by those who have been properly trained. The measurements should agree within 3 mm. A 5% error is expected in using skinfolds to estimate percentage of body fat; more occur when measurements are made on large or small skinfolds. Skinfold sites and methods of measurement are listed below.[9] All measurements should be taken on the right side of the body with the subject standing.

1. Chest—A diagonal fold is taken one half of the distance between the anterior axillary line and the nipple (in women, one third of the distance from the anterior axillary line).

2. Abdominal—A vertical fold is taken at a lateral distance of 2 cm from the umbilicus.
3. Thigh—Midway between hip and knee joints, a vertical fold is taken on the anterior of the thigh.
4. Triceps—Midway between the shoulder (acromial process) and elbow (olecranon) joint, a vertical fold is taken on the midline of the posterior side of the arm over the triceps muscle. The arm should be extended and relaxed.
5. Subscapular—Beneath or below the scapula, a fold is taken on a diagonal line coming from the vertebrae border 1 cm from the inferior angle of the scapula (a diagonal just below the lowest border of the scapula).
6. Suprailliac—A diagonal fold is taken 3 cm above the anterior superior iliac crest.

Grasp the skinfold between thumb and index finger. The skinfold should include two thicknesses of skin and subcutaneous fat, but not muscle. Apply the caliper perpendicular to the fold and 0.25 to 0.5 in. away from thumb and index finger. Release the caliper, exerting full tension on the skinfold, and read the dial 1 to 2 seconds after the grip has been released. A minimum of two measurements should be recorded on each site. Measurements should be at least 15 seconds apart to allow the skinfold site to return to normal. If repeated measurement varies more than 1 mm, a third measurement should be taken until there is consistency. Measurements should not be taken when skin is moist or after exercise. *Table 4.5* and *Table 4.6* are computer generated with the use of multiple regression equations derived from various combinations of anthropometric variables that measure body density and help expedite calculation of the percentage of body fat.

Example: Three measurements in a 31-year-old male

Chest	15 mm
Thigh	17 mm
Abdomen	27 mm
Sum of 3	**59 mm**

Using Table 4.5, locate 59 mm under the sum of skinfolds column, following across to the appropriate age column. The value is 17.9, or 17.9% body fatness.

To estimate the body composition of the adult from anthropometric measurements, the weight, age, and sum of three skinfolds are needed. The use of three skinfolds instead of more enhances technical feasibility. In clinical settings, subsequent measurements can be used to evaluate change over time.

Two new methodologies for estimating body fat that are suitable for use in the field have been introduced within the past five years. Both methods assume the body is divided into two compartments: (1) fat and (2) fat-free mass. Both methods estimate fat-free mass and derive body fat by subtraction.

Bioelectrical Impedance Analysis (BIA)*

BIA is based on the conduction of an applied electrical current in the body. Body fluids and electrolytes are primarily responsible for electrical conductance. Since fat tissue is largely anhydrous, conductance is attributed to the fat-free mass. Regression equations have been developed to predict total body water (TBW) from the impedance reading. These equations may also include body weight and gender. Concerns that TBW varies with degree of hydration, recent electrolyte intake, or stage of the menstrual cycle have not been adequately addressed. More research needs to be done on whether different regression equations are needed for estimating body fat in different populations, eg, patients who are elderly, athletic, pediatric, and so on.

*By Marilyn Schorin

Table 4.5
Percentage Fat Estimate for Men: Sum of Chest, Abdomen, and Thigh Skinfolds

	Age to Last Year								
Sum of Skinfolds, mm	Under 22	23–27	28–32	33–37	38–42	43–47	48–52	53–57	Over 57
8–10	1.3	1.8	2.3	2.9	3.4	3.9	4.5	5.0	5.5
11–13	2.2	2.8	3.3	3.9	4.4	4.9	5.5	6.0	6.5
14–16	3.2	3.8	4.3	4.8	5.4	5.9	6.4	7.0	7.5
17–19	4.2	4.7	5.3	5.8	6.3	6.9	7.4	8.0	8.5
20–22	5.1	5.7	6.2	6.8	7.3	7.9	8.4	8.9	9.5
23–25	6.1	6.6	7.2	7.7	8.3	8.8	9.4	9.9	10.5
26–28	7.0	7.6	8.1	8.7	9.2	9.8	10.3	10.9	11.4
29–31	8.0	8.5	9.1	9.6	10.2	10.7	11.3	11.8	12.4
32–34	8.9	9.4	10.0	10.5	11.1	11.6	12.2	12.8	13.3
35–37	9.6	10.4	10.9	11.5	12.0	12.5	13.1	13.7	14.3
38–40	10.7	11.3	11.6	12.4	12.9	13.5	14.1	14.6	15.2
41–43	11.6	12.2	12.7	13.3	13.8	14.4	15.0	15.5	16.1
44–46	12.5	13.1	13.6	14.2	14.7	15.3	15.9	16.4	17.0
47–49	13.4	13.9	14.5	15.1	15.6	16.2	16.8	17.3	17.9
50–52	14.3	14.8	15.4	15.9	16.5	17.1	17.5	18.2	18.3
53–55	15.1	15.7	16.2	16.8	17.4	17.9	18.5	19.1	19.7
56–58	16.0	16.5	17.1	17.7	18.2	18.8	19.4	20.0	20.5
59–61	16.9	17.4	17.9	18.5	19.1	19.7	20.2	20.8	21.4
62–64	17.6	18.2	18.8	19.4	19.9	20.5	21.1	21.7	22.2
65–67	18.5	19.0	19.6	20.2	20.8	21.3	21.9	22.5	23.1
68–70	19.3	19.9	20.4	21.0	21.6	22.2	22.7	23.3	23.9
71–73	20.1	20.7	21.2	21.8	22.4	23.0	23.6	24.1	24.7
74–76	20.9	21.5	22.0	22.5	23.2	23.8	24.4	25.0	25.5
77–79	21.7	22.2	22.8	23.4	24.0	24.6	25.2	25.8	26.3
80–82	22.4	23.0	23.6	24.2	24.8	25.4	25.9	26.5	27.1
83–85	23.2	23.9	24.4	25.0	25.5	26.1	26.7	27.3	27.9
86–88	24.0	24.5	25.1	25.7	26.3	26.9	27.5	28.1	28.7
89–91	24.7	25.3	25.9	26.5	27.1	27.6	28.2	28.8	29.4
92–94	25.4	26.0	26.6	27.2	27.3	28.4	29.0	29.6	30.2
95–97	26.1	26.7	27.3	27.9	28.5	29.1	29.7	30.3	30.9
98–100	26.9	27.4	28.0	28.6	29.2	29.8	30.4	31.0	31.6
101–103	27.5	28.1	28.7	29.3	29.9	30.5	31.1	31.7	32.3
104–106	28.2	28.8	29.4	30.0	30.6	31.2	31.8	32.4	33.0
107–109	28.9	29.5	30.1	30.7	31.3	31.9	32.5	33.1	33.7
110–112	29.6	30.2	30.6	31.4	32.0	32.5	33.2	33.8	34.4
113–115	30.2	30.8	31.4	32.0	32.6	33.2	33.8	34.5	35.1
116–118	30.9	31.5	32.1	32.7	33.3	33.9	34.5	35.1	35.7
119–121	31.5	32.1	32.7	33.3	33.9	34.5	35.1	35.7	36.4
122–124	32.1	32.7	33.3	33.9	34.5	35.1	35.8	36.4	37.0
125–127	32.7	33.3	33.9	34.5	35.1	35.8	36.4	37.0	37.6

Reprinted from Skinfolds and body density and their relation to body fatness: a review. *Hum Biol.* 1981;53:181 by Lohman TG. By permission of the Wayne State University Press.

Infrared Interactance (IRI)*

First described in 1984 by Conway et al,[10] IRI is a method in which a fiberoptic probe emitting a small quantity of electromagnetic radiation is placed at a particular site on the body. The energy that is reflected is scanned and read by a spectrophotometer. This energy is proportional to TBW.

*By Marilyn Schorin

Fifty-three subjects were scanned in the initial report, which indicated a high correlation between body fat determined by IRI and by deuterium dilution. A relatively inexpensive instrument that has been developed for use in the field is available. This instrument reportedly measures body fat with the accuracy of hydrodensitometry; however, no studies demonstrating this have been published to date. The energy at the biceps determined from the IRI device is incorporated into a regression equation that includes gender, weight, height, frame size, and exercise level (subjective). The regression equation has not been published and is considered proprietary information by the manufacturer. The lack of appropriate data about this instrument and concordance with other methods of body composition indicate that the instrument is still in the developmental stage.

Table 4.6
Percentage Fat Estimate for Women: Sum of Chest, Abdomen, and Thigh Skinfolds

	Age to Last Year								
Sum of Skinfolds, mm	**Under 22**	**23–27**	**28–32**	**33–37**	**38–42**	**43–47**	**48–52**	**53–57**	**Over 57**
23–25	9.7	9.9	10.2	10.4	10.7	10.9	11.2	11.4	11.7
26–28	11.0	11.2	11.5	11.7	12.0	12.3	12.5	12.7	13.0
29–31	12.3	12.5	12.8	13.0	13.3	13.5	13.8	14.0	14.3
32–34	13.6	13.8	14.0	14.3	14.5	14.8	15.0	15.3	15.5
35–37	14.8	15.0	15.3	15.5	15.8	16.0	16.3	16.5	16.8
38–40	16.0	16.3	16.5	16.7	17.0	17.2	17.5	17.7	18.0
41–43	17.2	17.4	17.7	17.9	18.2	18.4	18.7	18.9	19.2
44–46	18.3	18.6	18.8	19.1	19.3	19.6	19.8	20.1	20.3
47–49	19.5	19.7	20.0	20.2	20.5	20.7	21.0	21.2	21.5
50–52	20.6	20.8	21.1	21.3	21.6	21.8	22.1	22.3	22.6
53–55	21.7	21.9	22.1	22.4	22.6	22.9	23.1	23.4	23.6
56–58	22.7	23.0	23.2	23.4	23.7	23.9	24.2	24.4	24.7
59–61	23.7	24.0	24.2	24.5	24.7	25.0	25.2	25.5	25.7
62–64	24.7	25.0	25.1	25.5	25.7	26.0	26.2	26.4	26.7
65–67	25.7	25.9	26.2	26.4	26.7	26.9	27.2	27.4	27.7
68–70	26.6	26.9	27.1	27.4	27.6	27.9	28.1	28.4	28.6
71–73	27.5	27.8	28.0	28.3	28.5	28.8	29.0	29.3	29.5
74–76	28.4	28.7	28.9	29.2	29.4	29.7	29.9	30.2	30.4
77–79	29.3	29.5	29.8	30.0	30.3	30.5	30.8	31.0	31.3
80–82	30.1	30.4	30.6	30.9	31.1	31.4	31.6	31.9	32.1
83–85	30.9	31.2	31.4	31.7	31.9	32.2	32.4	32.7	32.9
86–88	31.7	32.0	32.2	32.5	32.7	32.9	33.2	33.4	33.7
89–91	32.5	32.7	33.0	33.2	33.5	33.7	33.9	34.2	34.4
92–94	33.2	33.4	33.7	33.9	34.2	34.4	34.7	34.9	35.2
95–97	33.9	34.1	34.4	34.6	34.9	35.1	35.4	35.6	35.9
98–100	34.6	34.8	35.1	35.3	35.5	35.8	36.0	36.3	36.5
101–103	35.3	35.4	35.7	35.9	36.2	36.4	36.7	36.9	37.2
104–106	35.8	36.1	36.3	36.6	36.8	37.1	37.3	37.5	37.8
107–109	36.4	36.7	36.9	37.1	37.4	37.6	37.9	38.1	38.4
110–112	37.0	37.2	37.5	37.7	38.0	38.2	38.5	38.7	38.9
113–115	37.5	37.8	38.0	38.2	38.5	38.7	39.0	39.2	39.5
116–118	38.0	38.3	38.5	38.8	39.0	39.3	39.5	39.7	40.0
119–121	38.5	38.7	39.0	39.2	39.5	39.7	40.0	40.2	40.5
122–124	39.0	39.2	39.4	39.7	39.9	40.2	40.4	40.7	40.9
125–127	39.4	39.6	39.9	40.1	40.4	40.6	40.9	41.1	41.4
128–130	39.8	40.0	40.3	40.5	40.8	41.0	41.3	41.5	41.8

Reprinted from Skinfolds and body density and their relation to body fatness: a review. *Hum Biol.* 1981;53:181 by Lohman TG. By permission of the Wayne State University Press.

Body-Fat Distribution*

Adipose tissue distribution is thought to be a risk factor for a number of chronic diseases. It is estimated from waist-to-hip ratio, which is calculated as follows: (1) For men, the waist at the navel is measured. Hips are measured at the top of the hip bone. (2) For women, the waist is measured midway between the bottom of the ribs and the top of the hip bone. Hips are measured at the widest point between the hips and buttocks. (3) The waist measurement (in inches) is divided by the hip measurement.

A waist-to-hip ratio greater than 0.8 in women places them at risk for diabetes, heart disease, and stroke; for men, a waist-to-hip ratio greater than 1.0 indicates increased risk for these diseases. These ratios (greater than 0.8 for women and greater than 1.0 for men) define android obesity. A waist-to-hip ratio that is less than these values (in association with excess body weight) characterizes gynoid obesity.[11]

ANTHROPOMETRIC ASSESSMENT FOR THE HOSPITALIZED PATIENT†

For patients hospitalized for extended periods of time or those who are at high risk for iatrogenic malnutrition (eg, patients who have or develop an infection or another illness, and elderly patients or persons with a complicating disease), anthropometric assessment is important. Measurements that can be made easily include height, weight, triceps skinfold, and upper-arm circumference, from which arm-muscle circumference is determined.

Knee height can be used to estimate the stature of a bedridden person. This computation requires the patient's knee height, age, and gender. Knee height is measured with a sliding, broad-blade caliper, similar to the one used to measure infants. The patient, lying supine, bends the left knee at a 90-degree angle. One blade of the caliper is placed under the heel of the left foot while the other is placed over the anterior surface of the left thigh, above the condyles of the femur and just proximal to the patella.[2] The shaft of the caliper must be parallel with the tibia. Pressure is applied to compress tissue. Two measurements are made; they should agree within 0.5 cm. The following formulas are used to compute stature[2]:

$$\text{Stature of men} = 64.19\text{ cm} - (0.04 \times \text{age}) + (2.02 \times \text{knee height})$$

$$\text{Stature of women} = 84.88\text{ cm} - (0.24 \times \text{age}) + (1.83 \times \text{knee height})$$

The nomogram (*Figure 4.2*) can also be used to determine stature from knee height, age, and gender.

Bed scales are available in most hospitals to weigh bedridden patients or patients whose activity is severely limited. Patients should be weighed regularly.

Triceps-skinfold and upper-arm-circumference measurements are used to calculate arm-muscle circumference, which is an index of the amount of muscle or lean tissue in the body. This information can be used to monitor lean-tissue loss, which is useful in determining drug doses and in estimating basal metabolic rate. While monitoring lean tissue status is not indicated for all patients, it is appropriate to assess lean-tissue catabolism for patients who are hospitalized for extended periods or for those who are at high risk of developing iatrogenic malnutrition.

*By Joyce Ann Gilbert
†By the Editors

Fig. 4.2
Nomogram to estimate stature from knee height.
Directions
1. Locate the person's age on the column farthest to the left.
2. Locate the person's knee height on the next column.
3. Lay a ruler or straightedge so that it touches these two points—age and knee height.
4. Note where the straightedge crosses the stature column for the appropriate sex. The stature column for women is the farthest right column. The stature column for men is between that column and the knee-height column. The point where the ruler crosses the appropriate column is the person's estimated stature.
5. Enter the estimated stature in the person's record.

Used with permission of Ross Laboratories, Columbus, OH 43216, from Nutritional Assessment of the Elderly Through Anthropometry. *© 1984 Ross Laboratories. (Adapted from* Am J Clin Nutr. *1981;34:2831.)*

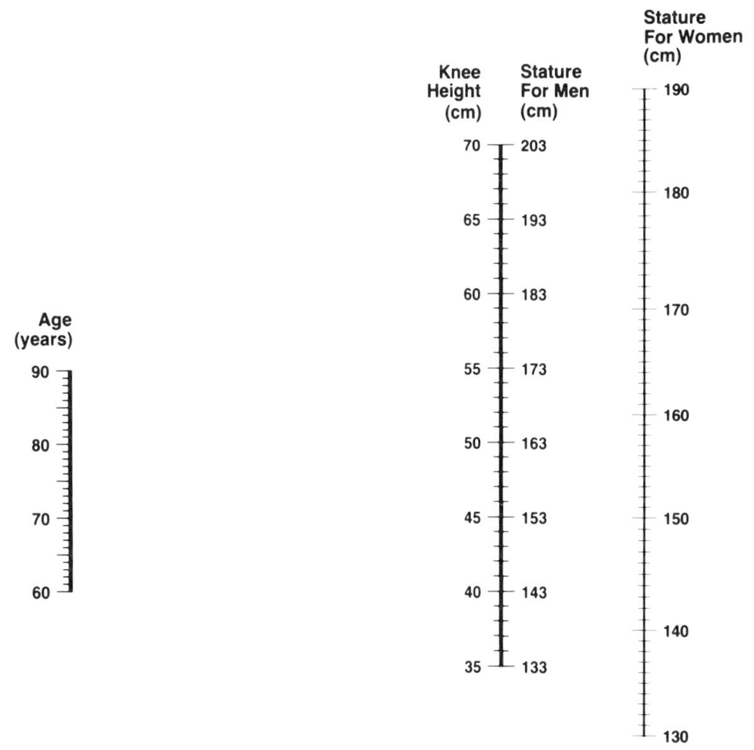

DIETARY ASSESSMENT*

For research purposes, it is important to assess the nutrient intake of both cardiac patients and persons at high risk for CHD. The accuracy of the dietary intake record (ie, the frequency of consumption, portion size, and knowledge of food composition) as well as the adequacy of the dietary assessment methodology (ie, the instrument and nutrient data base used) are also important. In clinical practice, however, precise food-intake information is not as important. Diet assessments need not have a high degree of precision, and approaches used to collect dietary information need not be rigorous. Several dietary-assessment methods are appropriate for practitioners. *Table 4.7* gives a list of the advantages and disadvantages of each method. Some methods are inexpensive, simple, and quick to administer to a large number of subjects. Others require more time and resources but may be more accurate and provide more useful information.

In a clinical or counseling situation a more comprehensive dietary assessment is usually preferred initially to facilitate nutrition intervention for the prevention and treatment of elevated plasma lipid levels. Less comprehensive dietary assessments may be more appropriate during follow-up.

Methods of Collecting Dietary Data†

24-hour recall. The client is asked to relate dietary intake during the previous 24 hours. This information is either recorded by a skilled interviewer or

*By the Editors
†By Lisa Martin

collected via a self-administered form with explicit directions. The major limitation of this method is reliance on the patient's memory. A skilled interviewer or a list of key questions will help a patient remember important information. In addition, accuracy in self-reports of intake has been shown to be improved by the aid of measuring devices or food models or photographs. The use of these aids is possible in an interview situation, but more difficult or impossible when respondents submit a written report or are interviewed by telephone without prior notice and preparation for the interview.

Table 4.7
Advantages and Disadvantages of Nutrition-Assessment Methods

Method of Nutrition Assessment	Advantages	Disadvantages
24-hour recall	Quick and easy. Appropriate when assessing diets of many people.	Limited by recall. Inappropriate for a research setting.
Food-frequency questionnaire (FFQ)	Easily administered to large numbers of people. Inexpensive. Can be mailed and self-administered. Can define current and past intake.	Actual intake is not known. If unquantified FFQs are used, assumptions are made about portion sizes. Recall method depends on memory. Difficult for persons with unusual diets to describe intake. Culture specific.
Food records	Higher degree of accuracy.	Study group must be trained to measure or weigh food. Participation rate tends to diminish when the instruments are difficult to use. Interviews using trained staff are expensive and time-consuming, not feasible with large populations. At least 3 days needed.
Food-scoring systems	Quick, easy method to estimate intake, by interviewer or subject. Increases effectiveness of dietary counseling by providing immediate feedback. Gives good approximation of intake. Possible use as a teaching tool for manipulating fat intake.	Based on self-reports (food records). Interviewer and subject must be trained in scoring method.
Computer-assisted assessment	Time efficient. Time saved if subject enters data on machine-readable cards.	Training time required for subjects to learn method. Limited by the size and accuracy of the data base.

While one 24-hour recall does not accurately represent a person's usual or habitual intake,[12-14] it can provide a general overview of diet if it is representative of a typical day's intake. If the previous day's intake is not representative of habitual intake, a subject can be asked to recall or record a representative intake instead. Sometimes a food-frequency questionnaire accompanies a 24-hour recall, and together the two methods provide more complete dietary intake information. For research purposes, a 24-hour recall is useful for estimating intake among a group of 50 or more.[12]

Large food intakes are frequently underestimated, whereas small food intakes are often overestimated.[15] Older people tend to report more inaccurately than younger people and women.[6] Periodic dietary assessment (over a one-year period) using the 24-hour recall method provides a reasonably good estimate of dietary intake compared to a single 24-hour recall.[14,16]

Food-frequency questionnaires. Food-frequency questionnaires (FFQs) are often used in epidemiological studies, clinical research situations, and clinical practice. For epidemiologic studies, FFQs permit investigators to rank subjects by their relative levels of nutrient intake to evaluate etiologic hypotheses and interactions.[17] For public health and clinical purposes, FFQs provide an estimate of calorie and nutrient intake, changes in intake, and patterns of intake.[17]

Block et al[17] identified important characteristics of FFQs. Most important, the FFQ must be representative of a subject's usual diet so that, for research purposes, associations between diet and health measures can be fully and accurately interpreted. For use in practice, an FFQ that is representative of usual intake has greater validity. Second, the instrument should be relatively brief—it should take no longer than 20 to 25 minutes to administer—so that dietary assessment is not burdensome to subjects or staff. Ideally, an FFQ should permit assessment of the total diet; assessment of nutrients as well as foods or food-group intakes should be possible. Moreover, the FFQ should permit the assessment of a broad range of nutrients. These latter two characteristics can be achieved if a data-based approach is used to develop the FFQ and if portion-size attributions are also included. The nutrient assignments made to foods listed on the FFQ are crucial to the success of the instrument. Finally, an FFQ should be capable of assessing the diet of a number of demographic groups.

There are many FFQs available. Some are unquantified FFQs, in which subjects indicate how frequently they consume specific foods, types of foods (eg, skim, low-fat, or whole milk), or food groups in unquantified amounts. In quantified or semiquantified FFQs, a typical portion size or other amount is specified with the food listed. It is important to note that many of the food-frequency instruments currently used for diet assessment have not been validated. This perhaps explains why the results obtained from FFQs have not correlated with information obtained from other methods of dietary assessment or various health parameters. Willett[18] and Block et al[17] have developed two FFQs that have been tested and shown to be valid.*

Unquantified FFQs are not useful for accurate assessments of intake. They are useful in obtaining general information (eg, whether a subject uses skim, low-fat, or whole milk), comparing the consumption of certain foods among subjects or before and after intervention in an individual subject or group, or even scoring intake using an acceptable scoring system and comparing it to a norm or reference score. Unquantified FFQs are used frequently in clinical practice. Food scores (frequency × nutrient/dietary factor in a specified amount of food) for individual foods can be added. The advantages and disadvantages of using FFQs to assess dietary intake are summarized in Table 4.7.

*Additional information about them, including their analysis, can be obtained by writing to: W. Willett and L. Sampson, 31 Braman Street, Danvers, MA 01923, 508/777-0744; and G. Block, National Institutes of Health, 9000 Rockville Pike, EPN Room 313, Bethesda, MD 20892, 301/496-8500.

Table 4.8
Ranges and Averages of Number of Days Required to Estimate True Average Intake for an Individual With Given Statistical Confidence*

	Range and Average Number of Days Required					
	Males ($n = 13$)			Females ($n = 16$)		
Component	**Minimum**	**Average**	**Maximum**	**Minimum**	**Average**	**Maximum**
Food energy	14	27	84	14	35	60
Iron	18	68	130	28	66	142
Vitamin A	115	390	1724	152	474	1372
Protein	23	36	72	23	48	70
Fat	34	57	131	32	71	114
Saturated fat	30	71	156	42	87	149
Oleic acid	35	68	163	31	85	145
Linoleic acid	77	145	225	82	166	237
Cholesterol	85	139	195	104	200	443
Carbohydrate	10	37	177	16	41	77
Crude fiber	43	82	146	51	86	138
Calcuim	30	74	140	35	88	168
Phosphorus	18	32	62	19	41	62
Potassium	17	34	67	25	48	83
Sodium	27	58	140	36	73	116
Thiamin	46	138	405	41	198	728
Riboflavin	13	57	135	31	90	231
Niacin	27	53	89	48	78	126
Vitamin C	90	249	900	83	222	328

*Estimated with intake from 1-year dietary intake study by the USDA's Beltsville Human Nutrition Center.

Reprinted with permission from Basiotis PP, Welsh SO, Cronin FJ, et al. Number of days of food intake: records required to estimate individual and group nutrient intakes with defined confidence. © *J Nutr.* 1987;117:1638. American Institute of Nutrition.

Food records. Written food records, in which foods consumed are weighed or measured, are generally considered the standard against which other methods of evaluating intake are measured. This method gives more specific information than the other methods previously discussed.[19]

When keeping a food record or diary, the client records the type and amount of food eaten immediately following a meal or snack. Ideally, all amounts are measured or weighed rather than estimated. Other information may be recorded, such as feelings and behaviors related to eating. Samples of food-record forms are given in the appendix (see Tables 14.10 and 14.11).

Food records have been shown to be an accurate measurement of both individual and group intake. The number of days of records needed depends on the degree of accuracy desired.[16] Recently Basiotis et al[20] reported the number of days of food-intake data needed to estimate the intake of food energy and 18 nutrients for males and females. The number of days required to estimate the true average intake for an individual client was more than that for groups (*Tables 4.8* and *4.9*). Different numbers of days of intakes were required for the nutrients studied. In a recent publication from the National Research Council, the issue of the number of days of diet records needed for an accurate assessment of nutrient intake is discussed.[21] While Tables 4.8 and 4.9 show that many days of food records are required to estimate intake accurately, collecting food-intake information for less time nonetheless provides valuable information that practitioners can use in prescribing a fat- and cholesterol-modified diet and monitoring the patient's progress. In practice, collecting and analyzing food records for many days for each patient is not possible for numerous reasons. Furthermore, such precision is usually not required in practice. It is important, however, for practitioners to be aware of the limitations of the information collected from the food records typically used.

Table 4.9
Number of Days Required to Estimate True Average Intake for Groups of Individuals With Given Statistical Confidence.*

Component	Estimated Number of Days Required for Each Group	
	Males ($n = 13$)	**Females ($n = 16$)**
Food energy	3	3
Iron	7	6
Vitamin A	39	44
Protein	4	4
Fat	6	6
Saturated fat	8	7
Oleic acid	6	7
Linoleic acid	13	12
Cholesterol	13	15
Carbohydrate	5	4
Crude fiber	9	9
Calcium	10	7
Phosphorus	4	5
Potassium	4	5
Sodium	6	6
Thiamin	13	16
Riboflavin	7	7
Niacin	5	6
Vitamin C	33	19

* Estimated with intake data from 1-year dietary intake study by the USDA's Beltsville Human Nutrition Research Center.

Reprinted with permission from Basiotis PP, Welsh SO, Cronin FJ, et al. Number of days of food intake: records required to estimate individual and group nutrient intakes with defined confidence. © *J. Nutr.* 1987;117:1638. American Institute of Nutrition.

For assessing individual intake, seven- to nine-day records have been found to estimate usual nutrient intake within 10%.[14,22,23] A three- to four-day record may be a reasonable compromise for a minimal assessment or for monitoring compliance. Often, interest in keeping a food record for seven to nine days wanes and shorter records (eg, covering three days) are more accurate. Three-day food records have been found to approximate the values obtained from seven- to nine-day records and may be acceptable for most uses.[13,22,24] At least one weekend day should be included in the shorter record as intake varies for most people on these days.[12,22]

The shorter (three- to four-day) record is most appropriate for clients with a fairly consistent intake, such as infants, school-aged children, and most adults. A seven- to nine-day food record is recommended for clients with a variable intake.[13] Practitioners often request a typical one-day food record when clients wish to not keep diet records for longer periods and/or for a quick diet assessment.

Clients (or, when working with young children, their caretakers) should be given specific instructions for completing food records. Some basic guidelines include[24]:

1. Record foods eaten and any other needed information as soon as possible after a meal or snack. Record amounts in household measures (eg, cups, tablespoons).
2. Include all beverages and anything added to them (eg, 1 cup coffee with 1 tbsp half-and-half). Include beverages taken with medication.
3. Include all condiments (eg, salad dressing, ketchup, butter, sugar, gravy).
4. Provide specific information about the food eaten (eg, whole-wheat bread, skim milk, canned peaches in heavy syrup).
5. Indicate how the food was prepared (eg, baked chicken, fried pork chop, breaded fish). Was fat on meat trimmed? Was poultry skinned before or after cooking?
6. Record all snacks, including beverages.
7. Keep the food diary accessible at all times.
8. Record supplement use.

Seasonal variation in diet is to be expected. Practitioners can collect information about this by assessing nutrient intake approximately four times per year.

To keep an accurate food diary, a client must be able to write and to measure food (or estimate food portions) accurately and consistently. The client's degree of accuracy and motivation may decrease the longer he or she keeps a food record.[14] A client must be trained to complete food records and measure food. While this requires time on the part of the interviewer, it increases the reliability of the results obtained. Simply observing a behavior such as eating will probably cause the behavior to change, whether the client is aware of it or not.[16]

Researchers have designed alternative methods of record keeping, such as use of a tape recorder, telephone interviews, intermittent 24-hour recalls, and use of itemized supermarket tapes.[22] For clients who are unable or unwilling to keep food records, such methods may be explored. One of these alternatives may be used along with another method such as a short food-frequency questionnaire to increase the accuracy of the information collected.

After the food-intake record is collected and checked, a nutrition analysis is done. A comprehensive or abbreviated analysis of specific nutrients (eg, total fat, saturated and unsaturated fatty acids, sodium, cholesterol) can be done, especially during the monitoring stage of intervention. A more comprehensive dietary analysis may be preferable initially and then intermittently during follow-up. It is important that the nutrient-analysis system and information are accurate, complete, and up-to-date.

Following the initial assessment, when specific problems have been defined, simpler food-record forms can be used. Involving the client in deciding what to record may be helpful. For example, recording only the evening meal and snacks for a week may be more acceptable to some people than more extensive record keeping.

Food records can be used to establish a baseline intake when a person begins nutrition counseling. They may be used intermittently during the counseling period to measure compliance, behavior modification, and the effectiveness of the nutrition care and intervention plan. They should be reviewed with the client with an emphasis on food intake and behavior modifications. It is important to recognize and praise positive behavior. Identify problems and ask the client to identify problems. Ask the client for suggestions for improvement. Together, the client and practitioner can negotiate the nutrition care plan. They can identify and prioritize problems, negotiate short- and long-term goals, decide on strategies to achieve the goals, and choose a follow-up plan.

DIETARY ANALYSIS AND INTERPRETATION*

Once information about food intake has been collected and checked for accuracy and completeness, it is most often translated into nutrition terms and compared against a standard. The standard frequently used is the Recommended Dietary Allowances (RDA). In addition, intake is compared to various recommendations that have been made by groups such as the American Heart Association, the Surgeon General, the National Cholesterol Education Program, and so on. Computerized nutrition assessments are growing in popularity. Food-record data are commonly entered into the computer via a terminal or can be recorded onto computer-readable cards. Many systems are user-friendly, but often some training is required. Many practitioners have purchased nutrient-analysis software program(s). Others pay for this service, which is provided by the private sector (individuals, businesses) or by universities. Some practitioners still use food-composition tables to analyze diet records. Both methods (computerized and noncomputerized) are acceptable if the nutrient data base and nutrient information are accurate and up-to-date. Most computerized analysis systems use the US Department of Agriculture (USDA) data base to which data from other sources are added.[25] It is important for practitioners to recognize how labor-intensive, time-consuming, and costly it is to keep any system or food-composition table up-to-date. Improved methodologies for quantifying nutrients and fiber, in particular, have made many data bases obsolete. Moreover, frequent food-production changes in industry as well as the introduction of many new food items on the market make updating a nutrient-analysis system important. In an interesting study reported by Adelman et al,[25] three computerized dietary analysis systems were compared. Significant differences were noted for calories, fat, saturated fatty acids, omega-6 fatty acids, cholesterol, and phosphorus.

Computerized Dietary Analysis for Cardiovascular Counseling†

The most efficient, accurate, and timely method for dietary assessment is a computerized dietary analysis program. The dietitian uses the dietary analysis program to enter foods that the patient recalls or has recorded in a food diary. The computer printout generated by the program allows both dietitian and patient to see the following information for that day's intake: number of calories; grams and percentages of calories from carbohydrate, protein, and fat; grams and percentages of calories from saturated fatty acids, monounsaturated fatty acids, and polyunsaturated fatty acids; and milligrams of dietary cholesterol. In addition, most nutrient-analysis programs will not only provide the total intake values for vitamins and minerals consumed, but will compare them to the RDAs for males and females in specific age categories. Some programs also provide amounts of specific fatty acids and amino acids. However, the user should examine the entire data base to be sure complete data are available for each entry. Based on the information in this personalized dietary analysis, the patient and the dietitian can immediately assess the patient's dietary intake with regard to specific dietary goals. If the computer program is designed to provide information about the amount of fat supplied in each serving of food, it

*By the Editors
†By Lynne W. Scott and Daniele Branchi

will be easier for the patient to see the contribution of a particular food to the total fat in the diet. This helps the patient and the dietitian pinpoint necessary changes in food choices.

Table 4.10
Comparison of Food-Record Analysis With and Without Fat Used in Preparation

Meal/Menu	Portion	Calories and Fat, Including Fat Used in Preparation		Calories and Fat, Not Including Fat Used in Preparation	
		cal	g fat	cal	g fat
Breakfast at home					
Orange, fresh	1 medium	62	< 1	62	< 1
Buttered cinnamon toast	1 slice	117	5	83	1
Scrambled egg with margarine	1	107	9	78	5
Skim milk	1 cup	86	< 1	86	< 1
Lunch at cafeteria					
Red fish, grilled, basted with unknown fat	4 oz	208	10	132	2
Tossed salad with Italian salad dressing	1 cup	81	7	12	< 1
Broccoli, seasoned with margarine	½ cup	39	2	22	< 1
Rice pilaf	½ cup	181	8	100	2
Sourdough roll	1 medium	124	< 1	124	< 1
Blueberry crisp	½ cup	346	13	238	1
Dinner, friend's house					
Grilled chicken breast marinated in oil and soy sauce mixture	3 oz	201	10	141	3
Mashed potatoes with unknown fat	½ cup	104	4	70	< 1
Green beans with margarine	½ cup	33	2	16	< 1
Gelatin molded salad with cream cheese	½ cup	153	10	94	5
Garlic bread with butter	1 med slice	98	3	70	< 1
Apple pie, single pastry, with butter added to filling	9-in. pie	232	10	218	8
Snack					
Popcorn, hot-air popped, seasoned with butter	1 cup	91	8	23	1
Total		**2263**	**104**	**1569**	**36**
Percentage calories from fat			41		17

Modified with permission from DeBakey MD, Gotto AM, Scott LW, et al. *The Living Heart Diet.* New York, NY: Raven Press Ltd; 1984.

Not all fat in a typical daily intake is clearly visible. It is not difficult to account for fat in foods such as cheese and milk. However, it is very important for a computerized nutrient-analysis program to account for all fat—including "hidden" fats that are added during food preparation.[26] A well-designed program should allow the person entering the dietary information to select the specific type of fat used in food preparation, eg, butter, magarine, bacon grease, or shortening. In order to assess total fat intake accurately, computerized dietary analysis programs should provide automated procedures that specify the addition of a standard amount of fat for various types of food preparations such as frying eggs, breading and frying meats, or seasoning vegetables.

Preparation fats are especially important when the patient has eaten food prepared away from home. Most restaurants routinely add fat to all vegetables and meat products. If the fat used in preparation is *not* part of the program, the analysis will not include all the fat actually eaten. This type of inaccurate information makes it difficult for the dietitian and patient to receive the full benefit from the analysis of food records. For example, typical vegetables served in a restaurant have 2 g of fat added per half-cup serving, and meat that is breaded and fried has an additional 4 g of fat per ounce of cooked weight. Therefore, a patient who has recorded eating two servings of vegetables and 5 oz of fried fish would have approximately 24 g of fat contributed by the fat used in preparation, in addition to the fat naturally occurring in the food. Other fat-related food preparation calculations, such as for fried eggs, stir-fried foods, meat salads, and vegetable salads, are important to use for increased accuracy in the analysis of patient food records.[27] *Table 4.10* compares the analysis of the same meal with and without the fat added in the food preparation. The type of counseling that would be done for a patient eating 17% of calories from fat is entirely different than that for a patient eating a diet with 41% of calories from fat.

To be effective, a computerized dietary analysis program needs to provide all the information necessary for in-depth nutrition counseling for the particular patient population. The most up-to-date and completely automated system—especially for fat, fatty acid, and cholesterol analysis—is located at the Nutrition Coordinating Center at the University of Minnesota. The system is described below.

Nutrition Data System*

With the rapid expansion in the number of foods available in the marketplace and the increase in the variety of foods in the American diet, data collection and coding procedures for meeting counseling and research needs have become increasingly complex and tedious. In an effort to increase the accuracy and standardization of these procedures and to reduce the time and cost of data processing, the Nutrition Coordinating Center (NCC) at the University of Minnesota† has developed a microcomputer-based system that provides interactive data collection and automatic coding of food-intake data. The system is based on the NCC Nutrition Data System, which has been used for collecting and analyzing dietary data in a number of multicentered clinical trials, including the Multiple Risk Factor Intervention Trial, the Lipid Research Clinics programs, the Diabetes Control and Complications Trial, and more than 90 other research studies.

The automated system standardizes the data-collection process by providing prompts that incorporate detailed probing for brand-name information, food-preparation methods, and variable ingredients in food combinations. Food descriptions and amounts are collected as reported by free-living persons using common terminology. The system automatically calculates nutrient intakes using the NCC nutrient-analysis system.

Special features of the automated system include code-free data entry; inclusion of over 3,000 brand-name products; calculation of percent of calories from carbohydrate, protein, fat, and alcohol; calculation of P/S ratio; and calculation of Cholesterol–Saturated-Fat Index (CSI). Amounts may be entered in any standard weight or volume unit, cooked or raw, with or without refuse, or in food-specific units such as slice, stalk, or piece. Edit checks for portion sizes and

*By Marilyn Buzzard
†Nutrition Coordinating Center (NCC), 2829 University Ave, SE, Suite 526, Minneapolis, MN 55414, 612/627-4871.

for daily totals of individual nutrients are incorporated into the system. Nutrient calculation options include a comparison with RDA levels and the ranking of foods by the amount consumed, number of times eaten, and contribution to a selected nutrient.

The NCC nutrient data base is routinely updated and is considered the most complete one available for calculating fat, fatty-acid, and sodium intakes. The current version of the data base (version 16) consists of 93 nutrients, including 23 individual fatty acids and 18 individual amino acids. Recent additions to the data base include dietary fiber fractions, individual sugars, selenium, aspartame, and saccharin. The data base also includes dietary supplements and medications containing caffeine and sodium.

A version of the automated system tailored to specifications of the National Center for Health Statistics is currently being used to collect 24-hour dietary recalls for 30,000 persons in the next National Health and Nutrition Examination Survey (NHANES III). This version of the system will produce food codes for the USDA Nationwide Food Consumption Survey (NFCS) nutrient data base.

The system operates on an IBM AT or compatible hardware with 640K memory and 10 megabytes of free hard-disk space.

Evaluation of Computerized Diet-Analysis Systems*

Many dietitians rely on computerized systems to design and analyze diets. However, there is considerable variation in the quality and usefulness of these systems. Furthermore, results can vary, in some cases widely, depending on the one selected. Thus, it is important to understand the limitations as well as the advantages of these tools. The following discussion presents ten questions to ask when evaluating computerized diet-analysis systems. Some questions focus on evaluating the precision and accuracy of a nutrient data base, while others concern the usefulness of the programs used for data entry and analyses. The final questions concern the documentation and cost-effectiveness of the system.

1. Are the needed nutrients on the nutrient data base? The number of nutrients on a nutrient data base can vary from less than 10 to over 100. It is important to ask if the diet-analysis system contains the nutrients of interest.

In addition to determining if the nutrients of interest are present, it may be important to ask about the form in which the nutrients are presented. For example, dietary fiber may be present in several forms: some data bases use total, some use only insoluble, and some have only crude fiber. Furthermore, the analytic methodology may vary within the different forms. It may be necessary to consider if the nutrient forms are the ones of physiologic importance for the user of the diet-analysis system.

2. What are the sources of the nutrient data? It is important to know the source of the nutrient values on a data base. The core of most data bases is from USDA *Handbook 8*.[28,29] However, many (probably most) data bases are augmented by other sources, which are of varying reliability. For example, analytic data published in journal articles and books can be reliable if from reputable labs, but if the data are for just a few samples and are not replicated, the values should be suspect. Information supplied by the food-processing industry is a good source of brand-name data, but often it is not complete for nutrients of

*By Suzanne P. Murphy and Patricia Booth

interest. Data from product labels are often low, since they represent minimum standards rather than the average amount present in the food. Adding data from other data bases is sometimes done, but care must be exercised to ensure that units and methods of analysis are compatible. Finally, unpublished lab values can be used to fill in missing data, but, once again, care must be exercised to ensure proper sampling, replications, methodology, and so forth.

Several researchers have approached the important issue of comparability between nutrient data bases. Hoover[30] sent the same one-day diet records (containing about 25 food items) to 11 different developers of nutrient data bases and then compared the results. Energy values ranged from 1,942 to 2,299 calories, a difference of 357 calories, or 18%. Protein was more homogeneous, varying by only 7%. Fat, on the other hand, varied by 45% from a low of 75 g to a high of 109 g. Taylor et al[31] calculated nutrient intake from 24 one-day diet records on three different systems. Mean intakes were not significantly different for proximate nutrients, but even the mean of 24 diets varied for less well-studied nutrients such as zinc (from 6.6 to 10.7 mg) and folacin (from 143 to 202 μg).

Thus, it is important to ask a data-base developer questions about the sources of nutrient values: Are the sources reliable? What methods were used to determine nutrient values? Was the development done by professionals who could evaluate the options correctly?

3. How often is the nutrient data base updated? The problems associated with keeping a data base current are enormous. Managers of large data bases can easily spend all of their time on this task alone. New sections of the revised USDA *Handbook 8* are being released approximately twice a year. These often contain major changes in nutrient values, as well as sizable increases in the number of nutrients for which data are presented. The previous *Handbook 8* was released in 1963 and is now over 25 years old. So it is important to be certain the new data are incorporated into the data base. In addition, many data bases contain information from manufacturers. Anyone who shops in a supermarket can appreciate the complexity of trying to stay current. Furthermore, the same product can change over the years (eg, in fortification levels). It is also important to inquire about the availability of updates after the system is purchased.

4. What validation procedures are used? There is always a problem in detecting clerical errors when setting up a nutrient data base. These errors are inevitable and happen in all of them. The problem increases as the size of the data base increases, but can be minimized by carefully checking each entry. However, checking takes time and patience, and it is frequently not a high priority for data-base developers. Even if values are taken from electronic sources such as tapes, programming errors are all too common. All data-base developers should have documented procedures to check that the values are correctly entered.

5. How prevalent are missing values and how are they handled? Missing data on the data base is also a major problem. If a nutrient value is missing on the nutrient data base, it often is assumed to be zero when the nutrients in a diet are totaled. At the very least, there should be a flag of some type indicating when a total contains missing data. The problem is particularly acute for brand-name items, since the manufacturer may only supply information about the major nutrients. For some data bases, values are imputed when analytical values are not available. This is the approach that the USDA is taking for their Survey Data Bases. However, it is not easy to impute nutrient values correctly.

Thus, it is important to know who imputed values, and how they did it. Furthermore, the values should be identified on the data base so that they can be examined.

6. Are the number and type of food items adequate? Determining the precision of a nutrient data base is a crucial task: How well do the food items on the data base match those actually consumed by the people whose diets are to be analyzed?

No matter how large the data base, the foods are still representative of many species, climates, growing conditions, storage methods, and so on. For example, some work done at the USDA[32] shows wide variation in the carotene content among cultivars of sweet potatoes grown in the same state—from 2,175 to 3,950 international units (IU) per 100 g (almost a twofold range). Even the same cultivar, grown in four different states, had a large variation (from 2,650 to 3,950 IU/100 g). A weighted average of all these values, based on the availability of the different products, is the number finally published in the food-composition tables. Thus, the sweet potato actually consumed will virtually never match the hypothetical "average" sweet potato in the food-composition table.

It is tempting to believe that the larger the data base, the higher the precision. However, this is not always the case—for example, there are almost 2,500 foods in USDA *Handbook 8*,[28] but some nutritionists find the new *Home and Garden Bulletin 72*,[33] with only 908 foods, more useful, because the foods are typical of those consumed today. Also, some data-base developers increase the apparent size of their data bases by counting multiple serving sizes as different foods (so a tablespoon of butter and an ounce of butter would be counted as two items). Therefore, the variety of foods is more important than the number. Some features to examine in evaluating the variety of foods include: (1) options to specify preparation method, since method of cooking (baked, fried, etc) may be important to the nutrient retention of cooked foods; (2) an option to specify the type of fat used in the preparation (which would be important if there is interest in fatty acids or cholesterol); (3) an option to specify whether items are salted or unsalted (important for information on the sodium content of a diet); (4) an option to specify whether enriched-grain products are used, and whether they are whole grain or refined; (5) the presence of ethnic foods and fast foods; and (6) the presence of brand name foods (but only if the data base is updated when product formulations change). The important point is to be certain that foods commonly consumed by the groups whose diets will be analyzed are on the data base. Even infrequently consumed food items should be present if they are sources of nutrients of interest for the users of the system.

7. Is the coding scheme easy to use? If a coding scheme is difficult to understand and use, the resulting diets may be improperly coded and the precision of the analysis will be affected. Furthermore, an awkward and time-consuming coding process can add substantially to the cost of analyzing diets. Numeric codes such as those used in USDA *Handbook 8* are common, but there are also alphabetic codes and hierarchical codes (where each digit or letter represents a food category). Many developers have put extensive effort into designing useful codes, so there is a wide variety from which to choose. To use the codes, a coding manual is necessary (an alphabetic list of food names and descriptions, along with corresponding codes). Perhaps the most time-consuming (and error-prone) part of dietary analyses is determining the correct code for a food item, so it is important that the coding manual be well organized and easy to use. In some cases, the coding manual is bypassed by the use of a menu-driven coding system—many dietitians find these a giant step forward. With the advent of video display screens, it is possible to show a variety of food items and let the user pick the proper one. The possibility of incorrect codes (or the inability to find codes) is thus minimized.

The ability to enter recipes can also facilitate the coding procedure. If the ingredients in commonly consumed recipes can be entered once and later referenced by a single code or name, coding time and errors can be reduced.

The method of specifying serving sizes may be important to system users. Most, but not all, systems allow specification of portions in gram weights. Many systems also allow the use of household measures such as cups, teaspoons, and so on. Some of the options are very elaborate and include features such as the use of food model codes. Data entry time, as well as accuracy, can be greatly affected by the method of specifying the portions.

8. Are results presented in the required format? There are several options for the presentation of the dietary results. Needs will vary depending on the application, but some or all of the following features may be important: (1) nutrients reported for each food item, for each meal, for each day, and as an average of multiple days; (2) totals compared to dietary standards, such as the RDA, the US Dietary Goals, or USDA Department of Health and Human Services (DHHS) Dietary Guidelines; (3) nutrients reported per kilogram of body weight; (4) percentage of nutrients from designated food groups or food items; (5) calculations such as percentages of calories from protein, fat, and carbohydrate; ratio of polyunsaturated to saturated fat; ratio of calcium to phosphorus; (6) a measure of overall diet quality, such as the Index of Nutritional Quality; (7) a report of food-group frequencies; (8) diet items saved for future reference; and (9) diet totals saved for future reference. If any of these features are critical for the users of the diet-analysis system, then it is important that they are present.

9. Is the system well documented? If a system does not have adequate documentation, the user will spend unnecessary time learning how to use the system properly. In addition, it may not be possible to determine, for example, the sources of nutrient values or the type of error checking that was applied. Therefore, it is crucial to ask about documentation before purchasing a diet-analysis system. At the very least, one would expect a user's guide for the diet-analysis program, and, if the nutrient data base has been developed (or modified in any way) by the vendor, a list of the sources of all nutrient values. A good developer should be willing to write clear and comprehensive documents that detail how the system was developed as well as how it is to be used.

10. Is the system cost-effective? Purchase prices of diet-analysis systems vary widely, depending to some extent on the size of the nutrient data base and the features of the diet-analysis software. Several basic systems are in the public domain, and are available for little more than the cost of duplicating and mailing. Other systems can cost several thousand dollars. It obviously is important to carefully consider the needs of the users of a diet-analysis system before deciding what features are critical. It is often possible to find relatively inexpensive systems that have all the required features.

The cost of the hardware must be considered also. Many users select systems that will run on microcomputers for this reason. Obviously, if a system will run on existing hardware the overall cost is substantially reduced. Finally, the cost of updates for the nutrient data base should be added to the overall cost of using the system.

If readers are interested in further pursuing some of these ideas to gain more information or share some thoughts and suggestions, there are several options. A number of review articles[34–53] contain useful information about the differences among various diet-analysis systems. In addition, several indexes of diet-analysis systems are published periodically, and can be a source of information on the general features of these systems.[54–56] The *Software Resource Manual* published in 1988 by the Sports and Cardiovascular Nutritionists Practice Group of The American Dietetic Association is an excellent resource for information on a number of commonly used software programs.* Since it is time-consuming to evaluate multiple systems personally, dietitians are urged to publicize their experiences and recommendations.

At meetings of professional societies exhibitors often demonstrate diet-analysis systems. This is a good opportunity to see firsthand how a system works and to ask questions. In addition, many vendors will provide demonstration disks for potential users to try in their own facilities at no cost, or sometimes for a small fee.

Two groups have been organized specifically to address some of the issues discussed here. One is the International Network of Food Data Systems (INFOODS).[57] This group is working on an international level to establish communications among and guidelines for developers of nutrient data bases. They welcome ideas and participation. A second group sponsors an annual conference—the National Nutrient Data Bank Conference—held in the spring or summer of each year.[58] It is an excellent place to learn about what both the government and the private sector are doing with nutrient data bases. There is ample time to discuss problems and new ideas. It is a volunteer group, and it welcomes your participation.†

Unfortunately, many people tend to believe that nutrient values that are calculated by a computer must be accurate. We all have an obligation as scientists to ask questions and ensure that the tools we use in our professions are as accurate as possible. There is no question that computers can be of enormous benefit to us, if used properly.

It is a challenge to evaluate nutrient-analysis software completely. An individual dietitian may lack the resources or time to acquire and compare several systems before purchase. Realistically, hands-on review of software may be impossible in many cases. Dietitians should ask for the names of the users of different software programs from nutrient data-base suppliers. It is very useful and important to collect unbiased information about a software program before making a large investment. The practicing dietitian must first decide what nutrients or food components are needed and what manipulations of the data are desired. Commonly used functions include nutrient totals; percentages of calories from protein, carbohydrate, fat, and alcohol; percentage of RDA for age- and sex-specified category; and a list of nutrients for each food in a diet. Special functions vary widely and their presence may or may not correlate with the cost of the software. The individual user should determine if the extra functions available with some software are important for the intended use. Most software packages are user-friendly, that is, they can be used without help beyond the documentation.

*Available through SCAN, c/o Joanne Milkereit, 7 Pitt St, Charleston, SC 29401, 803/792-3100.
†To have your name placed on the mailing list, contact the USDA's Human Nutrition Information Service, 304 Federal Building, Hyattsville, MD 20782.

The questions posed can be answered in the evaluation of software programs. However, information regarding software development may not be readily available. Validation procedures are generally not described in the documentation which accompanies the software. Correction and update policies for the data base seem to be on an as-needed basis for most of the software used.*

There are many software programs on the market for many different patient needs, including dietary analyses. It is important for dietitians to help patients choose a suitable program that will meet their individual needs. It is important to first ask whether a system is needed and then how and why it will be used. The ability of the patient to learn and use the system is an important consideration. Accuracy, updating capacity, service, and cost must also be considered. Finally, it is essential that patients know how to use the information that is generated from the software program.

Food-Scoring Systems†

Food records with accompanying comprehensive computer analyses may not be practical or efficient in all clinical settings. However, only a rapid or "eyeball" assessment of a food record may not detect small but significant changes in the intake of such nutrients as total fat, cholesterol, and so on.

Two food-scoring systems are useful for a quick estimation of the effect of diet on serum cholesterol in either groups or individual clients. One is the Food Record Rating (FRR) that was used in the Multiple Risk Factor Intervention Trial study. The other, the Dietary Achievement Score, was used in the Nutrition Education Project, Heart Saver Program of the Chicago Heart Association. Both methods are designed to estimate adherence and are thus indirectly predictive of serum cholesterol changes.[59] These tools can be used by both clients and dietitians. Both are useful for self-monitoring and for teaching clients how to select recommended foods.[59] Since the food score is an average of three days of records, it deemphasizes intake on one day.[24] The use of food-scoring systems in nutrition counseling has been described.[24]

Other methods to assess intake and evaluate compliance have been developed based on an exchange system. Both require that the patient keep a food record. Foods are converted into exchanges.[61,62] Another approach that is recommended for assessing the atherogenicity of foods is the Cholesterol–Saturated-Fat Index.

Cholesterol–Saturated-Fat Index (CSI)‡

The hypercholesterolemic and atherogenic effect of a given food depends on the amount of cholesterol and saturated fatty acids it contains. The more saturated fatty acids and cholesterol in a food, the greater its potential for raising the plasma total-cholesterol level.

Foods vary with regard to their cholesterol and saturated fatty-acid content, making it difficult to determine the exact hypercholesterolemic effect of a

*For information on specific software programs, contact Patricia Booth, Department of Nutritional Sciences, University of California, Berkeley, 415/642-6490; and Diane Ceja and Stephanie Chan, University of California Cooperative Extension Service, Oakland, 415/987-0505.
†By Lisa Martin
‡By Sonja L. Connor

particular food. For example, some foods are high in saturated fatty acids but contain no cholesterol. Some shellfish are high in cholesterol but are very low in saturated fatty acids. Egg yolk is especially rich in cholesterol and contains a moderate amount of saturated fatty acids. Other foods such as cheese and fatty red meats are relatively rich sources of both saturated fatty acids and cholesterol. Fish, poultry, extra-lean beef or pork, lamb, or regular cuts of beef contain comparable amounts of cholesterol but different amounts of saturated fatty acids.

To help clarify what is obviously confusing to a lot of people, an index has been developed—a single score that takes into account the respective amounts of cholesterol and saturated fatty acids in a given food and expresses the hypercholesterolemic and atherogenic potential of that food. It is known as the Cholesterol–Saturated-Fat Index or CSI.[63] The lower the CSI, the more desirable the food for a lipid-lowering diet. A list of fish, poultry, and red meat ranked by their CSIs appears in *Table 4.11.*

Table 4.11
The Cholesterol–Saturated-Fat Index (CSI) of Selected Fish, Poultry, and Red Meat

Fish, Poultry, Red meat (3.5 oz or 100 g cooked)	CSI
Whitefish (snapper, perch, sole, cod, halibut, etc), shellfish (clams, oysters, scallops), water-pack tuna	4
Salmon	5
Shellfish (shrimp, crab, lobster)	6
Poultry, no skin	6
Beef, pork, and lamb	
10% fat (ground sirloin, flank steak)	9
15% fat (ground round)	10
20% fat (ground chuck, pot roasts)	13
30% fat (ground beef, pork, steaks, lamb steaks, ribs, pork chops, lamb chops, roasts)	18

Adapted with permission from Connor SL, Gustafson JR, Artaud-Wild SM, et al. The cholesterol/saturated-fat index: an indication of the hypercholesterolaemic and atherogenic potential of food. *Lancet.* 1986;1:1229. © by The Lancet Ltd.

The CSI also helps explain why some new food products such as cheeses or frozen desserts (eg, Mini Chol cheese and Tofutti) in which the butterfat has been replaced by vegetable oil are better choices for blood cholesterol lowering than their counterparts that are high in saturated fat (cheddar cheese and ice cream). Butterfat is a source of cholesterol and saturated fatty acids. Vegetable oils used in these products contain virtually no cholesterol and little saturated fat; as a result the CSIs of these products are low.

Assessment of Sodium and Alcohol Intake*

Sodium. Multiple days of records are needed to quantify a client's sodium intake.[65] For population groups, a one-day food record will provide a reasonable estimate of intake. A method to assess sodium intake using a combination of methods has recently been developed.[66] Sodium intake can be estimated with a questionnaire that is based on regression equations that include: (1) the daily quantity of table salt actually used over a seven-day period; (2) the contribution of sodium from 17 high-sodium foods (based on a food-frequency checklist maintained for seven days); (3) an estimate of sodium

*By Lisa Martin

in drinking water; and (4) measurements of height and weight in order to estimate 24-hour energy needs. A sodium-assessment instrument appears in the appendix (see Table 14.14).

Alcohol. Alcohol intake is often difficult to assess accurately. Heavy users frequently underreport intake. Light users often forget to report intake, although probing helps in obtaining an accurate estimate of intake. An alcohol-assessment questionnaire appears in the appendix (see Table 14.13).

CLINICAL ASSESSMENT OF CARDIOVASCULAR DISEASE*

Clinical assessment is essential to establish the presence and severity of cardiovascular disease (CVD). Frequently used clinical protocols and noninvasive techniques include: history, physical examination, blood chemistry, 12-lead electrocardiography (ECG), chest x-ray films, echocardiography, cardiac nuclear imaging, graded exercise ECG treadmill testing, and respiratory profile. A number of other procedures have been developed but are not routinely used in clinical practice.

A medical history is essential in evaluating patients with CVD, establishing the diagnosis, determining the course of treatment, and evaluating subsequent therapy.

In the physical examination it is important to note that CVD can be associated with other diseases and that an accurate diagnosis of coexisting diseases is important in establishing the therapeutic protocol. The clinical examination is incomplete without the recording of a resting 12-lead ECG and chest x-ray films.[67] Both procedures are fundamentally important for evaluating the patient's clinical condition. The ECG is most useful in evaluating cardiac symptoms that may have an underlying arrhythmia as their basis or in the evaluation of chest pain in suspected cardiac origin.[68]

Echocardiography is extremely useful in clinical cardiology because the anatomy and function of the heart can be examined without pain or risk to the patient. Moreover, it can be repeated as often as necessary. Echocardiography uses ultrasound; several different approaches are used. Cardiac nuclear imaging is a noninvasive diagnostic technique that evaluates cardiac structure and function with radioactive tracers. The most widely used tracer techniques are: (1) myocardial imaging with thallium 201 to detect ischemia and infarction; (2) evaluation of ventricular function with technetium 99m human serum albumin or red blood cells to assess ventricular function; and (3) infarct avid imaging with technetium 99m pyrophosphate to detect acute myocardial infarction. The respiratory profile is examined for diagnostic purposes and to assess pulmonary function. It is derived from the results of a resting pulmonary test and a respiratory stress (exercise) test. Assessment of the pulmonary system provides information about concurrent lung and heart disease, pulmonary complications resulting from heart disease, pulmonary limitations that are reversible in nature, and limited and quantifiable exercise tolerance due to pulmonary limitations.[68]

Special Invasive Techniques Used in Clinical Cardiology

The most widely used invasive procedure is cardiac catheterization, which is used only after the patient has been comprehensively evaluated using noninvasive techniques. Therefore, these procedures typically are not used to establish the presence of CVD. Rather, they are used to make the diagnosis as

*By Dottie Dolezal

certain as possible. Cardiac catheterization and angiocardiography are used to define the presence of anatomic lesions within the coronary system, to assess the pathophysiology of cardiac disorders, and to provide information on left-ventricular function. The procedures available are chosen on the basis of the preliminary diagnosis.

The Graded Exercise Test

Exercise stress testing has become a well-accepted procedure for diagnosing coronary artery disease (for additional information, see chapter 9). Types of tests, purposes, procedures, safety precautions, and contraindications have been well documented by Ellestad[69] as well as the American College of Sports Medicine.[70] The treadmill is used most commonly (71% of the time), followed by bicycle ergometry (17%) and stair stepping (12%).[71] Treadmill testing is preferred for the following reasons: (1) it is familiar to most patients, (2) the work level can be easily controlled, (3) it can elicit maximal effort in the shortest period of time, and (4) it is very sensitive and specific in diagnosing coronary artery disease. Bicycle ergometry is preferred for patients who have difficulty ambulating on a treadmill (ie, those with peripheral vascular disease). Blood pressure monitoring and reading the ECG are easier with bicycle ergometry since the upper body is motionless. Step tests have become relatively obsolete due to (1) their difficulty in monitoring heart rate and blood pressure and (2) their relative lack of diagnostic capabilities due to inability to allow maximal cardiovascular response.[69]

Exercise tests may be continuous (ie, workload is periodically increased with no rest interval between work stages) or tests may be intermittent (ie, short rest periods are interspersed within work periods). Generally, no differences have been reported in diagnostic and exercise capacity of these two types of tests; however, continuous tests are usually preferred since they require less time.

The debate over the value of maximal* versus submaximal† testing continues. While submaximal testing may be preferred by the patient, maximal testing provides better diagnostic information for the physician.[71] For functional evaluation, prediction of maximal cardiovascular capacity from submaximal testing is fraught with errors.[69] Various protocols for exercise testing on motor-driven treadmills have been developed and evaluated. Three protocols are summarized in the appendix. Although slightly different, each protocol involves increases in workload at regular intervals which require progressively more work to be performed by the patient. (See Tables 14.31, 14.32, and 14.33.) Increases in workload are accomplished by increases in grade, speed, or both. The most popular protocols have been developed by Ellestad.[69] The advantage of the Bruce protocol is its ability to attain maximal exertion in a short period of time. The Balke protocol maintains a constant speed (3.0 mph) that is preferred by many patients followed by gradual increases in the grade by 1 metabolic equivalent (MET) per stage. One-MET increments have been recommended for cardiac patients, especially those with low functional capacity.[70] The Ellestad protocol, the most popular, increases the grade from 0% to 10% during the first 10 minutes of the test, while gradually increasing the speed. Walking up steep grades may be problematic for patients with low back pain or

*Maximal exercise test—one in which the test is terminated when the patient reaches maximum heart rate (usually estimated by 220 minus age), which is usually the point at which the patient can no longer continue.
†Submaximal exercise test—one in which the test is terminated before the patient reaches maximum heart rate or exhaustion.

extreme quadriceps weakness. There are reportedly no differences in the ability of these three protocols to elicit maximal heart rates or maximal oxygen consumption.[69]

In special cases, other types of stress tests are useful in diagnosing coronary artery disease. These include isometric handgrip, hypoxemia, atrial pacing, and arm ergometry. The sensitivity and specificity of these tests in diagnosing coronary artery disease are significantly less than the stress tests that require dynamic lower-extremity testing.[71,72] It is important that test specificity be maintained when stress tests are administered to athletes (ie, runners should be stress tested on a treadmill, cyclists should be stress tested on a bicycle ergometer, and so forth).

CLINICAL ASSESSMENT OF HYPERLIPIDEMIA*

When clinically assessing hyperlipidemia it is important to realize that hypercholesterolemia is the predominant disorder that presents readily discernible clinical signs. Patients have planar, tuberous, and tendon xanthomas (the presence of yellow nodules or slightly raised plates in the skin) during childhood. The tendon xanthomas typically involve the extensor tendons of the hand, the elbow tendon, the patellar tendon, and the Achilles tendon.[73,74] The presence of corneal arcus is another clinical sign of familial hypercholesterolemia. Children and young adults with heterozygous familial hypercholesterolemia frequently do not have any clinical signs. In some patients, however, there are small planar xanthomas that may be detected in the digital webs or behind the knees. As patients with heterozygous familial hypercholesterolemia become older, the tendon xanthomas become more discernible.

Patients with familial combined hyperlipidemia do not present with tendon xanthomas. Many patients with type III hyperlipoproteinemia do not present any clinical abnormalities; however, certain features may suggest type III hyperlipoproteinemia. The most characteristic xanthoma seen is xanthoma striatum palmare, which is present on the hands. These lesions vary from yellow to orange in color and may be found in the palmar crease of the hand. In the most severe form, tuberous xanthomas are present on the fingers and hands. In patients with severe elevations of plasma triglycerides (types I and V hyperlipoproteinemia), the color of the retina is opaque-red; the color of the retina in normotriglyceridemic patients is red.[74]

In patients with other plasma lipid disorders there are typically no clinical abnormalities presented during the physical examination.

BIOCHEMICAL ASSESSMENT†

The NCEP recommends that the plasma total-cholesterol level be determined first. If it is higher than 240 mg/dL and this value is confirmed, then a lipoprotein-cholesterol analysis is indicated. An LDL-cholesterol level of 130 to 159 mg/dL places a subject at risk, while a level of 160 mg/dL or more is indicative of high risk for CHD.[75] An HDL-cholesterol level of less than 35 mg/dL is a risk factor for CHD.[75] The Lipid Research Clinics' reference values for plasma total-cholesterol and lipoprotein-cholesterol levels that are gender and age specific are reported in the appendix (see Tables 14.1, 14.2, 14.3, 14.4, and 14.5).

Frequently the LDL-cholesterol/HDL-cholesterol and total-cholesterol/HDL-cholesterol ratios are used as an assessment of CHD risk. The LDL-

*By Dottie Dolezal
†By the Editors

cholesterol/HDL-cholesterol ratio provides information about the relative proportion of cholesterol transported in the undesirable and desirable lipoprotein fractions. A high LDL-cholesterol/HDL-cholesterol ratio is strongly associated with an increased risk of CHD.[76] The total-cholesterol/HDL-cholesterol ratio provides information about the proportion of total cholesterol carried in the HDL fraction. This ratio has been shown to be a consistent and important indicator of CHD risk.[77] (See *Table 4.12* for information on the relative atherogenicity of the lipoprotein classes.) Since LDL cholesterol parallels plasma total cholesterol, the ratios of LDL cholesterol to HDL cholesterol and total cholesterol to HDL cholesterol provide similar information. Gordon and associates[76] advise against using these ratios because some people may have similar ratios yet large differences in the concentration of plasma total cholesterol, LDL cholesterol, and HDL cholesterol. The ratios, presented alone, do not provide information on the LDL-cholesterol level, a significant risk factor for CHD.[75]

Table 4.12
Relative Atherogenicity of Lipoproteins

Lipoprotein	Atherogenicity
Chylomicrons	0
VLDL	+
Chylomicron and VLDL remnants	+++
LDL	
smaller	++++
larger	+++
Lp(a)	++++
HDL	Negatively correlated with atherosclerosis
HDL_2 HDL_3	Protective HDL particle

Reprinted with permission from Connor WE, Bristow JD. *Coronary Heart Disease: Prevention, Complications and Treatment.* Philadelphia, Pa: JB Lippincott; 1985.

Recently the Coordinating Committee of the NCEP, recognizing that HDL cholesterol is an independent risk factor for CHD, identified standards for risk. Using 45 mg/dL as a baseline level, the following HDL-cholesterol reference values are presented with the associated increase in risk of CHD: 40 mg/dL (increase 10% to 15%), 35 mg/dL (increase 20% to 30%), and 25 mg/dL (increase 40% to 60%).

Until recently it was generally believed that plasma triglyceride levels between 250 and 500 mg/dL in the presence of normal plasma total-cholesterol levels did not increase the risk of CHD.[74] Recent studies have raised questions about this (see chapter 1). Other studies have shown that HDL-cholesterol levels and plasma triglyceride levels are inversely related.[79] Thus, hypertriglyceridemic individuals are at increased risk of CHD because of low HDL levels.

There is increasing evidence that serum apolipoproteins may be better discriminators of CHD risk than plasma lipid and lipoprotein levels.[78] Currently, apolipoproteins A-I and B concentrations (individually and expressed as the ratio of A-I/B) have been used experimentally to assess the risk of CHD. The apolipoprotein A-I/apolipoprotein-B ratio appears to be the best consistent discriminator of the severity of CHD.[80] Apolipoprotein E has been shown to be higher, in some instances, in survivors of a myocardial infarction.[80] Serum apolipoprotein A-I and A-II concentrations are lower while apolipoprotein-B levels are higher in patients with CHD compared with control subjects.[80] Elevated plasma lipoprotein apolipoprotein-B levels may be due to defects in: (1) lipolysis, leading to hypertriglyceridemia; (2) apolipoprotein-E metabolism, leading to abnormal clearance of VLDL remnants (type III hyperlipoproteinemia); or (3) LDL receptors, leading to hypercholesterolemia.[81] In the future, it is likely that apolipoprotein concentrations will be used more widely in clinical practice to assess CHD risk.

When To Measure Plasma Total Cholesterol

The NCEP recommends that the plasma total-cholesterol level of all adults 20 years of age and older be measured. Blood cholesterol is classified as desirable (<200 mg/dL), borderline-high blood cholesterol (200 to 239 mg/dL), or high blood cholesterol (≥240 mg/dL). Others have recommended that the ideal plasma total-cholesterol level fall between 130 and 190 mg/dL ($\bar{X} = 160$ mg/dL). The average plasma total cholesterol of Americans is presently 210 mg/dL. A desirable LDL-cholesterol level is less than 130 mg/dL. Borderline-high-risk LDL cholesterol is 130 to 159 mg/dL and high-risk LDL cholesterol is 160 mg/dL or more.

Elevated cholesterol levels should be documented by at least two or three determinations since variations may occur due to measurement errors or day-to-day fluctuations in individuals.[82] Berenson reported a variation of 18 mg/dL for a single blood cholesterol analysis.[83] Therefore, for a reported value of 166 mg/dL, the "true" value most likely falls between 148 and 184 mg/dL.

The NCEP schedule for follow-up of serum cholesterol concentration appears in *Table 4.13*. An elevated blood cholesterol level is confirmed with a second test, followed by the measurement of plasma LDL cholesterol to estimate risk more precisely. Patients with a blood cholesterol of 200 mg/dL or greater should have the test repeated in one to eight weeks. If the second value is within 30 mg/dL of the first result, the first and second test values are averaged. Treatment and follow-up decisions are based on the averaged value. A third test is recommended within one to eight weeks if the first and second results differ by more than 30 mg/dL.

Patients with a borderline-high blood cholesterol level and no CHD and with less than two risk factors should be given information on the recommended diet and followed annually. Those who also have either CHD or two risk factors, such as a family history, hypertension, cigarette smoking, and diabetes mellitus, should have a lipoprotein analysis and their plasma LDL-cholesterol level assessed.

LDL cholesterol should be measured in patients with either high blood cholesterol levels or borderline-high levels with definite CHD or two other risk factors. Two to three LDL-cholesterol measurements are made (after a 12-hour fast) one to eight weeks apart. Patients with a desirable LDL-cholesterol level (<130 mg/dL) are tested again in five years. Those with a borderline-high-risk LDL-cholesterol level (130 to 159 mg/dL) who are free from CHD and have no other risk factors are reevaluated annually, while those with definite CHD or two risk factors should be clinically evaluated (ie, history, physical exam, and laboratory tests). Patients with a high-risk LDL-cholesterol level (>160 mg/dL) should always be evaluated clinically.

Approaches for Blood Cholesterol Measurement

The goal of the NCEP is to decrease the prevalence of elevated blood cholesterol in the United States. In order to do this, the majority of Americans (>90%) 20 years of age and older should know their blood cholesterol levels. Public screening programs will be required to achieve this objective. Recommendations regarding public screening for measuring blood cholesterol have been made by the National Heart, Lung, and Blood Institute. In brief, it recommends that public screening programs: (1) use appropriate recruitment approaches for adult groups; (2) accurately and precisely quantify blood cholesterol levels; (3) provide education materials to the participants; (4) use well-trained staff who are closely supervised; (5) create and maintain an environment that fosters public participation; (6) be affordable; and (7) provide referral and follow-up services as appropriate. Referrals should be based on NCEP guidelines (see Table 4.13).

Table 4.13
Initial Classification and Recommended Follow-up Based on Total Cholesterol

Classification	Recommended Follow-up
Total cholesterol < 200 mg/dL	Repeat within 5 years
Total cholesterol 200-239 mg/dL	
Without definite CHD or two other CHD risk factors (one of which can be male sex)	Supply dietary information and recheck annually
With definite CHD or two other CHD risk factors (one of which can be male sex)	Lipoprotein analysis; further action based on LDL-cholesterol level
Total cholesterol ≥240 mg/dL	Lipoprotein analysis; further action based on LDL-cholesterol level

From National Cholesterol Education Program Expert Panel. Report on detection, evaluation, and treatment of high blood cholesterol in adults. *Arch Intern Med.* 1988;148:36.

Blood cholesterol measurements for total-cholesterol determination can be made in nonfasted subjects at any time of day. Illness, weight loss or gain, pregnancy, myocardial infarction (within the previous three months), and a change in eating habits will affect blood cholesterol values.

An integral part of the program is the need to have accurate and precise methods for measuring blood cholesterol in small blood samples (eg, finger-stick). Furthermore, the method selected for cholesterol screening must be capable of measuring blood cholesterol in a large number of samples. The assay results must be obtained immediately.

The need for accuracy and precision in quantifying blood cholesterol levels are obvious for the success of the program. Accuracy is defined as "agreement with a true value." Precision is defined as "reproducibility of results." Many different methods are used for measuring blood cholesterol, based on different reagents, instruments, and so on. Thus, measurements must be accurate to avoid clinical misdiagnosis. The goal of the program is to achieve a precision (as coefficient of variation, CV) of 3% or less.[84] As shown in *Table 4.14*, there has been a marked improvement in the precision of blood cholesterol assays.

A number of portable, automated systems (eg, Reflotron, Kodak DT-60, Vision) are available for measuring blood cholesterol quickly and reliably in many cases. These will play an important role in achieving the objective of cholesterol screening by allowing cholesterol measurements to be done outside a clinical laboratory (eg, in physician's offices and at screening sites such as shopping malls, schools, and businesses). It is important to realize that these instruments cannot merely be plugged in and used. It is essential that users understand the performance characteristics and limitations of these new analyzers prior to adopting them for routine use. The accuracy and precision of the blood cholesterol assay by these analyzers must be established by appropriate calibration studies and proven quality-control measures. The accuracy of these instruments appears to meet the requirements of the program (CV ≤3%) when calibrated appropriately.[83] To assure good quality control the following steps are important:

1. Request documentation of instrument accuracy from the manufacturer.
2. Compare results of known standards with another reference method.
3. Check the accuracy of the instrument with calibrated standards that have low, medium, and high cholesterol concentrations.
4. Periodically, compare the blood cholesterol values with those obtained using another reference method.

Table 4.14
National Trends in Interlaboratory Comparability*

	1949	1969	1980	1983	1986
Cholesterol, %	23.7	18.5	11.1	6.4	6.2

*Mean precision (CV) after exclusion of outliers (values exceeding $x \pm 3$ SD).

From *Current Status of Blood Cholesterol Measurement in Clinical Laboratories in the United States.*[84]

To reduce CHD morbidity and mortality in the United States, Americans must first know their blood cholesterol levels. It is important that practitioners have an understanding of the procedures available for measuring blood cholesterol levels and the associated accuracy and precision of the selected assay.

Triglyceride and Apolipoprotein Measurement

Plasma total triglycerides should be measured after a 12- to 14-hour fast. The assays typically are done using an autoanalyzer or an enzymatic kit. Average levels appear in *Table 4.15.* Sometimes lipoprotein triglycerides (most often VLDL triglycerides) are measured when clinically indicated. Apolipoproteins are assayed by radioimmunoassay. Commercial kits are available to measure apolipoproteins A-I and B, but they are not typically measured in clinical practice. The kits are currently used for research purposes.

Lipoprotein Measurement

The separation of lipoproteins is achieved on the basis of differences in density using ultracentrifugation.[85] Another widely used method in clinical practice relies on precipitation techniques.[86] In this assay VLDL and LDL (the apolipoprotein-B–containing lipoproteins) are precipitated with heparin manganese. The supernatant is assayed for cholesterol, providing a direct assessment of HDL cholesterol. VLDL cholesterol and LDL cholesterol can be estimated indirectly. VLDL cholesterol is approximated by dividing the value obtained for plasma total triglycerides by 5. LDL cholesterol is the difference between plasma total cholesterol and the sum of VLDL cholesterol and HDL cholesterol.

Table 4.15
Average Levels of Plasma Triglycerides

Age, yr	Triglycerides, mg/dL
20–29	140
30–39	150
40–49	160
> 50	190*

*Any laboratory value over 260 with two reported measures needs further evaluation of the patient to find the cause of hypertriglyceridemia. The danger level for pancreatitis is over 1,000 mg/dL. Intensive treatment is recommended. Persons with plasma triglyceride levels above 500 mg/dL should be treated initially with diet.

Courtesy Raksha Shah, University of California, San Francisco, 1989.

Lipoproteins (and LDL cholesterol) can be assayed directly after separation by ultracentrifugation. This procedure is time-consuming and expensive. Results obtained are similar to indirect methods.

Experimentally, HDL_2 ($d = 1.063$ to 1.125) and HDL_3 ($d = 1.125$ to 1.21) are determined by ultracentrifugation. Interest in the quantification of the two subfractions has developed due to the emerging evidence demonstrating that HDL_2 cholesterol is protective against CHD. Electrophoresis is another technique used to separate plasma lipoproteins; however, it is not widely used except to diagnose type III hyperlipoproteinemia.

Biochemical Assessment After a Myocardial Infarct

Cholesterol and other plasma lipids can usually be measured in the first 24 hours after a myocardial infarction.[87] Thereafter, plasma total-cholesterol and lipoprotein-cholesterol levels should not be measured until at least two to three months after a myocardial infarct.

The measurement of serum enzymes is useful in making the diagnosis and establishing the severity of the myocardial infarction, although there may be other causes for elevated enzymes.[66] Hence, elevated serum enzyme levels are not a definitive diagnosis of a heart attack. With cell necrosis of the myocardium, enzymes such as creatine phosphokinase (CPK), serum glutamic-oxaloacetic transaminase (SGOT), lactate dehydrogenase (LDH), and 3-hydroxybutyrate dehydrogenase are released into the blood. The rise in serum enzymes is reflective of the size of an acute myocardial infarction and/or other factors such as perfusion of the infarcted area, clearance of the enzyme from the plasma, and the presence of serum enzyme inhibitors. SGOT begins to rise within 6 to 12 hours after acute myocardial infarction, reaches a maximum within one to three days, and remains elevated for four to eight days. Serum LDH may be elevated for as long as ten days after the myocardial infarction. Measurement of the myocardial band (MB) isoenzyme of CPK is sensitive and specific for myocardial infarction. MB-CPK levels return to normal within four to eight days. Serum myoglobin levels are also elevated in patients following an acute myocardial infarction. The specificity and sensitivity of this measurement for diagnosing myocardial infarction are currently under investigation. However, myoglobinuria often precedes the increase in serum enzymes. This measurement has been shown to be a more sensitive indicator of cardiac muscle necrosis and may reflect the size of the myocardial infarction.

CLASSIFICATION OF HYPERLIPIDEMIA*

Hyperlipidemia refers to an elevation of one or both of the commonly determined individual components of lipoproteins, cholesterol, and triglycerides. In general, persons classified as hyperlipidemic have cholesterol and/or triglyceride levels above the 90th percentile for age and gender. The diagnosis usually implies that a lipoprotein abnormality is present as well, since cholesterol and triglycerides are major constituents of lipoprotein particles.

Table 4.16
Classification of Hyperlipidemias Based on Lipoprotein Concentrations

Type	Lipoprotein Abnormality	Lipid Profiles	Typical Values, mg/dL
I	Chylomicrons markedly increased; VLDL and LDL both normal or low	TC* increased TG† significantly increased	320 4000
IIa	LDL increased; VLDL normal	TC increased TG N‡	370 90
IIb	LDL increased; VLDL increased	TC increased TG increased	350 400
III	Abnormal cholesterol—enriched VLDL present in excess	TC increased TG increased	500 700
IV	VLDL increased; LDL normal	TC N TG increased	220 400
V	Chylomicrons markedly increased; VLDL increased; LDL normal or low	TC increased TG significantly increased	700 5000

*TC = cholesterol.
†TG = triglycerides.
‡N = normal.

Adapted from Beaumont JL, Carlson LA, Cooper GR, et al[88]; Fredrickson DS, Levy RI, Lees RS, et al.[89]

The classification of hyperlipidemias is most commonly based on the plasma lipoprotein patterns. *Table 4.16* presents the classification scheme used to characterize hyperlipidemias based on lipoprotein concentrations.[88,89] In addition to the conditions listed, one in which plasma lipid levels are normal but HDL-cholesterol levels are low is known as *hypoalphalipoproteinemia.* A newly discovered lipoprotein phenotype called *hyperapobetalipoproteinemia* (hyperapo B) presents with an elevated level of apolipoprotein B of LDL in the presence of a normal concentration of LDL. Hyperapo B is strongly associated with premature CHD in adults, and one third of the children born to such patients have hyperapo B.[90]

The causes of hyperlipidemia may be primary (genetic), secondary, or a combination of the two. Primary hyperlipidemia may be polygenic or monogenic. Most of the hyperlipidemias appear to be the result of three different metabolic defects: (1) overproduction of VLDL, (2) reduced lipolysis of triglyceride-rich lipoprotein, and (3) decreased clearance of LDL and IDL (by the B100/E receptor).[91]

The secondary causes of hyperlipidemia include diet (excessive saturated fat, cholesterol, and calories), uncontrolled diabetes, alcohol, hypothyroidism, nephrotic syndrome, renal dialysis and transplantation, biliary obstruction, estrogens, corticosteroids, thiazide diuretics, beta-blockers, retinoic acid, dysglobulinemia, autoimmune disease, glycogen-storage disease, porphyria, and

*By the Editors

anorexia nervosa. In patients with cholestasis, an abnormal lipoprotein accumulates in the plasma (LPX), although occasionally a patient may have an abnormally elevated HDL-cholesterol level. Secondary causes of lipid abnormalities should be ruled out through the history, physical examination, and laboratory tests.

Certain drugs have been shown to elevate lipid levels. These include oral contraceptives, alcohol, most antihypertensive drugs, and beta-adrenergic blocking agents.[92] Oral contraceptives (estrogen and, to a lesser extent, progestins) can elevate serum triglycerides via increased hepatic VLDL production. Little significant change in VLDL actually occurs due to a compensatory increase in lipoprotein lipase. Some women, however, experience an elevation in both VLDL and chylomicron triglycerides, most likely due to their genetic predisposition for hypertriglyceridemia.[92] The type and dosage of hormone used and the particular route of administration can produce distinct changes in lipoprotein profiles.[92]

Thiazide-type diuretic agents have been shown to elevate VLDL-triglyceride levels.[92] Plasma total cholesterol may be elevated or unchanged while HDL-cholesterol levels may decrease. The mechanism of these changes is unknown but may be due to hemoconcentration of lipids as plasma volume decreases with diuresis, or they may be due to thiazide-induced diabetes leading to increased triglyceride synthesis. Beta-adrenergic blocking drugs such as propranolol, metoprolol, and atenolol tend to elevate serum triglyceride and decrease HDL-cholesterol levels without affecting the plasma total-cholesterol level. However, the impact of beta-blockers on serum lipids is not consistent and may be less pronounced at small doses.[92] A summary of the affect of selected drugs on plasma lipids is summarized in chapter 11.

Alcohol consumption has been shown to affect HDL-cholesterol levels positively.[93,94] Research on alcohol's influence on HDL_2 and HDL_3 concentration has produced conflicting results, perhaps because of the different methods used to isolate the HDL subfractions (see chapter 2 for additional information). Excessive intake of alcohol usually elevates VLDL-triglycerides as well. In persons with underlying familial hypertriglyceridemia, even small amounts of alcohol can result in massive increases in both VLDL and chylomicron triglycerides.[92]

BIOCHEMICAL ASSESSMENT OF THE HOSPITALIZED PATIENT*

In addition to monitoring plasma lipid levels and various enzymes in the plasma, it is advisable to assess the nutritional status of the patient to prevent clinical malnutrition. Many routine laboratory tests are useful; key tests are: serum albumin (or transferrin, due to its shorter half life) to assess visceral protein status; total lymphocyte count, which provides information about cellular defense mechanisms and visceral protein status; and hemoglobin and hematocrit, which are both indicators of iron status. Assessing the immune-system response to skin-test antigens is useful in assessing both protein and energy status.

*By the Editors

ASSESSMENT OF HYPERTENSION STATUS*

Hypertension, or high blood pressure, is one of the three major risk factors for heart disease, stroke, and kidney failure. A primary reason for the 35% decrease in mortality from CVD is due to the decrease in the incidence of uncontrolled hypertension. It is called the silent killer because it has no symptoms. Therefore, awareness, prevention, and treatment are critical in controlling hypertension. The following information is excerpted from *The 1984 Report of Detection, Evaluation, and Treatment of High Blood Pressure.*[95]

Thirty percent of adults in the United States have high blood pressure. Prevalence increases with age and is higher in blacks than in whites. The principal causes of hypertension are not known in 80% of the cases; genetics and environment are causally linked to the remaining 20%. Overall, only 25% of persons who are diagnosed with hypertension follow the recommended treatment program. Health professionals need to be aware of this and encourage compliance as much as possible. The major objective is to maintain arterial pressure at a level that does not exceed 140/90 mm Hg.

Table 4.17 contains the classification of blood pressure based on diastolic and systolic readings. *Table 4.18* shows recommendations for the follow-up criteria for initial blood pressure measurement.

Table 4.17
Classification of Blood Pressure* in Adults Age 18 Years or Older

Range, mm Hg	Category†
Diastolic	
< 85	Normal blood pressure
85–89	High normal blood pressure
90–104	Mild hypertension
105–114	Moderate hypertension
≥115	Severe hypertension
Systolic, when diastolic blood pressure is < 90	
< 140	Normal blood pressure
140–159	Borderline isolated systolic hypertension
≥160	Isolated systolic hypertension

* Classification is based on the average of two or more readings on two or more occasions.

† A classification of borderline isolated systolic hypertension (SBP 140 to 159 mm Hg) or isolated systolic hypertension (SBP ≥160 mm Hg) takes precedence over high normal blood pressure (diastolic blood pressure, 85 to 89 mm Hg) when both occur in the same person. High normal blood pressure (DBP 85 to 89 mm Hg) takes precedence over a classification of normal blood pressure (SBP < 140 mm Hg) when both occur in the same person.

From *The 1984 Report of the Joint National Committee on Detection, Evaluation, and Treatment of High Blood Pressure.*[95]

ASSESSMENT OF CHD RISK STATUS†

Three methods for calculating CHD risk are presented. The first method, taken from the NCEP, is preferred. It can be used to determine whether a person is at low risk, borderline-high risk, or high risk for CHD. The other two methods presented, taken from the American Heart Association and the Framingham Study, can be used to estimate the probability of CHD development.

*By Patricia Volz-Clarke
†By the Editors

Table 4.18
Follow-up Criteria for Initial Blood Pressure Measurement for Adults Age 18 Years or Older

Range, mm Hg	Recommended Follow-up*
Diastolic	
<85	Recheck within 2 years
85–89	Recheck within 1 year
90–104	Confirm within 2 months
105–114	Evaluate or refer promptly to source of care within 2 weeks
≥115	Evaluate or refer immediately to source of care
Systolic, when diastolic blood pressure is <90	
<140	Recheck within 2 years
140–199	Confirm within 2 months
≥200	Evaluate or refer promptly to source of care within 2 weeks

* If recommendations for follow-up of diastolic and systolic blood pressure are different, the shorter recommended time for recheck and referral should take precedence.

From *The 1984 Report of the Joint National Committee on Detection, Evaluation, and Treatment of High Blood Pressure.*[95]

The NCEP CHD risk-classification procedure has been described previously. Initial classification is based on the plasma total-cholesterol level (see Table 4.13). As noted, in addition to assessing the blood cholesterol level, the presence of other risk factors should be assessed (*Table 4.19*). Someone with either definite CHD or two of the other listed risk factors is considered to be at high CHD risk.

Table 4.19
Initial Classification Based on Total Cholesterol

- The total blood cholesterol level is the basis for initial patient classification.
- All blood cholesterol levels above 200 mg/dL should be confirmed by repeat measurements, with the average used to guide clinical decisions.
- Other CHD risk factors should be taken into account in selecting appropriate follow-up measures for patients with borderline-high cholesterol levels.
- All patients with a blood cholesterol level of 240 mg/dL or above, which is classified as high blood cholesterol, should receive a lipoprotein analysis. Patients with borderline-high blood cholesterol levels (200–239 mg/dL) who in addition have definite CHD or two other CHD risk factors should also have a lipoprotein analysis performed.
- CHD risk factors as defined in the report include:
  - male sex
  - family history of premature CHD (definite myocardial infarction or sudden death before age 55 in a parent or sibling)
  - cigarette smoking (currently smokes more than ten cigarettes per day)
  - hypertension
  - low HDL-cholesterol concentration (below 35 mg/dL confirmed by repeat measurement)
  - diabetes mellitus
  - history of definite cerebrovascular or occlusive peripheral vascular disease
  - severe obesity (≥30% overweight)
- In public screening programs, all patients with a level about 200 mg/dL should be referred to their physicians for remeasurement and evaluation.

From the National Cholesterol Education Program Expert Panel. Report on detection, evaluation, and treatment of high blood cholesterol in adults. *Arch Intern Med.* 1988;148:36.

The probability of CHD's developing in six years can be calculated using the following information: systolic blood pressure, the presence or absence of left ventricular hypertrophy, glucose intolerance, and cigarette smoking (the AHA method), age, serum total-cholesterol level, and gender.[95] This information has been used to compile the probability tables that appear in the appendix. (See tables 14.8 and 14.9.)

ASSESSMENT OF HEALTH AND CHD RISK: USE OF A HEALTH-RISK APPRAISAL INSTRUMENT*

In the past decade, health-risk appraisal (HRA) has become increasingly popular as a means of assessing a person's health status. HRAs provide an estimate of the likelihood of mortality or morbidity based on information about such risk factors as blood pressure, weight, smoking habits, and medical history. According to recent estimates, between 5 million and 15 million Americans have completed HRAs.[96]

Appraisal questionnaires have been widely touted as an educational tool for making people aware of the implications of their life-style and health habits.[97] A growing number of organizations are administering HRAs to their employees to help design health insurance and benefits packages. HRA results have even been used in attempts to evaluate the effectiveness of health promotion programs.

There are differences among HRAs in the way risk is defined and estimated. The computations required to predict risk levels are usually so complex that they must be scored by computer, but there are also many HRAs that can be self-scored. In general, four major types of HRAs can be distinguished on the basis of risk outcome and scoring methodology.

Most common are HRAs that forecast the probability of dying from each of the leading causes of death over a certain time period, typically ten years. Separate estimates for heart disease and stroke are almost always included. Mortality risk estimates are usually derived from an actuarial approach known as the Geller-Gesner method, although many developers are turning to more sophisticated statistical techniques. A second category of HRAs consists of questionnaires that focus exclusively on heart attacks and heart disease. Instead of probabilities, these HRAs contain arbitrary scales divided into low, average, and high risk ranges. These pencil-and-paper tests are scored by adding together the point values associated with a variety of individual risk factors. In the third HRA category, years of life expectancy serves as a surrogate for risk. These HRAs usually contain most of the major factors affecting CHD risk. They can also be scored by hand, but the computations tend to be lengthier and more complicated than for the questionnaires in the second category. The final category consists of questionnaires providing broad measures of overall health, variously described as life style, wellness, stress, or simply health risk. These questionnaires are the simplest to score by hand, but often contain crude measures of risk factors and neglect many important determinants of CHD.

There is also considerable variation in the extent to which HRAs use information about diet and nutrition. Many HRAs do not contain any questions about dietary habits. Others include one or two brief dietary items, but do not use the data in their risk computations. Instead, the responses simply trigger recommendations for improving dietary practices. Another approach adopted by some HRAs is to substitute questions about fat and sodium consumption only when blood pressure or plasma total-cholesterol or lipoprotein-cholesterol levels are unavailable.

*By Kevin W. Smith and John B. McKinlay

There are several reasons why nutrition has not been a central element in health-risk appraisal. First of all, dietary status is difficult to measure. Using 24-hour dietary recalls to assess self-reported weekly consumption patterns may be unreliable in some subjects, but there is little consensus regarding how to summarize frequency of intake across food groups. Comprehensive dietary inventories are too lengthy to include in most HRAs.[98] Second, due in part to the measurement problem, extensive evidence is not available about the independent (and direct) effects of nutrition on long-term mortality. In the case of CHD, for example, risk computations are usually derived from prospective surveys such as the Framingham Heart Study. Since many of these longitudinal surveys do not contain adequate dietary data, the unique influence of nutrition on disease over an extended period cannot be determined. Third, most HRA risk methodologies focus on physiological precursors of death and disease. Habits like diet and exercise affect more immediate precursors such as blood pressure, plasma cholesterol, lipid fractions, and body mass. Therefore, in terms of the casual linkages among risk factors, these habits are considered to have indirect rather than direct effects on risk status.

Guidelines for Selecting an HRA

It is estimated that there are more than 200 types of HRA available in the United States. Choosing among these may seem a daunting task, but several guidelines may be helpful.

One of the primary considerations should be the validity, or accuracy, of the risk estimates produced by an HRA. Due to the diversity of scoring methods and sources of data, different HRAs can give widely discrepant estimates of risk for a single subject. In a recent study of 41 of the most common appraisal instruments, the validity of HRA risk estimates was evaluated for CHD through comparisons with the projections made by epidemiological models from the Framingham Heart Study and the UCLA Risk Factor Update Project.[99] The closest approximations to epidemiologic estimates of heart disease mortality were found for HRAs based on logistic regression equations, followed by the Geller-Gesner method and additive scales. An important indicator of validity is the comprehensiveness of the items appearing in an appraisal questionnaire. Instruments that fail to include major risk factors, that ignore important nonmodifiable characteristics such as gender and age, or that use only two or three broad categories to measure a factor will tend to have lower correlations with epidemiologic models.

A second consideration is the nature of the results that are to be reported to HRA respondents. What type of feedback is most appropriate for clients? In some cases, simple classifications of lower-than-average, average, and higher-than-average risk categories may suffice. Other applications may require more detailed estimates of life expectancy or the probability of dying during the next ten years. Another popular approach is to contrast a person's actual age with his or her "appraised" age—the average age at which members of the general population have the same risk of death as the respondent. In addition to overall risk results, in some cases it may also be desirable to provide data about the risks associated with specific factors such as smoking or physical activity. Research applications, particularly those in which HRA data are to be used to evaluate a health promotion or dietary intervention, may also place certain demands on the nature of the risk results.

A third consideration when choosing an HRA is cost. The least expensive alternative is to select an HRA that respondents can score themselves. Self-scored questionnaires can usually be purchased in bulk from local and national health organizations at a nominal charge. With the proliferation of personal computers, many developers have begun marketing HRA software. For prices ranging from $50 to several hundred dollars, this software can perform sophisticated risk analyses either interactively or in batch mode. Finally, there are several corporations that conduct HRA assessments for a fee. These services typically produce personalized booklets for individual respondents filled with charts and detailed explanations of the results, as well as summary reports for subgroups of clients. While this is the most expensive option, it can be cost-effective when entire worksites or large populations are to be evaluated.

Limitations of an HRA

While a health-risk appraisal is a promising tool, it is subject to several limitations that may decrease its usefulness in practice. First, clients may find it difficult to comprehend and interpret HRA results. Many people are uncomfortable with probability estimates and may fail to grasp the meaning of abstract concepts such as one's "appraised" age. Uncertainty about the meaning of the results undercuts an HRA's educational and motivational potential. A second drawback is that respondents may not know some of the information required for an accurate appraisal. Blood pressure and cholesterol levels for determining CHD risk are two common examples. If these values are missing and cannot be supplied by a laboratory analysis, most HRAs simply assign an average risk weight. This practice produces risk estimates that are closer to the population norm than they should be. To mitigate this bias, some HRAs contain "substitution rules" specifying estimates for unknown values. A third limitation is that self-scored HRAs are subject to mathematical errors on the part of respondents. Computational errors when adding and subtracting point values are not uncommon, even in the shortest questionnaires, and will sometimes mislead respondents about their actual status. Finally, the usefulness of health appraisals is also affected by the context in which they occur. Many practitioners feel that HRAs should only be administered in supervised settings where health professionals are available to answer questions and explain scores. In the absence of some form of counseling, HRA results may provoke needless fear and anxiety. The American Institutes for Research is conducting a field test of several major HRAs to determine the implications of some of these limitations. One risk-factor assessment instrument that is considered to be very good is available from the Carter Center. It is a 45-question, four-page questionnaire that requires the purchase of special software. As such, it cannot be self-scored, and it is probably more useful in a corporate or structured clinical setting than as an individual teaching tool.*

References

1. Grant A, DeHoog S. *Nutritional Assessment and Support.* 3rd ed. Seattle, Wash: North Gate Station; 1985.
2. Chumlea WC, Roche A, Mukkerjee D. *Nutritional Assessment of the Elderly Through Anthropometry.* Columbus, Ohio: Ross Labs; 1984.
3. Metropolitan Life Insurance Company, Health and Safety Education Division. New weight standards for men and women. *Stat Bull Met Life Insur.* 1959;40:3.
4. Himes JH, Brouchard C. Do the new Metropolitan Life Insurance weight-height tables correctly assess body frame and body fat relationships? *Am J Public Health.* 1985;75:1076.
5. Burton BT, Foster WR, Hirsch J, et al. Health implications of obesity. *Int J Obesity.* 1985;9:155.

*For more information, contact Dr. Ed Hutchins, Carter Center Health Risk Appraisal Project, 1989 N. Williamsburg Dr, Suite E, Decatur, GA 30033.

6. Burton BT, Foster WR. Health implications of obesity. *J Am Diet Assoc.* 1985;85:1117.
7. Olmstead Schulz L. Obese, overweight, desirable, ideal: where to draw the line in 1986. *J Am Diet Assoc.* 1986;86:1702.
8. Lukaski HC. Methods for the assessment of human body composition: traditional and new. *Am J Clin Nutr.* 1987;46:537.
9. Lohman TG. Skinfolds and body density and their relation to body fatness: a review. *Hum Biol.* 1981;53:181.
10. Conway JM, Norris KH, Bodwell CE. A new approach for the estimation of body composition: infrared interactance. *Am J Clin Nutr.* 1984;40:1123.
11. Bjorntorp P. Regional patterns of fat distribution. *Ann Intern Med.* 1985;103:994.
12. Todd K, Hudes M, Calloway DH. Food intake measurement: problems and approaches. *Am J Clin Nutr.* 1983;37:139.
13. Suitor CW, Crowley MF. *Nutrition, Principles and Application in Health Promotion.* New York, NY: JB Lippincott Co; 1984.
14. Krantzler NJ, et al. Methods of food intake assessment: an annotated bibliography. *J Nutr Educ.* 1982;14:108.
15. Guthrie HA. Selection and quantification of typical food portions by young adults. *J Am Diet Assoc.* 1984;84:1440.
16. Lee J, Koloel LN, Hankin J. Cholesterol intake as measured by unquantified and quantified food frequency interviews: implications for epidemiological research. *Int J Epidemiol.* 1985;14:249.
17. Block G, Hartman AM, Dresser CM, et al. A data-based approach to diet questionnaire design and testing. *Am J Epidemiol.* 1986;124:453.
18. Willet WC, Reynolds RD, Cottrell-Hoehner S, et al. Validation of a semi-quantitative food frequency questionnaire: comparison with a 1-year diet record. *J Am Diet Assoc.* 1987;87:43.
19. Sampson L. Food frequency questionnaires as a research instrument. *Clin Nutr.* 1985;4:171.
20. Basiotis PP, Welsh SO, Cronin FJ, et al. Number of days of food intake: records required to estimate individual and group nutrient intakes with defined confidence. *J Nutr.* 1987;117:1638.
21. National Research Council. *Nutrient Adequacy: Assessment Using Food Consumption Surveys. A Report of the Subcommittee on Criteria for Dietary Evaluations.* Washington, DC: National Academy Press; 1989.
22. Jackson B, Dujovne CA, DeCoursey S, et al. Methods to assess relative reliability of diet records: minimum records for monitoring lipid and calorie intake. *J Am Diet Assoc.* 1986;86:1531.
23. White EC, McNamara DJ, Ahrens EH. Validation of a dietary record system for the estimation of daily cholesterol intake in individual outpatients. *Am J Clin Nutr.* 1981;34:199.
24. *Heart to Heart.* Public Health Service, National Institutes of Health; 1983. US Dept of Health and Human Services NIH publication 83-1528.
25. Adelman MO, Dwyerm JT, Woods M, et al. Computerized dietary analysis systems: a comparative view. *J Am Diet Assoc.* 1983;83:421.
26. Feskanich MS, Buzzard IM, Welch BT, et al. Comparison of a computerized and a manual method of food coding for nutrient studies. *J Am Diet Assoc.* 1988;88:1263.
27. DeBakey MD, Gotto AM, Scott LW, et al. *The Living Heart Diet.* New York, NY: Raven Press Ltd; 1984.
28. Watt BK, Merrill AL. *Composition of Foods: Raw, Processed, Prepared.* Washington, DC: US Govt Printing Office; 1963. US Dept of Agriculture handbook 8.
29. *Handbook 8* (revised). Washington, DC: US Govt Printing Office; 1976-1987. Sections 8-1 through 8-15.
30. Hoover LW. Computerized nutrient data bases, I: comparison of nutrient anaylsis systems. *J Am Diet Assoc.* 1983;82:501.
31. Taylor ML, Kozlowski BW, Baer MT. Energy and nutrient values from different computerized data bases. *J Am Diet Assoc.* 1985;85:1136.
32. Goodard MS, Matthews RH. Current knowledge of nutritive values of vegetables. *Food Tech.* 1979;33:71.
33. Gebhart SE, Matthews RH. *Nutritive Value of Foods.* Washington, DC: US Govt Printing Office; 1986. Home and Garden bulletin 72.
34. Adelman MO, Dwyer JT, Woods M, et al. Computerized dietary analysis systems: a comparative view. *J Am Diet Assoc.* 1983;83:421.

35. Bagu K, Rutishauser IHE. Comparison of computerized nutrient analysis programs based on Australian, British and American tables of food composition. *J Food Nutr.* 1984;41:17.
36. Bright-See E, Jaxmaji V, Benda CA. Computerized food and nutrient calculation for research. *J Can Diet Assoc.* 1986;47:14.
37. Brown JE. Computer software. *Community Nutritionist.* 1983;2:24.
38. Brown JE, Hoover LW, Bross JK. Shopping for computers. *Community Nutritionist.* 1982;1:18.
39. Cook RA, Quatromoni PA, Cook CM. Use of two short data bases adapted to the microcomputer. *Nutr Rep Int.* 1985;32:1303.
40. Dare D, Al-Bander SY. A computerized diet analysis system for the research nutritionist. *J Am Diet Assoc.* 1987;87:629.
41. DuBois D, Jacobson M, Moyer G. Eat by numbers? *Nutr Action.* November 1983:10.
42. Dwyer J, Suitor CS. Caveat emptor: assessing needs, evaluating computer options: evaluating mail order and microcomputer diet analysis programs. *J Am Diet Assoc.* 1984;84:302.
43. Frank GC, Pelican S. Guidelines for selecting a dietary analysis system. *J Am Diet Assoc.* 1986;86:72.
44. Frank GC, Farris RP, Berenson GS. Comparison of dietary intake by two computerized analysis systems. *J Am Diet Assoc.* 1984;84:818.
45. Hoover LW. *Computers in Nutrition, Dietetics and Foodservice Management: A Bibliography.* Columbia, Mo: Dept of Human Nutrition, Foods and Food Systems Management, University of Missouri-Columbia; 1985.
46. Hoover LW, Perloff BP. Computerized nutrient data bases, II: development of model for appraisal of nutrient data base system capabilities. *J Am Diet Assoc.* 1983;82:506.
47. (Theme issue devoted to computers.) *Journal of Nutrition Education.* June 1984.
48. Karkeck JM. Computer applications in clinical nutrition. *J Can Diet Assoc.* 1985;46:41.
49. Nieman DC, Nieman CN. A comparative study of two microcomputer nutrient data bases with the USDA Nutrient Data Base for Standard Reference. *J Am Diet Assoc.* 1987;87:930.
50. Samonds KW. Computerization of nutrient data for dietary evaluation. In: Beal VA, Laus MJ, eds. *Proceedings of the Symposium on Dietary Data Collection, Analysis, and Significance.* Amherst, Mass: Massachusetts Agricultural Experiment Station; 1982:50. Research bulletin 675.
51. Shanklin D, Endres JM, Sawicki M. A comparative study of two nutrient data bases. *J Am Diet Assoc.* 1985;85:308.
52. Slavin JL, Wilson A, Willey D. Take the proper "byte" when selecting microcomputer nutrient analysis software. *Food Tech.* 1985;39:74.
53. Willard R. Computers in dietetics. *Diet Currents.* 1982;9:7.
54. Hoover LW. *Nutrient Data Bank Dir.* Columbia, Mo: Department of Human Nutrition, Foods and Food Systems Management, 217 Gwynn Hall, University of Missouri-Columbia; 1987.
55. *Annual Journal of Dietetic Software.* 1986-87. PO Box 2565, Norman, OK 73070.
56. Hildebrandt DM, Huskey J. *Computer Programs and Databases in the Field of Nutrition.* Seattle, Wash: Computing Information Center, University of Washington; 1985.
57. Rand WM. Food composition data: problems and plans. *J Am Diet Assoc.* 1985;85:1081.
58. *Proceedings of the National Nutrient Data Bank Conference.* For proceedings of conferences 1–10 (1976–1985) contact: National Technical Information Service, 5285 Port Royal Road, Springfield, VA 22161. For proceedings of the 11th conference contact: Georgia Center for Continuing Education, The University of Georgia, Athens, GA 30602.
59. Anderson JT, Jacobs DR, Foster N, et al. Scoring systems for evaluating dietary pattern effect of serum cholesterol. *Prev Med.* 1979;8:525.
60. Remmel PS, Benfari RC. Assessing dietary adherence in the Multiple Risk Factor Intervention Trial (MRFIT), II: food record rating as an indicator of compliance. *J Am Diet Assoc.* 1980;76:357.
61. Boyar AP, Loughridge JR. The fat portion exchange list: a tool for teaching and evaluating low fat diets. *J Am Diet Assoc.* 1985;85:589.

62. Ney D, Fischer C. A tool for assessing compliance with a diet for diabetes. *J Am Diet Assoc.* 1983;82:287.
63. Connor SL, Gustafson JR, Artaud-Wild SM, et al. The cholesterol-saturated fat index for coronary prevention: background, use, and a comprehensive table of foods. *J Am Diet Assoc.* 1989;89:807.
64. Connor SL, Gustafson JR, Artaud-Wild SM, et al. The cholesterol/saturated-fat index: an indication of the hypercholesterolaemic and atherogenic potential of food. *Lancet.* 1986;2:1229.
65. Caggiula AW, Wing RR, Norwalk MP, et al. The measurement of sodium and potassium intake. *Am J Clin Nutr.* 1985;42:391.
66. Sowers M, Stumbo P. A method to assess sodium intake in populations. *J Am Diet Assoc.* 1986;86:1196.
67. Sokolow M, McIlroy MB. *Clinical Cardiology.* Los Altos, Calif: Lange Medical Books; 1981.
68. Acierno LJ. *Comprehensive Cardiac Rehabilitation and Prevention: A Model Program.* New York, NY: Immergut and Siolek Publishers; 1985.
69. Ellestad MH. *Stress Testing.* 2nd ed. Philadelphia, Pa: FA Davis Co; 1980.
70. American College of Sports Medicine. *Guidelines for Exercise Testing and Exercise Prescription.* 3rd ed. Philadelphia, Pa: Lea & Febiger; 1986.
71. Jopke T. Choosing an exercise testing protocol. *Phys Sports Med.* 1981;9:141.
72. Balady G. Value of arm exercise testing in detecting coronary artery disease. *Am J Cardiol.* 1985;55:37.
73. Castelli WP. Epidemiology and risk in coronary artery disease. In: *The Clinical Significance of Hyperlipidemia, Proceedings of an International Symposium.* Morris Plains, NJ: Warner-Lambert; 1984.
74. Grundy SM. Pathogenesis of hyperlipoproteinemia. *J Lipid Res.* 1984;25:1611.
75. National Cholesterol Education Program Expert Panel. Report on detection, evaluation, and treatment of high blood cholesterol in adults. *Arch Intern Med.* 1988;148:36.
76. Gordon T, Castelli WP, Hjortland MC, et al. High density lipoprotein as a protective factor against coronary heart disease: the Framingham Study. *Am J Med.* 1977;62:707.
77. Castelli WP, Garrison RJ, Wilson PWF, et al. Incidence of coronary heart disease and lipoprotein cholesterol levels: the Framingham Study. *JAMA.* 1986;256:2835.
78. Connor WE, Bristow JD. *Coronary Heart Disease: Prevention, Complications and Treatment.* Philadelphia, Pa: JB Lippincott; 1985.
79. Kane JP, Malloy JM. Disorders of lipoprotein metabolism. In: *Basic and Clinical Endocrinology.* Los Angeles, Calif: Appleton-Lane; 1988:559.
80. Naito HK. New diagnostic tests for assessing coronary heart disease risk. In: Widhalm K, Naito HK, eds. *Recent Aspects of Diagnosis and Treatment of Lipoprotein Disorders.* New York, NY: Alan Liss; 1986.
81. Shepard J, Packard CJ, Patsch JR, et al. Effect of dietary polyunsaturated and saturated fat on the properties of high density lipoproteins and the metabolism of apoprotein A-1. *J Clin Invest.* 1978;61:1582.
82. Marshall WJ, Ballantyne FC. Current clinical laboratory practice: investigation of plasma lipids—which test and when? *Br Med J.* 1986;292:1652.
83. Berenson GS, McMahan CA, Voors AW, et al. *Cardiovascular Risk Factors in Children.* New York, NY: Oxford University Press; 1980.
84. *Current Status of Blood Cholesterol Measurement in Clinical Laboratories in the United States.* US Dept of Health and Human Services; 1988.
85. Nelson GJ. *Blood Lipids and Lipoproteins: Quantitation, Composition and Metabolism.* New York, NY: John Wiley & Sons; 1972.
86. Bachorik PS, Albers JL. Precipitation methods for quantification of lipoproteins. *Methods Enz.* 1986;129:79.
87. Ryder RE, Hayes TM, Mulligan LP, et al. How soon after myocardial infarction should plasma lipid values be assessed? *Br Med J.* 1984;289:1651.
88. Beaumont JL, Carlson LA, Cooper GR, et al. Classification of hyperlipoproteinemias. *Bull WHO.* 1970;43:891.
89. Fredrickson DS, Levy RI, Lees RS. Fat transport in lipoproteins: an integrated approach to mechanism and disorders. *N Engl J Med.* 1967;276:34, 94, 148, 215, 273.
90. Kwiterovich P. *Beyond Cholesterol.* Baltimore, Md: Johns Hopkins University Press; 1989:150-158.

91. Breslow JL. Apolipoprotein genetic variation and human disease. *Physiol Rev.* 1988;68:85.
92. Powers D, Morre AD. *Food-Medication Interactions.* 3rd ed. Tempe, Ariz: FMI Publishers; 1983.
93. Haskell WL, Camargo C, Williams PT, et al. The effect of cessation and resumption of moderate alcohol intake on serum high-density lipoprotein subfractions. *N Engl J Med.* 1984;310:805.
94. Crouse JR, Grundy SM. Effects of alcohol on plasma lipoproteins and cholesterol and triglyceride metabolism in man. *J Lipid Res.* 1984;25:486.
95. *The 1984 Report of the Joint National Committee on Detection, Evaluation, and Treatment of High Blood Pressure.* US Dept of Health and Human Services, National Institutes of Health; 1984. NIH publication 84-1088.
96. Kannel WB, Schatzkin A. Risk factor analysis. *Prog Cardiovasc Dis.* 1983;26:309.
97. Schoenbach VJ. Appraising health risk appraisal. *Am J Public Health.* 1987;77:409.
98. Willet W. Nutritional epidemiology: issues and challenges. *Int J Epidemiol.* 1987;16:312.
99. Smith KV, McKinlay SM, Thorington BD. The validity of health risk appraisal instruments for assessing coronary heart disease risk. *Am J Public Health.* 1987;77:419.
100. Krause MV, Mahan LK. *Food, Nutrition and Diet Therapy.* 7th ed. Philadelphia, Pa: WB Saunders Co; 1984:197.

5. PREVENTION AND TREATMENT OF CHD BY DIET

The dietitian's role is to translate scientific evidence into practice and to help people adopt dietary plans that promote health and well-being and prevent morbidity and mortality from coronary heart disease (CHD). This means encouraging the general public to modify their eating habits to reduce their serum cholesterol levels and other diet-related risk factors associated with CHD. In addition, dietitians play an important role in developing and implementing individual nutrition care plans for CHD prevention and treatment.

PREVENTION*

Revised dietary recommendations for the prevention of CHD were released by the American Heart Association in December 1986.[1] Intended to reduce hyperlipidemia (especially hypercholesterolemia) and hypertension, these prudent diet recommendations are as follows:

1. Dietary saturated fatty acids should be less than 10% of calories.
2. Total fat should be less than 30% of calories.
3. Cholesterol intake should be less than 100 mg per 1,000 calories, not to exceed 300 mg per day.
4. Protein should contribute approximately 15% of calories.
5. Carbohydrate should contribute 50% to 55% or more of calories, with an emphasis on complex carbohydrates.
6. The sodium intake should be reduced to 1 g per 1,000 calories, not to exceed 3 g per day.
7. If alcoholic beverages are consumed, intake should be limited to 15% of total calories, not to exceed 50 mL of ethanol per day.
8. Total calories should be sufficient to maintain a desirable body weight.
9. A variety of foods is recommended.

The average American diet contains 13% of calories from saturated fatty acids.[2] Reducing saturated-fatty-acid intake to 10% of calories will lead to reductions in the plasma total-cholesterol and LDL-cholesterol levels.

Fats are calorically dense. A reduction in total fat facilitates a decrease in both calories and saturated fatty acids. Even unsaturated fatty acids, which favorably affect plasma lipid levels, should be limited for most people for reasons related primarily to weight control.

Dietary cholesterol, at intakes greater than 200 mg per 1,000 calories, affects the plasma total-cholesterol level. Hence, the suggested cholesterol intake is based on individual calorie requirements.

Protein requirements are based on body weight. Americans currently consume 15% of their calories from protein. In general, dietary protein comprises 10% to 20% of calories, despite manipulations in carbohydrate and fat.

Complex carbohydrates are emphasized in the prudent diet. Populations that consume 60% to 70% of their calories from complex carbohydrates have a low prevalence of atherosclerosis. Foods high in complex carbohydrates usually are low in calories and high in vitamins, minerals, and fiber. Soluble fibers such as those found in pectin, guar gum, and oat bran lower the serum cholesterol level.[3]

*By Bela Lauber

Most Americans have a high sodium intake. While only 0.2 g is required daily, Americans presently consume 4 to 5 g. Both epidemiologic studies and controlled clinical trials provide support for recommending a sodium intake of 1 g per 1,000 calories, not to exceed 3 g daily, to help prevent hypertension in sodium-sensitive people.

For those who choose to consume alcohol, intake should not exceed 50 mL per day (there is 1 oz of ethanol in two drinks of distilled spirits, two 4-oz glasses of wine, or two 12-oz bottles of beer). The incidence of high blood pressure increases significantly with the consumption of three or four drinks per day.[4]

Calories consumed in excess can be a nutritional risk factor for CHD. Consumption of excess calories may lead to an increase in body fat, which increases the prevalence of high blood pressure, an elevated serum cholesterol level, and diabetes mellitus. Ideal body weight should be established and calorie needs determined so that a desirable body weight can be achieved and maintained.

A variety of foods is recommended to achieve an adequate nutrient intake. Variety also adds palatability and interest to meals and decreases adverse reactions to certain foods that some may experience.

Recently the National Research Council's Committee on Diet and Health (which is part of the Food and Nutrition Board for the Commission on Life Sciences) proposed dietary guidelines for maintaining health and reducing chronic disease risk based on a critical examination of the scientific evidence.[5] These guidelines are similar to those of the American Heart Association (AHA) and the National Cholesterol Education Program (NCEP). The committee's dietary recommendations are as follows:

- Reduce total fat intake to 30% or less of calories. Reduce saturated-fatty-acid intake to less than 10% of calories and the intake of cholesterol to less than 300 mg daily. The intake of fat and cholesterol can be reduced by substituting fish, poultry without skin, lean meats, and low-fat or nonfat dairy products for fatty meats and whole-milk dairy products; by choosing more vegetables, fruits, cereals, and legumes; and by limiting oils, fats, egg yolks, fried foods, and other fatty foods.
- Every day eat five or more servings of a combination of vegetables and fruits, especially green and yellow vegetables and citrus fruits. Also, increase intake of starches and other complex carbohydrates by eating six or more daily servings of a combination of breads, cereals, and legumes.
- Maintain protein intake at moderate levels.
- Balance food intake and physical activity to maintain appropriate body weight.
- The committee does not recommend alcohol consumption. For those who drink alcoholic beverages, the committee recommends limiting consumption to the equivalent of less than 1 oz of pure alcohol in a single day. This is the equivalent of two cans of beer, two small glasses of wine, or two average cocktails. Pregnant women should avoid alcoholic beverages.
- Limit total daily intake of salt (sodium chloride) to 6 g or less. Limit the use of salt in cooking and avoid adding it to food at the table. Salty, highly processed salty, salt-preserved, and salt-pickled foods should be consumed sparingly.
- Maintain adequate calcium intake.
- Avoid taking dietary supplements in excess of the RDA in any one day.
- Maintain an optimal intake of fluoride, particularly during the years of primary and secondary tooth formation and growth.

The newly released Population-Based Recommendations for the entire American population* are consistent with the recent dietary recommendations of the American Heart Association and the Food and Nutrition Board. The panel recommends the following nutrient intakes for healthy Americans (including healthy women and persons age 65 and older):

- Less than 10% of total calories from saturated fatty acids
- An average of 30% of total calories or less from all fat
- Dietary energy levels needed to reach or maintain a desirable body weight
- Less than 300 mg of cholesterol per day

TREATMENT†

Diet is the primary treatment for elevated blood cholesterol levels. While the initial classification of CHD risk and follow-up decisions are based on the plasma total-cholesterol level (see chapter 4, Nutrition Assessment), treatment decisions are based on the LDL-cholesterol level (*Figure 5.1*). The minimal goal of therapy is to lower LDL-cholesterol levels to below 160 mg/dL, or below 130 mg/dL if definite CHD or two other CHD risk factors are present. The schematic for recommended dietary treatment appears in *Figure 5.2*.

A two-step diet-therapy approach for cholesterol lowering is recommended by both the American Heart Association and the NCEP. The goal of the recommended dietary therapy is to provide a nutritionally adequate intake, to reduce saturated fatty acids and cholesterol progressively, and to promote weight loss when indicated. The Step One and Step Two diets are defined in *Table 5.1.* On the Step One Diet, total fat is less than 30% of calories, saturated fatty acids are less than 10% of calories, and cholesterol is less than 300 mg/day. Saturated fatty acids are reduced further to less than 7% of calories and cholesterol is less than 200 mg/day on the Step Two Diet. Since the Step One Diet can be achieved with the reduction of major sources of saturated fatty acids and cholesterol in the diet, significant changes in dietary habits are often not required. In the Step Two Diet, saturated fatty acids and cholesterol are reduced further and more significant dietary changes are required.

The Step One Diet is most frequently prescribed by and explained by a physician or the physician's staff or both. However, if a registered dietitian is available, he or she is the most qualified to teach the Step One Diet. The plasma total-cholesterol level as well as dietary adherence should be assessed at four to six weeks and again at three months. If the plasma total-cholesterol goal is achieved, the LDL-cholesterol level should also be measured to assure that the LDL-cholesterol goal has also been met.[6] If successful, the patient is monitored four times yearly during year 1 and twice yearly thereafter. If the plasma total-cholesterol goal has not been achieved, the patient is referred to a registered dietitian for either assistance with the Step One Diet or progression to the Step Two Diet. The plasma total-cholesterol level and dietary adherence should be monitored after four to six weeks and three months of therapy. Long-term monitoring begins if the plasma total-cholesterol and LDL-cholesterol goals have been achieved. At least six months (or less for patients with severely elevated— > 225 mg/dL—LDL-cholesterol levels) of intensive dietary therapy is recommended before drug therapy is initiated in people who do not achieve the plasma total-cholesterol and LDL-cholesterol goal. For patients on lipid-lowering drugs, dietary therapy is also indicated. Dietary therapy along with drug therapy will enhance the effectiveness of the treatment. Often dietary therapy allows the drug dose administered to be lower, thereby reducing the number and severity of side effects as well as the cost of the therapy.

*Taken from the draft of the *NCEP Report of the Expert Panel on Population Strategies for Blood Cholesterol Reduction,* February 15, 1990.
†By Cindy Ragin

Fig 5.1
Classification and treatment decisions for LDL-cholesterol levels. From National Cholesterol Education Program Expert Panel. Report on detection, evaluation, and treatment of high blood cholesterol in adults. **Arch Intern Med.** ***1988;148:36.***

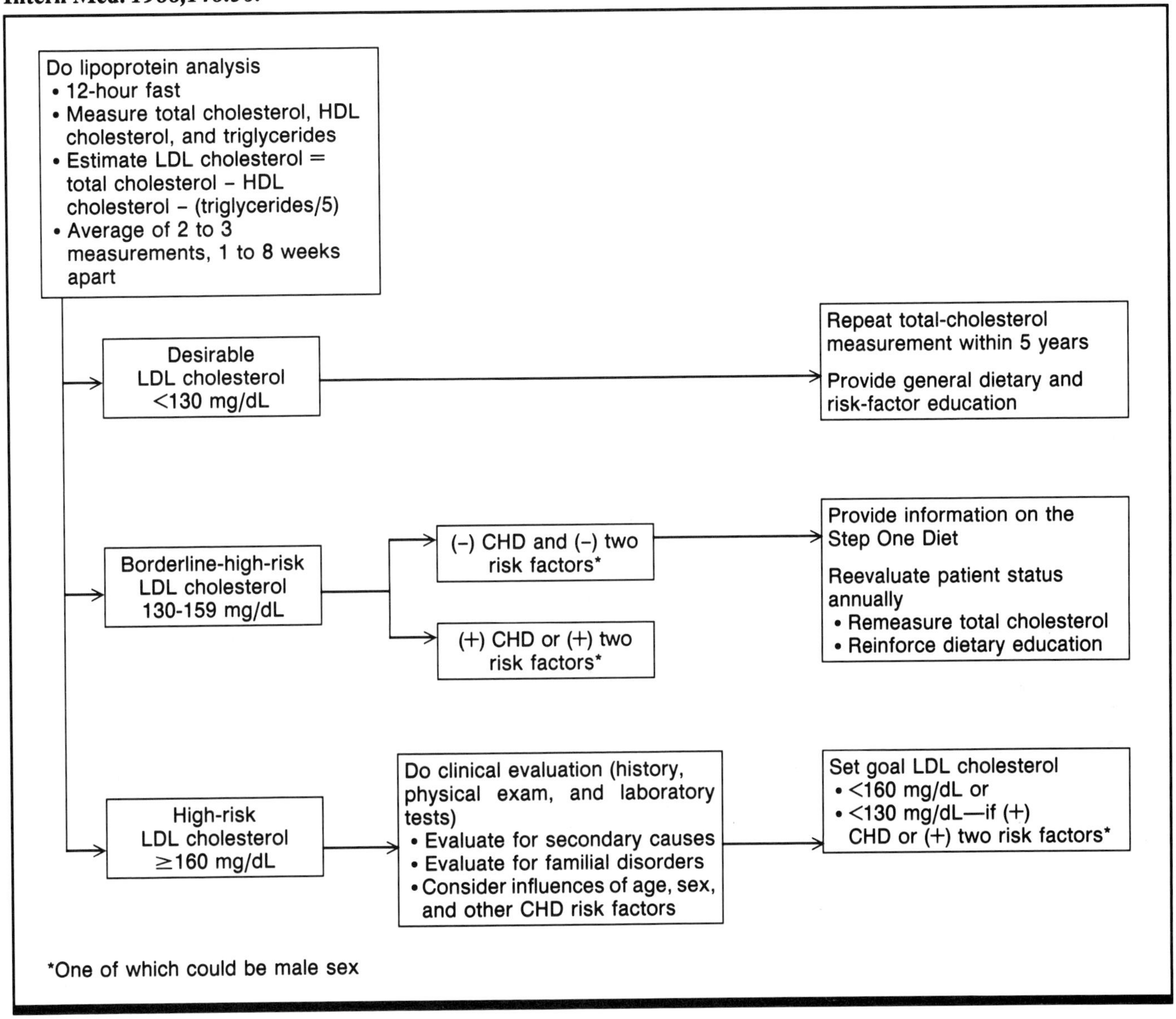

Fig 5.2
Classification of dietary treatment based on total cholesterol and LDL cholesterol. From National Cholesterol Education Program Expert Panel. Report on detection, evaluation, and treatment of high blood cholesterol in adults. **Arch Intern Med.** ***1988;148:36.***

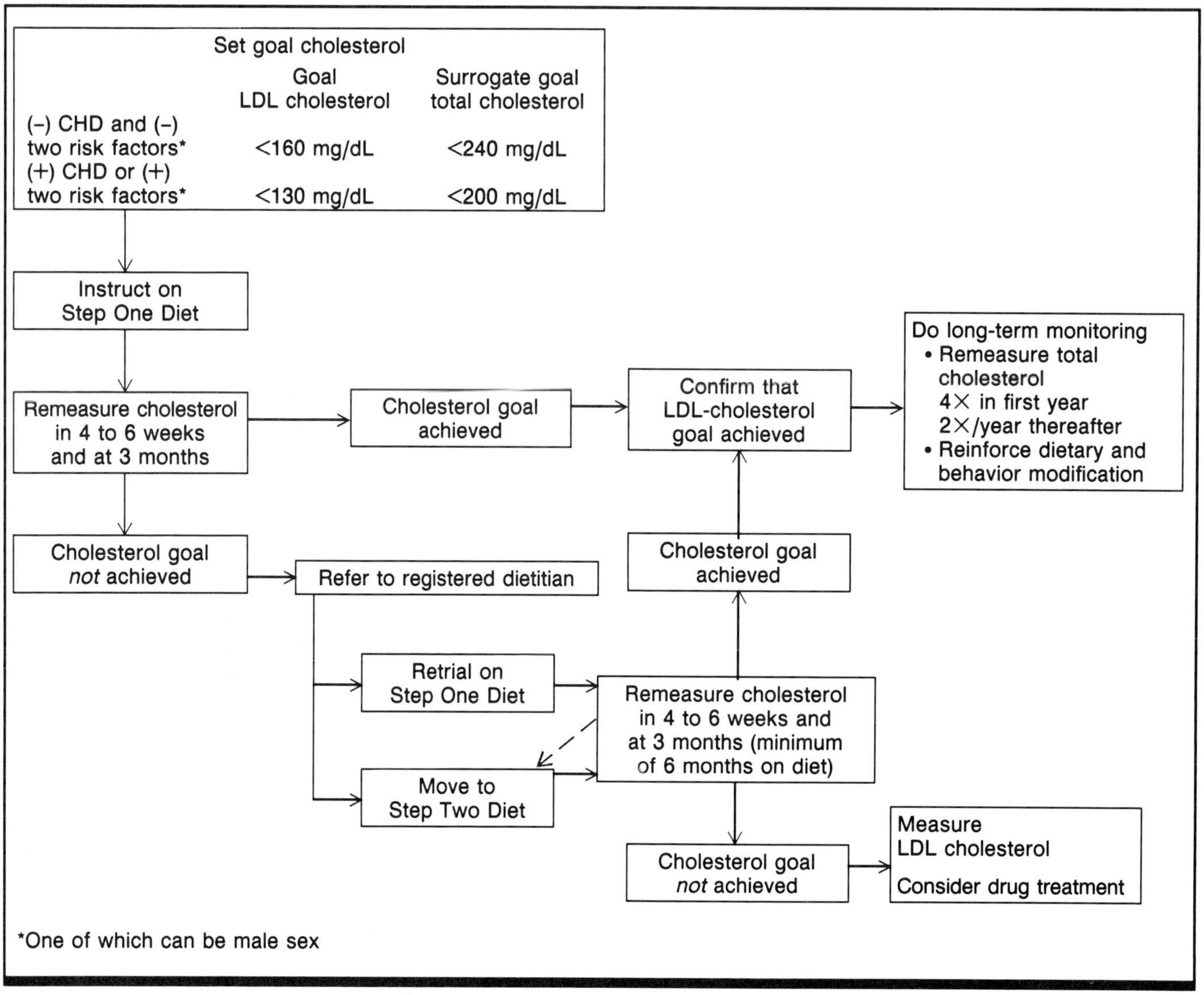

Table 5.1
Dietary Therapy for High Blood Cholesterol

Nutrient	Recommended Intake: Step One Diet	Step Two Diet
Total fat	Less than 30% of total calories	Less than 30% of total calories
Saturated fatty acids	Less than 10% of total calories	Less than 7% of total calories
Polyunsaturated fatty acids	Up to 10% of total calories	Up to 10% of total calories
Monounsaturated fatty acids	10% to 15% of total calories	10% to 15% of total calories
Carbohydrates	50% to 60% of total calories	50% to 60% of total calories
Protein	10% to 20% of total calories	10% to 20% of total calories
Cholesterol	Less than 300 mg/day	Less than 200 mg/day
Total calories	To achieve and maintain desirable weight	To achieve and maintain desirable weight

From National Cholesterol Education Program Expert Panel. Report on detection, evaluation, and treatment of high blood cholesterol in adults. *Arch Intern Med.* 1988;148:36.

The rationale for the recommended diet-therapy approach appears in the NCEP Expert Panel report on the detection, evaluation and treatment of high blood cholesterol in adults.[6] The following is a brief summary.

Nutritionally Adequate Diet

Therapeutic diets must be nutritionally adequate. They must meet the RDAs for vitamins, minerals, and protein. They should also contain a variety of foods from all four food groups. The diets should be palatable and acceptable.

Total Fat

In both Step One and Step Two diets, total fat should not exceed 30% of calories. The purpose of decreasing total fat from 37% of calories (the average intake) is to facilitate the reduction of saturated fatty acids and to promote weight reduction when indicated. A further reduction in fat is not required for reducing plasma total-cholesterol and LDL-cholesterol levels to desirable levels if unsaturated fatty acids are emphasized. For persons who are highly motivated and who require a greater lipid-lowering response than attainable by the Step Two Diet, there is another diet option: A very-low-fat ($\leq$20% of calories), low-saturated-fat and low-cholesterol diet ("phase III"), referred to as a near-vegetarian diet, is described in this chapter.

Saturated Fatty Acids

Saturated fatty acids are the most hypercholesterolemic dietary constituent. The hypercholesterolemic saturated fatty acids are $C_{12:0}$, lauric acid; $C_{14:0}$, myristic acid; and $C_{16:0}$, palmitic acid. Stearic acid, $C_{18:0}$, found in chocolate (cocoa butter) and meat, does not raise the plasma total-cholesterol level. Since

Americans consume approximately 13% to 16% of calories from saturated fatty acids, the Step One and Step Two diets require a one-third to one-half reduction, respectively, in saturated fatty acids. Animal fats, palm oil, palm kernel oil, and coconut oil are rich sources of saturated fatty acids.

Polyunsaturated Fatty Acids: (Omega-6 and Omega-3 Fatty Acids)

Americans presently consume approximately 7% of their calories as polyunsaturated fatty acids including both omega-6 and omega-3 fatty acids. It is recommended[6] that therapeutic diets contain at least this amount and preferably more (up to and not exceeding 10% of calories from omega-6 and omega-3 fatty acids). Omega-6 fatty acids should replace, in part, saturated fatty acids in the diet. Higher intakes are not recommended since the long-term safety of diets high in omega-6 acids is not known. Diets high in omega-6 fatty acids can be calorically dense and cause weight gain.

The major categories of polyunsaturated fatty acids are omega-6 and omega-3 fatty acids. Vegetable oils (including safflower oil, sunflower seed oil, soybean oil and corn oil) are rich in linoleic acid, the major omega-6 fatty acid in the diet. Omega-6 fatty acids lower plasma total-cholesterol and LDL-cholesterol levels. Given in amounts that exceed recommended levels, omega-6 fatty acids may also lower plasma HDL-cholesterol levels. Accordingly, omega-6 fatty acids do not appear to lower HDL-cholesterol levels at intakes that are within recommended ranges. Fish oils are the major source of omega-3 fatty acids, of which eicosapentenaenoic acid (EPA) and docosahexaenoic acid (DHA) are the major fatty acids. Large doses have been shown to lower plasma triglyceride consistently but not consistently lower plasma total-cholesterol levels. Replacing fatty meats and cheese with fish is recommended to provide omega-3 acids and as a means by which saturated fatty acids (and total fat) can be reduced. At least two fish meals are recommended weekly. Fish-oil supplements are not recommended.

Monounsaturated Fatty Acids

Monounsaturated fatty acids should contribute 10% to 15% of calories in both the Step One and Step Two diets. Americans presently consume 14% to 16% of their calories as monounsaturated fatty acids, much of which comes from animal products that are also high in saturated fatty acids. Oleic acid is the major monounsaturated fatty acid in the diet. Other sources include olive oil, rapeseed (canola) oil, and high-oleic acid sunflower seed and safflower oil. When animal-fat intake is reduced to lower saturated-fatty-acid intake, it is appropriate to use vegetable oils high in monounsaturated fatty acids.

Recently, monounsaturated fatty acids have been shown to be as potent as omega-6 fatty acids in reducing plasma total-cholesterol and LDL-cholesterol levels. Unlike large amounts of omega-6 fatty acids, however, they do not lower the HDL-cholesterol level. Monounsaturated fatty acids may be a more desirable lipid-lowering fat than omega-6 fatty acids. More work is needed in this area since the independent cholesterol-lowering effect of monounsaturated fatty acids compared with omega-6 fatty acids is being questioned.

Dietary Cholesterol

Dietary cholesterol is hypercholesterolemic and elevates both plasma total-cholesterol and LDL-cholesterol levels. The recommendation of an upper limit of 300 mg/day of cholesterol is both practical and reasonable for the Step One Diet. A further restriction (200 mg/day) is required on the Step Two Diet. Further reductions would result in a greater plasma cholesterol-lowering effect.

Protein

The level of protein in the diet is generally consistent, ranging from 10% to 20% of calories despite significant modifications in fat quantity and quality. There are no specifications regarding the source of protein in the Step One and Step Two diets.

Carbohydrate

The Step One and Step Two diets recommend that carbohydrate intake contribute 50% to 60% of calories. Sources of carbohydrate are simple sugars, complex digestible carbohydrate (starch), and complex indigestible carbohydrate (fiber). To help ensure that the diet is nutritionally adequate, complex carbohydrates should contribute more than half of the digestible carbohydrate. An increase in dietary carbohydrate may raise the plasma triglyceride level transiently or permanently (although current research suggests that plasma triglyceride levels begin to normalize with long-term consumption of a high-carbohydrate diet).

Total Calories

In overweight people, weight reduction will lower elevated (and normal) LDL-cholesterol and triglyceride levels; in some people, it will raise HDL-cholesterol levels. In fact, normalizing body weight alone will normalize the LDL-cholesterol level in some people. Exercise is beneficial in losing and controlling weight, and it favorably affects plasma lipid levels (it decreases serum triglycerides, increases HDL-cholesterol levels, and sometimes lowers LDL-cholesterol levels).

Fiber

While insoluble fiber contributes to normal colon function and adds bulk to the stools, it has little or no effect on plasma lipid levels. Soluble fibers (pectin, gums, and psyllium) have been shown to lower the plasma total-cholesterol level. Beta-glucans, present in oat products and beans, lower plasma cholesterol 5% to 15% when 15 to 25 g/day are consumed. Improved gastrointestinal tolerance has been reported with prolonged fiber usage.

Alcohol

Alcohol increases plasma triglyceride and HDL-cholesterol levels. Epidemiologically, alcohol consumption is a negative risk factor for CHD. Since alcohol abuse causes social, physiological, and psychological problems, a recommendation to increase alcohol consumption is inappropriate, but moderate alcohol intake need not be discouraged unless there is an indication to do so.

EXPECTED LDL-CHOLESTEROL RESPONSE TO DIETARY THERAPY*

The response to diet therapy is affected by the patient's habitual diet and inherent responsiveness.[6] The greatest reduction in LDL-cholesterol levels (absolute decrease) occurs most frequently in patients with higher, rather than relatively low, cholesterol levels.[6] A 30 to 40 mg/dL reduction in total cholesterol can be expected when a patient with a typical American diet follows the Step One Diet. A further reduction of 15 mg/dL can be expected when advancing to the Step Two Diet. Diets even lower in cholesterol and saturated fatty acids and higher in fiber would produce greater reductions in plasma total cholesterol and LDL cholesterol. Most of the decrease in the plasma total-cholesterol level occurs as a result of reduction in LDL cholesterol.[6] Some people will have greater or lesser responses than expected.

IMPLEMENTATION OF THE STEP ONE AND STEP TWO DIETS*

In-depth information appears in two sources: the NCEP Expert Panel report on the detection, evaluation and treatment of high blood cholesterol in adults[6] and the American Heart Association's handbook.[8] A brief summary follows. *Table 5.2* summarizes the diet modifications recommended to lower blood cholesterol levels for the Step One Diet. To reduce total fat, saturated fatty acids, and cholesterol, the intake of butterfat (found in butter, cheese, chocolate, ice cream, whole milk, and low-fat milk) should be reduced. Only lean meat is recommended. Visible fat should be removed, and fat should be allowed to drain from the meat during cooking. Chicken skin should be removed. Fish should be frequently substituted for meat. Rich sources of cholesterol in the diet (eggs and organ meats) should be limited. Consumption of vegetable oils rich in saturated fatty acids (coconut, palm kernel, palm, and hydrogenated vegetable oils) should be decreased. Skim milk and skim-milk products are recommended.

Specific Subgroup Recommendations

Table 5.2 provides recommended dietary modifications for the Step One Diet. Additional information about food groups is listed below.

Meats. It is not necessary to limit red-meat consumption severely. Lean cuts of beef, pork, lamb and veal are acceptable. Lean cuts of beef include: sirloin tip, round steak, rump roast, arm roast or center-cut ham, loin chops, and tenderloin. A list of 30 different cuts of lean meat appears in the appendix (see Table 14.26).

High-fat processed meat products (such as bacon, bologna, salami, sausage, and hot dogs) and organ meats (such as liver, sweetbreads, kidneys, and brain) should be used only occasionally or eliminated. The skin and underlying fat layers of chicken and turkey should be removed, and poultry should not be prepared with fats rich in saturated fatty acids. Fish should not be prepared with fats rich in saturated fatty acids. Shellfish is generally low in fat. Some shellfish are relatively high in cholesterol (see Table 14.24 in the appendix); they can be included in the diet within the recommended cholesterol intake. A total of 6 oz of lean meat, poultry, and fish can be included in the diet daily.

Dairy products. Skim milk is recommended. The consumption of natural and processed cheeses should be limited; low-fat (1% or 2%) cottage cheese, low-fat cheese that contributes less than 6 grams of fat per ounce, or synthetic cheeses made from vegetable oils can be substituted for high-fat cheese. Nonfat or low-fat yogurt are recommended. Heavy cream and sour cream should be avoided. Two servings of low-fat or nonfat dairy products (eg, 16 oz of skim

*By the Editors

Table 5.2
Recommended Diet Modifications to Lower Blood Cholesterol: The Step One Diet

Food Group	Choose	Decrease
Fish, chicken, turkey, and lean meats	Fish; white-meat poultry without skin; lean cuts of beef, lamb, pork or veal; shellfish	Fatty cuts of beef, lamb, pork; spare ribs; organ meats; regular cold cuts; sausage; hot dogs; bacon; sardines; roe
Skim and low-fat milk, cheese, yogurt, and dairy substitutes	Skim or 1% fat milk (liquid, powdered, evaporated); buttermilk; substitute 1 cup skim milk alone or with up to 1 cup nonfat dry-milk powder added instead of whole milk (for consistency in cooking); For acceptable whipped topping: combine 1/3 cup ice water, 1 tbsp lemon juice, 3/4 tsp vanilla, and 1/3 cup nonfat dry-milk powder; beat 10 minutes or until stiff; add 2 tbsp sugar	Whole milk (4% fat): regular, evaporated, condensed; cream; half and half; 2% milk; imitation milk products; most nondairy creamers; whipped toppings
	Nonfat (0% fat) or low-fat yogurt	Whole-milk yogurt
	Low-fat cottage cheese (1% or 2% fat)	Whole-milk cottage cheese (4% fat)
	Low-fat cheeses, farmer, or pot cheeses (all of these should be labeled no more than 2–6 g fat/oz)	All-natural cheeses, (eg, blue, roquefort, camembert, cheddar, Swiss)
		Low-fat or "diet" cream cheese, low-fat or "diet" sour cream
		Cream cheese, sour cream
	Sherbet, sorbet	Ice cream
Eggs	Egg whites (2 whites = 1 whole egg in recipes), or mix together 1 egg white, 2 tsp nonfat milk powder, and 2 tsp acceptable oil*; cholesterol-free egg substitutes	Egg yolks
Fruits and vegetables	Fresh, frozen, canned or dried fruits and vegetables	Vegetables prepared in butter, cream, or other sauces
Breads and cereals	Homemade baked goods using unsaturated oils sparingly, angel food cake, low-fat crackers, low-fat cookies	Commercial baked goods: pies, cakes, doughnuts, croissants, pastries, muffins, biscuits, high-fat crackers, high-fat cookies
	Rice, pasta, barley, bulgur, legumes	Egg noodles
	Whole-grain breads and cereals (oatmeal, whole wheat, rye, bran, multigrain, etc)	Breads in which eggs are a major ingredient, cereals with coconut oil or palm oil or palm kernel oil
Fats and oils	Acceptable unsaturated vegetable oils*	Butter, coconut oil, palm oil, palm kernel oil, bacon fat, hydrogenated vegetable shortening
	Margarine or shortening made from one of the acceptable unsaturated oils	
	Reduced-fat margarine	
	Mayonnaise, salad dressings made with acceptable unsaturated oils	Dressings made with egg yolk
	Low-fat dressings	
	Seeds and nuts, nonhydrogenated, old-fashioned-style peanut butter (100% peanuts)	Coconut, hydrogenated peanut butter

*Acceptable oils include canola, corn, cottonseed, olive, safflower, sesame, soybean, and sunflower.

From National Cholesterol Education Program Expert Panel. Report on detection, evaluation, and treatment of high blood cholesterol in adults. *Arch Intern Med.* 1988; 148:36.

milk) should be included daily as a source of calcium. A list of low-fat cheeses appears in the appendix (see Table 14.30).

Fats and oils. The consumption of fats high in saturated fatty acids and cholesterol (butter fat, lard, beef fat) and saturated fatty acids (coconut oil, palm oil, palm kernel oil) should be reduced. The latter are used in baked products, processed foods, popcorn oils, and nondairy creamers, although many industries are removing tropical oils from their products. Consumers are encouraged to read labels.

Six to 8 tsp of unsaturated vegetable oils can be included in the diet daily. Recommended vegetable oils include canola, olive, cottonseed, corn, safflower, sesame, soybean, and sunflower. Small amounts of peanut oil are acceptable. Regular stick-type margarine should be limited. A reduced-fat and reduced-calorie tub margarine should be recommended over a regular stick-type margarine. However, a variety of unsaturated fat and oils should be included in the 6 to 8 tsp recommended daily. Other fats made from recommended unsaturated fat (mayonnaise and salad dressings) can be included in the diet within the recommended fat allowance.

Table 5.3
Number of Portions per Day from Food Groups of Diets With Different Calorie Levels

	Calories per Day							
	Step One Diet				**Step Two Diet**			
Food Group	**2500**	**2000**	**1600**	**1200**	**2500**	**2000**	**1600**	**1200**
Meat, poultry, and seafood	6 oz	6 oz	6 oz	6 oz	6 oz	6 oz	6 oz	6 oz
Eggs (per week)	3	3	3	3	1	1	1	1
Dairy products	4	3	3	2	3	2	2	2
Fat	8	6	4	3	8	7	5	3
Bread, cereal, pasta, and starchy vegetables	10	7	4	3	10	8	5	4
Vegetables	4	4	4	4	5	4	4	4
Fruit	5	3	3	3	7	4	3	3
Optional foods*	2	2	2	0	2	2	2	0
Calories	2499	1964	1625	1192	2459	1986	1596	1213
Fat, % calories†	29%	30%	30%	32%	25%	27%	28%	27%
Saturated fatty acids, % calories	8%	8%	9%	10%	6%	6%	7%	7%
Monounsaturated fatty acids, % calories	10%	11%	11%	12%	9%	10%	10%	10%
Polyunsaturated fatty acids, % calories	6%	6%	6%	6%	6%	7%	7%	5%
Cholesterol, mg	311	300	299	286	217	208	208	205
Protein, % calories	19%	21%	23%	25%	18%	20%	22%	26%
Carbohydate, % calories	52%	49%	47%	43%	57%	53%	50%	47%
Sodium, mg	2772	2179	1737	1356	3025	2419	1955	1682
Calcium, mg	1322	1012	943	669	1149	825	744	687
Iron, mg	21	17	13	11	22	18	14	12

*If foods from the "optional foods" group are not used, add two portions from the "bread, cereal, pasta, and starchy vegetables" group plus one portion from the "fat" group. See Table 5.5 for optional foods composite.
†The values for total fat in the eating plans are greater than the sum of saturated, monounsaturated, and polyunsaturated fatty acids, since total fat includes not only fatty acids but also other fatty substances and glycerol.

Reproduced with permission, *Dietary Treatment of Hypercholesterolemia: A Handbook for Counselors,* 1988. American Heart Association.

Eggs. On the Step One Diet, egg yolks should be limited to three to four per week. On the Step Two Diet, egg yolks should be limited to two per week.

Fruits and vegetables. Fruits and vegetables should be included with meals and snacks. They contribute vitamins, fiber, and minerals to the diet.

Breads, cereals, pasta, rice, legumes. Foods low in fat should be substituted for foods higher in fat. Small amounts of meat, poultry, and fish can be eaten with larger amounts of pasta, rice, legumes, and vegetables in order to lower fat, saturated fatty acids, cholesterol, and calories.

Nuts. While high in fat, nuts are generally rich in unsaturated fatty acids. Limiting the intake of nuts and peanut butter will be necessary to keep the diet within fat allowance.

Other suggestions. Good choices for snacks include graham crackers, RyKrisp, melba toast, soda crackers, bagels, English muffins, fruit, cereals, vegetables, and skim-milk dairy products. Snacks high in fat such as most candy, snack crackers, french fries, and chips should be limited. For desserts, fruit, nonfat yogurt, fruit ice, sherbet, angel food cake, Jello, frozen low-fat (1%) or nonfat yogurt and, occasionally, ice milk are acceptable.

Table 5.4
Number of Portions per Day from Food Groups of Diets With Different Calorie Levels (5 oz of Meat)

	Calories per Day		
Food Group	**2000**	**1600**	**1200**
Meat, poultry, and seafood	5 oz	5 oz	5 oz
Eggs (per week)	1	1	1
Dairy products	3	3	3
Fat	7	5	4
Bread, cereal, pasta, and starchy vegetables	8	5	4
Vegetables	4	4	4
Fruit	4	3	3
Optional foods*	2	2	0
Calories	2005	1616	1197
Fat, % calories†	27%	27%	29%
Saturated fatty acids, % calories	6%	7%	7%
Monounsaturated fatty acids, % calories	10%	10%	11%
Polyunsaturated fatty acids, % calories	7%	7%	6%
Cholesterol, mg	192	192	181
Protein, % calories	19%	22%	23%
Carbohydrate, % calories	54%	51%	48%
Sodium, mg	2605	2141	1660
Calcium, mg	1041	959	684
Iron, mg	17	13	11

*If foods from the "optional foods" group are not used, add two portions from the "bread, cereal, pasta, and starchy vegetables" group plus one portion from the "fat" group. See Table 5.5 for optional foods composite.
†The values for total fat in the eating plans are greater than the sum of saturated, monounsaturated, and polyunsaturated fatty acids, since total fat includes not only fatty acids but also other fatty substances and glycerol.

Reproduced with permission, *Dietary Treatment of Hypercholesterolemia: A Handbook for Counselors,* 1988. American Heart Association.

Table 5.5
Optional Foods Composite

Food Name	Weight g	Energy cal	Fat g	Sat Fatty Acid g	Mono Fatty Acid g	Poly Fatty Acid g	Chol mg	Prot g	Carb g	Na mg	Ca mg	Iron mg
Alcohol composite	173.0	112.0	0.00	0.00	0.00	0.00	0.0	0.38	5.70	8.7	22.3	0.26
Sweets composite	79.5	72.7	0.28	0.12	0.11	0.03	0.5	0.65	17.91	21.5	8.6	0.10
Modified-fat dessert	49.7	143.0	4.41	0.69	1.22	2.24	0.2	1.86	25.08	90.5	18.1	0.44
Total for composite	**302.2**	**327.7**	**4.69**	**0.81**	**1.33**	**2.27**	**0.7**	**2.89**	**48.69**	**120.7**	**49.0**	**0.80**
Total for one portion	**101.0**	**109.0**	**1.56**	**0.27**	**0.44**	**0.76**	**0.2**	**0.96**	**16.23**	**40.2**	**16.3**	**0.27**

Sat, Mono, and Poly Fatty Acid = saturated, monounsaturated, and polyunsaturated fatty acids; Chol = cholesterol; Prot = protein; Carb = carbohydrate; Na = sodium; Ca = calcium.

Reproduced with permission, *Dietary Treatment of Hypercholesterolemia: A Handbook for Counselors,* 1988. American Heart Association.

Table 5.6
One-Day Sample Menus for Step One and Step Two Diets (approximately 2,000 Calories)

	Step One Diet	Step Two Diet
Breakfast	6 oz orange juice	6 oz orange juice
	1/2 c blueberries	1/2 c blueberries
	1 c oatmeal	1 c oatmeal
	1 slice whole wheat toast	2 slices whole-wheat toast
	1 tsp tub margarine	1 tsp tub margarine
	8 oz skim milk	8 oz skim milk
	Coffee	Coffee
	2 tsp sugar or jelly	2 tsp sugar or jelly
Lunch	Turkey sandwich	Turkey sandwich
	3 oz turkey (no skin)	3 oz turkey (no skin)
	2 slices bread	large Kaiser roll*
	1 tsp mayonnaise	1 tsp mayonnaise
	1/2 c potato salad with 1 tsp oil and 1 tsp vinegar	1/2 c potato salad with 1 tsp oil and 1 tsp vinegar
	1/2 c cole slaw with low-calorie dressing	1/2 c cole slaw with low-calorie dressing
	Small apple	Small apple
	Tea with lemon and honey	Tea with lemon and honey
Snack	8 oz skim milk	1 large tangerine
Dinner	3 oz lean roast beef	3 oz lean roast beef
	1 c stir-fry rice	1 c stir-fry rice
	1/2 c rice	1/2 c rice
	1/2 c mixed vegetables	1/2 c mixed vegetables
	2 tsp oil	2 tsp oil
	1/2 c cauliflower	1/2 c cauliflower
	1/2 c tossed salad with 1 tbsp Italian dressing	1/2 c tossed salad with 1 tbsp Italian dressing
	8 oz skim milk	8 oz skim milk
Snack	1 c air-popped corn	1 c air-popped corn

*3 bread exchanges. See Table 5.3 for food exchange information.

Basic Eating Plans

Basic eating plans for the Step One and Step Two diets have been published in The American Heart Association's handbook. These are presented in *Tables 5.3* and *5.4*. A list of optional foods and their nutrient information is in *Table 5.5*. Also included in the American Heart Association publication[8] are eating plans for people with special needs (ie, Step One Diet and Step Two Diet Eating Plans without dairy products; Step One Diet and Step Two Diet Eating Plans without desserts, sweets, or alcoholic beverages; and Step One Diet Eating Plans without eggs). One-day sample menus are presented in *Table 5.6*.

ALTERNATIVE APPROACHES TO THE STEP ONE AND STEP TWO DIETS

Two alternative approaches for the management of high blood cholesterol will be discussed. They are being used in practice on an individual basis. It is important to note that the diet high in monounsaturated fatty acids and the very-low-fat, high-carbohydrate diet are not officially endorsed by The American Dietetic Association, the American Heart Association, or SCAN.

High Monounsaturated Fatty-Acid Diet*

An alternative dietary approach suggested for cholesterol-lowering is the use of diets higher in total fat (approximately 35% of calories), high in monounsaturated fatty acids (approximately 20% of calories), and low in saturated fatty acids (< 10% of calories). Studies have shown that monounsaturated fatty acids are as effective in lowering plasma cholesterol levels as diets high in omega-6 fatty acids or low-fat diets.[9-12] These studies have shown that diets high in monounsaturated fatty acids and moderately high in total fat (approximately 35% of calories) can be as effective as the Step One and Step Two diets, provided that saturated fatty acids (primarily lauric, $C_{12:0}$; myristic, $C_{14:0}$; and palmitic, $C_{16:0}$) are decreased to less than 10% of calories. For some patients, diets high in monounsaturated fatty acids may be more popular for cholesterol lowering because they are effective and because some patients consider them to be more palatable than low-fat diets. Therefore, patient compliance with the cholesterol-lowering diet may be better. It is important to note, however, that diets high in monounsaturated fatty acids may make weight control more difficult than diets lower in total fat. Thus, a diet high in monounsaturated fatty acids and total fat is not suggested for persons who are attempting to lose weight.

Table 5.7
Percentage of Calories Consumed as Oleic Acid by Adults

Age	< 9.8%	9.9% to 15.1%	> 15.2%
18–24	22.6	51.1	26.3
25–34	19.9	50.0	30.1
35–44	17.8	48.1	34.1
45–54	19.6	47.5	32.9
55–64	19.9	47.4	32.7
65–74	23.6	47.5	28.9

Adapted from Abraham S, Dresser CM.[2]

Americans now consume 10% to 15% of their calories from oleic acid, the main source of monounsaturated fatty acids in the diet *(Table 5.7)*. Food patterns published by the American Heart Association[8] indicate that as calories from total fat and saturated fatty acids decrease, the percentage of calories from

*By Lynne W. Scott and Mary C. McMann

monounsaturated fatty acids also decreases. The decrease is from the 13% to 14% of calories from monounsaturated fatty acids in the typical American diet[12] to 10% to 11% in the AHA diet.

The primary source of monounsaturated fatty acids are olive oil and canola oil (see chapter 2, Table 2.5). Meat is also a source of monounsaturated fatty acids; however, it also contains appreciable quantities of saturated fatty acids. In the future, high-oleic-acid safflower and sunflower oils will likely be available on the retail market.

In the American culture, olive oil is not commonly used except in small amounts because of its distinctive flavor. Although peanut oil is a source of monounsaturated fatty acids, it contains almost 17% saturated fatty acids, and its use is not recommended as a way of increasing monounsaturated fatty acids in the diet. The principal way to add monounsaturated fatty acids to the diet is by using them in food preparation and via salad dressings.

If future research indicates that Americans should increase their intake of monounsaturated fatty acids, more products low in saturated fatty acids and high in monounsaturated fatty acids will need to be developed for consumer use. These products should include foods for both home and commercial uses.

The primary dietary guideline for reducing hypercholesterolemia is the reduction of saturated-fatty-acid intake to lower plasma LDL-cholesterol levels. When total fat and saturated fatty acids are reduced to less than 30% and less than 10%, respectively, up to 10% of calories can be provided by omega-6 fatty acids and the remainder from monounsaturated fatty acids. At this time, data are insufficient to make broad dietary recommendations for increasing monounsaturated-fatty-acid intake for the treatment of hypercholesterolemia.

Patients should be told about the additional lipid-lowering effects of a very-low-fat, near-vegetarian diet. In many cases, poor adherence by the patient with this type of diet may simply be from a lack of knowledge about implementing the diet and/or a lack of support from health care professionals, family, and friends.

A Very-Low-Fat, High-Carbohydrate Diet for Maximal Dietary Treatment and Prevention of Hyperlipidemia and Cardiovascular Disease*

A very-low-fat, high-carbohydrate diet (VLFHC) may be a safe and effective alternative to medical (pharmaceutical) intervention for treating hyperlipidemia in a patient who still has high plasma total-cholesterol and LDL-cholesterol levels after following the Step Two Diet advocated by the NCEP. On average this dietary approach may lower serum cholesterol nearly twice as much as the NCEP's Step Two Diet. Preliminary evidence also suggests that a VLFHC diet may be a viable alternative therapy to drugs and surgical intervention for some patients with angina or other evidence of advanced athero-scelerosis or both.

The diet advocated by Connor and Connor[7] has been referred to as the phase III diet. In this diet, fat provides no more than 20% of the calories, and saturated fatty acids are limited to 5% to 6% of calories. Less than 100 mg of dietary cholesterol is recommended per day. Carbohydrates supply at least 65% of calories. *Table 5.8* compares the phase III diet with a typical American diet.

*By James J. Kenney

Table 5.8
Chemical Composition of the Present American Diet, the New American Diet, and the Pritikin Therapeutic Diet—Alternative Approaches for Possible Use With Selected Patients

Nutrient	American Diet†	New American Diet (Phase III)†	Pritikin Therapeutic Plan‡
Cholesterol, mg*/day	300–435	100	25
Fat, percentage (%) of total calories	37	20	10
Saturated fat, % calories	13	5	2
Monounsaturated fat, % calories	14	8	4
Polyunsaturated fat, % calories	7	7	4
P/S value	0.5	1.3	2
Vegetable fat, % fat	40	75	95
Animal fat, % fat	60	25	5
Protein, % calories	16	15	15
Vegetable protein, % protein	32	56	75
Animal protein, % protein	68	44	25
Carbohydrate, % calories	46	65	75
Starch, % calories	17	40	50
Sugars added to food, % calories	20	10	0
Sugars naturally present in food, % calories	9	15	30
Dietary fiber, g*	12–18	45–60	60–90
Sodium, mEq*	200–300	75–100	15–70
Potassium, mEq	60–85	100–140	100–150

*mg = milligrams; g = grams; mEq = milliequivalent.
†Adapted from Connor SL, Connor WE.[7] Copyright © 1986 by Sonja L. Connor, MS, RD, and William E. Connor, MD. Reprinted by permission of Simon & Schuster, Inc.
‡From Kenney J (unpublished); not officially endorsed by SCAN.

Diets even lower in fat, saturated fatty acids, and cholesterol have been advocated by Pritikin,[13] Ornish,[14] McDougall,[15] and more recently by Kenney.[16] All of these books recommend limiting dietary fat to about 10% of calories and emphasize the consumption of minimally processed foods of vegetable origin.

These authors all advocate considerably more dietary change than that required by the NCEP dietary guidelines. Major dietary changes make adherence to these diet plans much more difficult. Nevertheless, the dietary and life-style changes these authors advocate are likely to prove safer and more cost-effective than pharmaceutical or surgical intervention. Clinicians must be careful not to confuse potential problems with compliance with a lack of efficacy.

While all patients should be informed of this approach before instituting drug therapy, only those patients who are sufficiently educated and motivated to maintain these dietary changes for a prolonged period are likely to benefit. Patient selection for this approach must consider the candidate's motivation and attitudes toward drugs, surgery, and life-style change. For patients who wish to avoid drugs and surgery for personal or monetary considerations, the VLFHC diet is likely to prove more efficacious than the NCEP's Step Two Diet.

In patients with CHD, the ultimate goal of therapy is not simply to reduce the plasma total-cholesterol level moderately. It is to prevent or reverse the progression of the underlying disease process (atherosclerosis). Unfortunately, there is still no definitive data that would enable the clinician to accurately predict the extent to which plasma cholesterol and other risk factors must be reduced in order to successfully treat (regress) atherosclerotic lesions in a given patient. Nevertheless, the bulk of the scientific evidence strongly suggests that the greater the reduction in plasma cholesterol, the greater the likelihood that atherosclerotic lesions will regress or stabilize rather than progress.

If regression of atherosclerotic lesions is the goal, the lowest possible plasma cholesterol attainable by a nutritionally adequate diet would seem more rational than a less-ambitious reduction in plasma cholesterol. A plasma cholesterol level less than 160 mg/dL and an LDL-cholesterol level less than 100 mg/dL are achievable goals in many persons with life-threatening atherosclerotic lesions. This goal frequently can be achieved without drugs only with the adoption of a VLFHC diet.

Dietary intervention to lower the plasma total-cholesterol level should also favorably affect other independent CVD risk factors (ie, hypertension, obesity, diabetes, low HDL cholesterol, and so on). The overall efficacy of any dietary approach should also consider its likely impact on other diet-related diseases (eg, diverticulosis, cancer, gout, gallstones, and kidney stones) as well as other coexisting pathologies (eg, renal disease, ulcers, and Crohn's disease). In general, a VLFHC diet would likely have a favorable impact on other CVD risk factors and diet-related diseases.[5,17]

The expert panel for the NCEP has estimated that switching from the typical American diet to the Step One Diet will lower plasma cholesterol "on average by 5% to 7% and the Step Two Diet could be expected to cause a further decline of approximately 5% to 7%."[6] For the Step Two Diet, this would correspond to about a 10% to 14% decrease in plasma cholesterol. Most people with a high plasma total-cholesterol level will be unable to attain the NCEP's "desirable" cholesterol level (< 200 mg/dL) or LDL-cholesterol level (< 130 mg/dL) using the Step Two Diet. Few would be able to achieve a level of plasma cholesterol that would promote regression of atherosclerosis (< 160 mg/dL).

Since about one in four Americans has a plasma total-cholesterol level in excess of 240 mg/dL, the current NCEP guidelines will inevitably require many patients to take hypocholesterolemic drugs for the rest of their lives in order to achieve and maintain a minimally acceptable cholesterol level. The long-term health consequences of taking most lipid-lowering drugs have not been adequately studied. Even if detrimental long-term side effects prove to be rare, the cost-benefit ratio of massive drug intervention is likely to be very high.[18] It is reasonable to explore promising alternatives that are likely to prove less expensive.

Epidemiological evidence has shown that populations consuming a VLFHC diet have an average plasma cholesterol below 160 mg/dL and a very low incidence of CVD. For example, the average plasma total-cholesterol and LDL-cholesterol levels of adult Tarahumara Indians are 134 mg/dL and 87 mg/dL, respectively.[19] The Tarahumara diet provided about 10% fat and 75 mg of dietary cholesterol daily. A group of strict vegetarians living in the Boston area had average plasma total-cholesterol and LDL-cholesterol levels of 133 mg/dL and 78 mg/dL, respectively.[20] Their diet contained about 15% calories from fat and only 14 mg of cholesterol per day. These studies suggest that it is possible to achieve and maintain a plasma total-cholesterol level below 160 mg/dL and an LDL-cholesterol level below 100 mg/dL on a VLFHC diet.

Clinical studies have demonstrated very beneficial effects of a VLFHC diet on the plasma lipids of hyperlipidemic individuals. In a three-month trial in hyperlipidemic patients (mean plasma total cholesterol = 305 mg/dL) with severe CVD, total cholesterol and LDL cholesterol decreased 41% on a diet containing 10% calories from fat and about 75 mg of cholesterol per day. Long-term follow-up of subjects closely adhering to a low-fat (8% of calories) and low-cholesterol (35 mg/day) diet for an average of 5.9 years found that plasma total-cholesterol and LDL-cholesterol levels were 34% and 40% lower, respectively, than age-matched controls.[21] These studies suggest that a VLFHC can achieve and maintain considerably greater reductions in plasma total cholesterol and LDL cholesterol than the NCEP's Step Two Diet. However, recent evidence suggests that the additional lipid-lowering benefits of diets with less than 26% calories from fat and less than 7% calories from saturated fatty acids are not significantly greater than that achieved by the Step Two Diet (R. Knopp, personal communication). At this time, additional information is needed to establish the lipid-lowering effectiveness of diets low in fat that vary in fat quantity (10% to 26% of calories from fat).

It seems likely that the greater reduction in blood lipids that can be achieved by a VLFHC diet compared with the Step Two Diet would have a more-favorable effect on the underlying cause of most CVD, namely atherosclerosis. Research in nonhuman primates has clearly shown that switching from a diet high in fat and cholesterol to a VLFHC diet not only dramatically reduces plasma total-cholesterol and LDL cholesterol, but also regresses atherosclerosis lesions.[22] It has also been demonstrated in monkeys that a diet that considerably lowers the plasma total-cholesterol level will be most likely to regress atherosclerotic lesions produced by a diet high in fat and cholesterol.[23]

The results of animal research coupled with epidemiological evidence suggests that a VLFHC diet will produce a maximal plasma cholesterol-lowering response in patients with hyperlipidemia or advanced atherosclerosis or both. Preliminary clinical trials have been encouraging. A five-year follow-up study of 64 patients with documented CVD who were instructed to follow a VLFHC diet observed a death rate only slightly higher than expected for men their age.[24] At follow-up, only 32% reported angina compared with 80% initially, even though compliance was a problem for about one in four. More recently, regression of atherosclerotic lesions has been reported in patients with advanced coronary artery disease (who refused bypass surgery) using a VLFHC diet and other life-style changes.[25] One year later, Ornish reported more evidence of regression on a VLFHC diet, while patients following the AHA diet continued to show progression of atherosclerotic lesions.[26] More recently Blankenhorn et al found that the intake of both polyunsaturated and monounsaturated fatty acids positively correlated with the progression of atherosclerotic lesions, while regression of plaques was more likely to occur when carbohydrates or protein replaced saturated fatty acids in the diet. These findings, if confirmed, would support a VLFHC diet for the treatment of advanced atherosclerosis.[27]

The use of a VLFHC diet to treat hyperlipidemia and CVD remains limited. The primary reasons given for not advocating a VLFHC diet are concerns about its nutritional adequacy and possible deleterious effects along with the assumption that long-term compliance is not possible in a population exposed to a highly refined diet emphasizing animal products.

The nutritional adequacy of diets high in fiber and limited in animal products has been questioned repeatedly. Considerable scientific evidence, however, suggests that such diets do not routinely create nutritional deficiencies. Two long-term studies found no evidence of either vitamin or mineral deficiencies in free-living subjects closely adhering to a VLFHC diet for more than two years[28] and more than five years.[21] "It is the position of The American Dietetic Association that vegetarian diets are healthful and nutritionally adequate when appropriately planned."[17]

The nutritional adequacy of any therapeutic diet, however, should be monitored periodically. If, on occasion, a nutritional deficiency is found, dietary changes or the use of an appropriate supplement or both would appear to be a more rational response than abandoning an effective therapeutic diet that, in at least some cases, can be expected to regress atherosclerotic lesions. The risk associated with more-aggressive dietary intervention must be weighed against the risks associated with the increased use of pharmaceutical agents and surgical intervention.

VLFHC diets for treating or preventing atherosclerosis have been questioned primarily because they are claimed to increase serum triglyceride levels and lower HDL-cholesterol levels[9,10] and promote hyperinsulinemia and hyperglycemia.[29] Hyperinsulinemia has also been associated with sodium retention and hypertension.[30] VLFHC diets have also been criticized because they lack satiety[31] and may trigger binge eating.[32] These criticisms have been based on short-term clinical studies. Population studies, however, have shown that VLFHC diets are associated with lower incidences of CVD, obesity, and diabetes than high-fat diets.[33,34] Nor is there evidence that serum triglycerides, insulin, or blood pressure are clinically elevated in people consuming VLFHC diet for prolonged periods.

In addition, eating disorders reportedly have been triggered by low-carbohydrate diets,[35] and obesity appears to be better correlated with dietary fat intake than caloric intake.[36,37] It is not clear that high-carbohydrate diets might trigger binge eating when most bulimics report that their binge eating was initially triggered by a carbohydrate-restricted diet.

How can these and other contradictory claims and observations be explained? Inappropriate experimental controls imposed by researchers during short-term clinical trials are the most likely explanation. Some short-term clinical trials have found increased serum insulin and triglycerides on high-carbohydrate versus high-fat diets. In short-term trials when a high-carbohydrate diet is compared to high-fat diet, calories or body weight or both are held constant.

It has been argued that caloric intake and fiber intake must be identical when comparing high-fat diets with high-carbohydrate diets.[38] However, if weight loss is a natural consequence of increasing the carbohydrate-to-fat ratio, then these experimental controls create an artificial situation that may not apply in the long run to free-living subjects.

When calorie intake is not controlled, human subjects markedly reduce their calorie intake on low-fat (15% to 20%) diets, rather than high-fat (45% to 50%) diets (2,087 versus 2,714 calories/day, respectively) even when palatability and fiber are similar on both diets.[39] Since most high-fat foods have little or no fiber, and most vegetable foods that are low in fat (unless refined) contain an appreciable amount of dietary fiber, under normal circumstances dietary fiber intake will decrease in response to increasing dietary fat. Switching from a diet high in refined carbohydrates to one that is less refined with more fiber results in lower insulin levels and improved blood lipids in type II diabetics.[40] When a high-carbohydrate, high-fiber diet was compared to a high-fat, low-fiber diet, the difference in ad libitum caloric intake was even greater (1,570 versus 3,000 calories/day, respectively).[41]

There are reasons why switching from a high-fat, low-fiber diet to one very low in fat and high in fiber leads to a reduced calorie intake and spontaneous weight loss.[16,42–45] If dietary fat does promote increased calorie intake and weight gain, it appears that the results of experiments that require subjects to consume the same calorie level (and/or maintain the same body weight) on both low-fat and high-fat diets might not be applicable to free-living subjects. Specifically, plasma triglyceride, insulin, and HDL-cholesterol levels (all of which have been shown to be adversely affected on a low-fat diet) may respond differently to less-controlled but more-typical (real-world) conditions.

These observations help to explain why epidemiological data show that persons with diabetes and normal subjects subsisting on low-fat, high-fiber diets have lower plasma total-cholesterol and LDL-cholesterol levels and higher HDL-cholesterol levels. They also experience far less atherosclerosis than persons with diabetes who consume a high-fat, low-fiber diet,[46] despite suggestions that reducing dietary fat would compromise diabetic control and have adverse effects on blood lipids. While it is most important to limit saturated fatty acids and cholesterol in the diabetic diet, it appears that replacing monounsaturated fatty acids with unrefined carbohydrate foods would incur additional benefits.[47]

Since it appears that weight loss is a normal consequence of adopting a VLFHC diet, one should expect this weight loss to mitigate the drop in HDL cholesterol reported in many short-term studies where carbohydrate is substituted isocalorically for fat. This may be why the relatively large drops in HDL cholesterol reported during short-term clinical studies (with fiber and calories carefully controlled) do not necessarily occur when subjects consume the very-low-fat diet ad libitum over several months.[48] There is also some evidence that replacing animal protein with vegetable protein may lower LDL-cholesterol levels but raise HDL-cholesterol levels.[49]

Other potential advantages of VLFHC diets include their decreased caloric density. This leads to increased meal frequency. A recent study suggests that increasing meal frequency and decreasing meal size may lower HDL cholesterol by more than 10%.[50] In addition, an increase in dietary fiber associated with a VLFHC diet (particularly soluble fiber) will not only help lower LDL cholesterol[51] but it may also reduce calorie intake and promote spontaneous weight loss.[52]

In conclusion, a VLFHC diet appears to be an effective dietary strategy for lowering plasma total-cholesterol and LDL-cholesterol levels. It has shown some promise for regressing atherosclerotic lesions without the adjunctive use of pharmaceutical agents. It also appears to be effective for weight loss, lowering blood pressure (especially if sodium is also restricted), and improving glycemic control. Furthermore, there is no compelling evidence that VLFHC diets create nutritional deficiencies or eating disorders, as has been suggested. It is also likely that a VLFHC diet might reduce the risk of developing some common cancers (eg, breast, colon, prostate, and female reproductive tract).[53]

At the present time, a VLFHC diet remains a viable therapeutic option for treating hypercholesterolemia or atherosclerosis or both. It should be seriously considered for patients who wish to avoid drug therapy for hyperlipidemia when the NCEP dietary guidelines fail to lower plasma total-cholesterol and LDL-cholesterol levels sufficiently. A VLFHC diet may also be efficacious in preventing restenosis after angioplasty or in reducing occlusion of bypass grafts. The widespread use of this diet would certainly reduce the need for pharmaceutical and/or surgical interventions in treating and preventing CVD. A VLFHC diet coupled with regular aerobic exercise appears to have more-favorable risk-benefit and cost-benefit ratios than current medical options.

One type of VLFHC is the Pritikin Plan. Recommended food choices and amounts are outlined in the Pritikin Lifetime Eating Plan brochure.* A summary follows.

Grains and starchy foods—Four or more servings of whole grains are recommended daily. These include wheat, oats, rye, corn, brown rice, barley and buckwheat (as cereal, pasta, bread, etc). Chestnuts, beans, peas, and starchy vegetables (potatoes, yams, winter squash, corn) are included in this group.

Table 5.9
Sample Menus for a Very-Low-Fat, High-Carbohydrate (VLFHC) Diet

Day 1	Day 2	Day 3	Day 4	Day 5	Day 6	Day 7
Cantaloupe Raisin bran cereal Skim milk English muffin with jam	Orange juice Whole-wheat pancakes topped with unsweetened applesauce	Plain lowfat yogurt with banana Cereal Bran muffins	Berries Shredded wheat Skim milk Whole-grain toast	Grapefruit half Potatoes (hash-browned with small amount of oil in non-stick pan) Whole grain toast with marmalade	Blueberries Hot whole-grain cereal Skim milk English muffin	Fresh melon German oven pancakes
Tuna sandwich (water-packed tuna mixed with tangy dressing or imitation mayonnaise) Carrot sticks Fresh fruit	Chili bean salad in whole-wheat pocket bread Tomato soup (Campbell's low-sodium) Fresh fruit Graham crackers	Lentil soup Lowfat crackers Laughing Cow reduced-calorie cheese Fresh fruit	Bean burritos Lettuce and sliced tomato Fresh fruit	Salad bar (greens topped with kidney beans, tomato, radishes, garbanzo beans, and cucumbers) Low-calorie commercial or Western dressing Bagel Fruit	Peanut butter and jelly sandwich Vegetable sticks (carrot, celery, etc) Fresh orange Whole-wheat fig bar	Minestrone soup Wheat-berry rolls Low-fat cottage cheese Fresh fruit
Bean lasagna Tossed salad with Western dressing French bread Fresh berries	Cashew chicken Steamed rice Fresh pineapple slices Wheat-berry rolls Hot-fudge pudding cake	Easy tuna noodle casserole Steamed broccoli Confetti apple slaw Wheat rolls Strawberry ice	Pizza rice casserole Green peas Green salad with low-calorie dressing Sourdough rolls Gingersnaps	Baked herbed fish Baked potato with mock sour cream Steamed zucchini Waldorf salad Caraway puffs	Corn chips with bean dip Creamy enchiladas Meatless Spanish rice Shredded lettuce and tomato Fresh fruit	Spaghetti with marinara sauce Tossed salad with low-calorie dressing Steamed green beans seasoned with lemon and pepper French bread Fresh fruit

Courtesy James Kenney, PhD, RD.

*This eating plan is not officially endorsed by SCAN; however, for more information contact The Pritikin Plan, 1910 Ocean Front Walk, Santa Monica, CA 90405.

Vegetables—Four or more servings (1 cup raw; 0.5 cup cooked) are recommended daily. Dark green and yellow or orange vegetables are recommended daily.

Fruit—Three or more servings of whole fruit are recommended daily. A half-cup serving of fruit juice is equivalent to a one-third serving of fruit.

Dairy—Two servings of nonfat dairy products are recommended daily.

Fish, shellfish, lean fowl or lean red meat—Up to 3.5 oz can be included daily. The portion size for crayfish, conch, crab, shrimp, and squid is 2 oz. Cooked beans (1.5 cup) and/or tofu (6 oz) may be substituted for meat, fish, or poultry. The "therapeutic plan" limits animal-protein foods to just 3.5 oz per week, with fish and shellfish being the preferred sources of animal protein; two servings of legumes per day are then recommended. In addition, all added fats and oils, refined carbohydrates, egg yolks, organ meats, and seeds and nuts (except chestnuts) are excluded on the "therapeutic plan." Sodium is limited to a maximum of 1.6 g per day.

Another type of VLFHC is the phase III diet defined by Connor and Connor,[54] in which egg-yolk consumption is minimal, and meat, poultry, and fish are limited to reduce saturated-fatty-acid and cholesterol intake. To reduce total fat, added fat should be limited to 3 tsp per day for women and 5 tsp per day for men. Fried foods should be avoided and the fat added to baked products should be reduced by one third. Peanut butter should be used as part of a meal rather than as a snack, and nuts should be used sparingly. To reduce saturated fatty acids, lean red meat or low-fat cheese is recommended no more than twice weekly. Snack foods high in saturated fatty acids should be avoided and soft margarine and oils should be used sparingly. To increase carbohydrate intake, Connor and Connor recommended consuming at least two complex-carbohydrate–containing foods at each meal. Snacks high in complex carbohydrate (eg, air-popped corn) are recommended. Additional recommendations include: 3 to 5 cups of legumes weekly, 2 to 4 cups of vegetables per day, three to five pieces of fruit per day. To decrease refined-sugar intake by 50%, sweets (soda pop, candy, desserts) are limited to one serving per day. Sample very-low-fat, high-carbohydrate menus appear in *Table 5.9.*

SUGGESTIONS FOR PATIENTS ON FAT-MODIFIED DIETS

The following information will be useful to patients who are on a Step One or Step Two Diet. Additional information that will be useful to dietitians appears in Table 5.2 and in the appendix. Some reduced-fat products are relatively high in sodium and will not be appropriate for patients on a sodium-restricted diet.

Eating Out*

When dining out, food selections should be in keeping with the Step One Diet or Step Two Diet. The following recommendations are appropriate for patients following these diets. They will help formalize a plan for dining out.

1. Skipping meals in order to indulge while dining out is counterproductive. Avoid excessive hunger when dining out.
2. Control consumption of alcoholic beverages. Limit drinks to one to two per day.

*By Cindy Ragin

3. Order an appetizer portion of fish, chicken, or beef in place of a main entree, or share an entree.
4. Before ordering, ask the server how the food is prepared and served. Request all sauces and dressings on the side.
5. Be assertive. If food is not served properly, ask to have it corrected.
6. Most bread and crackers served with meals are acceptable. Request margarine instead of butter and use it sparingly, or do not use it at all.
7. Keep a list of restaurants that serve acceptable food.
8. Many airlines will provide low-cholesterol, low-sodium, low-calorie, diabetic, vegetarian, or Kosher meals if the request is made 24 hours in advance.

See *Tables 5.10* and *5.11* for tips on menu selection in restaurants.

Table 5.10
Tips for Restaurant Menu Selections*

Main dishes and accompaniments

- Order "light meals" or petite sizes to control serving size.
- Eat half the meat or entree served and take the rest home. Try to keep the serving size to 3 oz (or the amount equal in size to a deck of cards), and eat no more than *6 oz of meat per day.*
- Order foods baked, broiled, steamed, or grilled rather than fried.
- Choose dinner rolls, breads, bread sticks, saltines, or melba toast instead of croissants, butter-toasted breads, or Texas toast.

Salads

- At the salad bar, choose salad greens, tomatoes, cucumbers, radishes, cauliflower, broccoli, green pepper, onion, carrots, sprouts, and fruits. Bacon, olives, avocados, nuts, coconut, croutons, and cheese are high in fat, so use them sparingly.
- Prepared salads such as potato, tuna, and chicken salads may be high in fat. Eat them only occasionally and limit the serving size to a half-cup.
- Order salad dressings to be served on the side. If possible, order low-calorie salad dressings, or use only 1 tbsp of regular dressing.

Appetizers

- Enjoy broth or vegetable soup, raw vegetables, or fresh fruit as an appetizer.

Desserts

- Choose sherbet, ice milk, fresh fruit, or low-fat yogurt.

Sandwiches

- Order a sandwich of lean meat, fish, or poultry that is baked, broiled, or grilled. Use mustard when possible as a spread and ask that spreads such as margarine, mayonnaise, and sauces be served on the side—then use them sparingly. For extra flavor and texture, ask for lettuce, tomatoes, or sprouts with the sandwich.
- Ask for garnishes of fruit or vegetables rather than potato chips or french fries.

Soups

- Order broths, consomme, or vegetable, rice, meat, or pasta soups. Cream soups are often high in fat.

Breakfast

- Order cereals served with skim milk or 1% milk.
  - Choose toast, English muffins, and bagels with margarine, jam, or jelly (instead of butter) on the side.

*By Rebecca M. Mullis.

Table 5.11
Specialty Restaurant Menu Choices*

	Chinese
Best choices	
Selections	Tofu, chicken, fish, vegetables, lean beef, and pork
Preparation	Clear chicken broth, garlic, scallions, vegetables, ginger sauce, oyster sauce
Menu listings	Tofu with vegetables Steamed chicken with wine Steamed fish with ginger Beef with mushrooms White rice, plain
Second best	
Selections	Shellfish, lean beef
Preparation	Brown-bean sauce, soy sauce, peanuts
Menu listings	Chicken with Chinese vegetables Shrimp with black-bean sauce Beef with green pepper, mushrooms, and snow peas Hot and sour soup
Avoid	
Selections	High-fat duck, pork
Preparation	Oyster sauce, sweet and sour sauce, cream sauce
Menu Listings	Sweet and sour chicken Shrimp with lobster sauce Beef chow mein, beef with oyster sauce Pork fried rice
	French
Best choices	
Selections	Veal, fish, chicken, frog legs
Preparation	Tomato sauce, mushrooms, garlic, vegetables, grapes
Menu listings	Truite au vin blanc (trout in white wine) Fricadelles de veau niçoise (veal meatballs with tomato/onion/brown sauce)
Second best	
Selections	Shellfish and lean lamb, ham, or pork
Preparation	Cheese, butter, almonds, sherry/orange sauce, breading
Menu listings	Truite au bleu (boiled trout, vinegar/butter) Escalope de veau à l'anglaise (breaded veal with parsley/lemon/butter)
Avoid	
Selections	Brains, liver, sweetbreads, duck, or goose
Preparation	Cream sauce, hollandaise, bacon
Menu listings	Truite au hollandaise Côtes de veau aux herbes de Provence (2 small veal chops with herbs, hollandaise sauce)

*By Cindy Ragin.

Table 5.11
Specialty Restaurant Menu Choices*—(cont.)

	Italian
Best Choices	
Selection	Chicken, fish, veal, pasta
Preparation	Wine, tomato, mushrooms, onions, lemon, broiled, marinara, primavera
Menu listings	Baked chicken with prosciutto, garlic, wine
	Linguini with red clam sauce
Second Best	
Selection	Shellfish, pasta
Preparation	Butter, oil, breaded
Menu listings	Sauteed chicken, floured with butter, wine
	Shrimp scampi, oil, garlic
	Shrimp marinara
	Linguini with white clam sauce (prepared without cream)
Avoid	
Selections	High-fat cuts of beef and pork, sausage
Preparation	Parmigiana, meat sauce, cream sauce, anchovies, fried dishes
Menu listings	Chicken parmigiana, breaded chicken with mozzarella, tomato sauce
	Shrimp parmigiana, mozzarella, tomato sauce
	Fettuccine Alfredo, cream, butter, parmesan
	Mexican
Best Choices	
Selections	Chicken, vegetable, and bean dishes, limit cheese
Preparation	Onion, sherry, garlic, tomato, pepper
Menu listings	Pollo en salsa verde (chicken with green tomatoes, chilis, onion, garlic, coriander, sherry)
	Chicken taco (with chilis, onion, tomato, lettuce)
	Chicken tostada (onion, tomato, lettuce, and chili sauce)
	Bean tostada, limit cheese
Second Best	
Selections	Nonmeat entrees that emphasize legumes
Preparation	Chili sauce
Menu listings	Bean taco with chilis, tomato, and lettuce
	Bean tostada with guacamole
	Bean burrito, limit cheese
Avoid	
Selections	Ground beef, nachos
Preparation	Sour cream, cheese, deep-fried foods
Menu listings	Beef super taco with cheese, onions, lettuce, sour cream
	Beef super tostada, beans, sour cream
	Beef super burrito, cheese, sour cream

*By Cindy Ragin.

COOKING TIPS FOR PATIENTS ON BLOOD CHOLESTEROL-LOWERING DIETS*

To prepare meat, fish and poultry, trim all visible fat and skin prior to cooking. When roasting (cooking in an uncovered pan in the oven), always place the meat on a rack to allow fat to drip away. Use low cooking temperatures (350 °F) to increase the fat drip-off (high temperatures sear the meat and seal in the fat). Use baking for less-fatty meats, fish, and poultry (preferably broilers or fryers rather than roasters), and lean pork chops. Baking helps to retain moisture. Braising or stewing (cooking in a closed container in the oven or on the stove-top) can be used to tenderize meat. To reduce unwanted fat, cook the meat a day ahead of serving time, refrigerate it until the fat hardens, and

*By Peg Seng

remove the fat (this is more effective than skimming fat during cooking when the liquid is hot). Broiling or grilling (cooking by exposure to direct heat) allows the fat in meats to drip away. When sautéing, use a low-calorie nonstick spray or another fat substitute to reduce total fat, or use a small amount of liquid (broth, wine, or juice) in place of the fat. Sautéing does not optimize fat loss.

Chill meat drippings and remove the solid fat. The remaining broth can be used for sauces and gravies or to season meats. When a recipe calls for basting the meat with its drippings, try basting with wine, tomato juice, or lemon juice instead. Use reduced-sodium soy sauce in place of regular soy sauce.

When making gravy, use defatted broth or bouillon. To one-half cup cold liquid, add 1 tbsp cornstarch or 1 to 2 tbsp browned flour (browned flour can be made by heating flour in a shallow pan over low heat, stirring frequently, until the flour turns brown); heat, and boil 1 minute.

Always refrigerate soups, stews and gravies until the fat solidifies, then remove it by skimming. Ice cubes can be added to broths, gravies, or stews to harden the fat for removal. Also, an ice cube can be wrapped in a paper towel and skimmed over the surface to remove fat (but this method is not as effective as refrigeration).

When using skim milk in soups and puddings, add extra nonfat dry-milk powder for richer flavor. A drop of vanilla extract per cup will make cream soups or custards taste richer, too. Instead of using cream in soup, thicken homemade chicken or beef broth with flour, arrowroot, grated raw potato, or another pureed vegetable.

When using ground meat in recipes, first cook the meat, then put it in a strainer and rinse thoroughly with hot water. Use extra-lean ground beef or ground turkey only occasionally. Processed foods should be rinsed for 1 minute to reduce their salt content. To reduce salt in canned fish, rinse with water.

Use plain (low-fat) yogurt as a substitute for sour cream. Use low-fat milk, skim milk, or buttermilk in place of whole milk in recipes. To prevent yogurt from separating during cooking, mix 1 tbsp cornstarch with 1 tbsp yogurt and stir it into 1 cup plain yogurt. Stir over medium heat until thickened. For a sour-cream substitute, blenderize 1 cup low-fat cottage cheese with 1 tbsp skim milk and lemon juice to taste. Use low-fat cottage cheese or part-skim ricotta in place of cream cheese in a recipe. Try the following low-fat dip for raw vegetables and baked potatoes: Puree 12 oz low-fat cottage cheese and 1/2 cup skim milk in a blender. Add 1 tbsp chopped chives, 1 tbsp chopped green peppers, 1/4 cup chopped onion, a pinch of salt and pepper, and paprika.

SHOPPING TIPS FOR PATIENTS ON BLOOD CHOLESTEROL-LOWERING DIETS*

1. Make a shopping list and plan meals for the week. This helps reduce impulse buying.
2. Eat before grocery shopping. Shopping when hungry often leads to unnecessary purchases.
3. Dried beans, peas, lentils, and legumes are low in fat and contain no cholesterol. They are also a good source of protein and fiber.
4. When choosing ground meat:
   - Use only occasionally.
   - Purchase extra-lean ground beef or lean ground turkey.
   - Buy ground round (usually very lean).

*By Peg Seng

- Select a well-trimmed steak, lean stewing meat, or lean chuck roast, and have it ground.

5. Read the label before selecting a margarine:
   - A liquid vegetable oil should be the first ingredient listed.
   - Partially hydrogenated oil may be the second ingredient but not the first (hydrogenation reduces the unsaturated fatty acids to saturated fatty acids).
   - Tub margarines are usually more unsaturated than stick margarines (but not always).
   - Reduced-fat (diet) margarines contain water and provide less fat; some have limited usefulness for cooking and baking. Compare the product with its regular variety to determine the fat and calories.
   - Always read the label—ingredients often change.
6. Read labels on packaged foods:
   - *Vegetable fat* or *vegetable oil* may still mean that a product is appreciably high in a saturated fat
   - *No cholesterol* or *no animal fat* does not mean that the product is acceptable, because it can still be high in saturated fatty acids.
   - Ingredients are listed in decreasing order according to weight; the first item used is present in the greatest amount.
7. Avoid the following commercial products, because they contain dried egg yolk, whole milk, and a significant amount of fat and saturated fatty acids: biscuits, muffins, donuts, egg bread, cheese bread, sweet rolls, and cake mixes. Packaged products that contain no fat are generally acceptable.
8. Convenience foods (premixed, packaged, frozen, dehydrated, instant) can be used if they are low in cholesterol and saturated fatty acids. Limit ready-made foods (microwave or other), potato chips, french-fried potatoes, frozen dinners and pot pies, ready-to-eat canned or frozen foods (desserts, bread products, side dishes, entrees, etc). Dehydrated foods (potatoes) or mixes (pancake) to which fat is added during preparation are usually acceptable, but check the label to be sure.
9. Nondairy creamers—avoid those with coconut or palm oil.
10. Self-basting turkeys generally should be avoided because butter or coconut oil are often used for basting (check the label) and some are basted with corn oil, which adds extra calories.

RECOMMENDATIONS FOR INCREASING DIETARY FIBER*

Dietary fiber and, specifically, simple food choices may significantly prevent or qualitatively manage the four major diet-related CHD risk factors: hyperlipidemia, hypertension, diabetes, and obesity.[55] Americans presently consume 13 to 18 g of dietary fiber per day.[56] Types of fiber to include in the diet, the amount of fiber recommended, and realistic ways to add fiber to the diet are discussed.

Types of Fiber

Fiber types are distinguished by their physiological properties and systemic effects. There are two types of dietary fiber: water soluble and water insoluble.[57] Water-soluble fiber will dissolve in hot water; insoluble fiber will not.

Examples of soluble fiber include gums, pectin, certain hemicelluloses, and storage polysaccharides. Fruits, some vegetables, oats, barley, and legumes contain a significant amount of soluble fiber. Insoluble fiber includes cellulose,

*By Sarah E. Whitis

lignin, and many hemicelluloses. Many vegetables, wheat, and most grain products contain primarily insoluble fibers.[58,59] The fiber content of selected foods appears in the appendix (see Table 14.28).

Soluble fiber and insoluble fiber function differently in the body.[60] Soluble fiber increases intestinal transit time, delays gastric emptying, and slows glucose absorption, leading to lower postprandial blood glucose concentrations and a decrease in the plasma total-cholesterol level, and other metabolic effects.[61] Insoluble fiber decreases intestinal transit time, increases fecal bulk, delays glucose absorption, and slows the rate of starch hydrolysis. These effects alter gastrointestinal function but do not lower plasma glucose or cholesterol levels.

Current Fiber Recommendations

Because of the hypocholesterolemic action of soluble fiber, it appears prudent to recommend that fiber intake be increased especially for persons at risk for cardiovascular disease (CVD). The Surgeon General's 1988 report on nutrition and health recommends low-fat, low-cholesterol dietary patterns that emphasize the consumption of vegetables, fruits, and whole-grain products—foods rich in complex carbohydrates and fiber and relatively low in calories.[62]

Several national health organizations have made recommendations for fiber intake. Although the American Heart Association does not recommend a specific fiber intake,[63] the Step One Diet usually provides approximately 23 g fiber per 2,000 calories, while the Step Two Diet contains 27 g. The National Cancer Institute recommends an intake of 25 to 35 g fiber per day[64] and the British National Advisory Committee on Nutrition Education[65] recommends 30 g/day of total dietary fiber with an emphasis on cereal fiber. Other national health organizations recommending specific fiber intakes per day include the American Diabetes Association[66] (25 g fiber per 1,000 calories) and the HCF Diabetes Foundation[67] (20 to 35 g fiber per 1,000 calories).

Fiber intake guidelines for patients with various metabolic conditions are virtually nonexistent. Scientists in fiber research such as James Anderson, MD, at the University of Kentucky recommend 20 to 25 g/day of total dietary fiber and a maximum of 60 g/day[61] for persons under medical supervision for metabolic conditions such as diabetes, obesity, and hyperlipidemia. Dietary fiber intake at this level provides 6 to 7.5 g of soluble fiber per 1,000 calories.

Implementing a High-Fiber, High-Carbohydrate Diet

Intensive nutrition intervention with diets high in complex carbohydrates and water soluble fiber reduces the plasma total-cholesterol level 10% to 30% and fasting serum triglycerides 10% to 20%.[68-72] With weight loss, plasma lipid changes are at the upper range reported. Further research shows supplementation of soluble fiber such as psyllium hydrophilic mucilloid can reduce plasma total-cholesterol by 15% and LDL cholesterol by 20% in persons with mild to moderate hypercholesterolemia.[73]

Meeting recommended therapeutic levels of fiber intake can be achieved by increasing consumption of foods such as legumes, fruits, vegetables, and whole grains while decreasing intake of high-fat meats and dairy products, eggs, and fat. An additional 5 g of soluble fiber is recommended for the reduction of blood cholesterol levels and may be achieved by selecting the foods listed in *Table 5.12*.

Table 5.12
Selected Foods High in Soluble Fiber

Item	Serving	Total Fiber, g	Soluble Fiber, g
Oat bran	1/3 cup dry (28 g)	4.4	2.0
	1/2 cup dry (42 g)	6.6	3.0
Oat meal	1/3 cup dry (27 g)	2.8	1.3
	1/2 cup dry (41 g)	4.3	2.0
Oat-bran muffin	1 medium	3.3	1.6
Beans	1/2 cup cooked	6.7	2.0

Adapted with permission from Anderson JW. *HCF Exchanges: A Sensible Plan for Healthy Eating.* HCF Nutrition Research Foundation, Inc, PO Box 22124, Lexington, KY 40522; 1989.

The High-Carbohydrate, High-Fiber (HCF) exchange system developed at the University of Kentucky by Anderson et al[74] may be used to tailor guidelines to meet individual food preferences and health status. *Table 5.13* outlines the basic steps for calculating the HCF diet for hyperlipidemic individuals. *Table 5.14* illustrates an 1,800-calorie sample HCF daily menu.

Practical suggestions to help patients increase their fiber intake are listed in *Table 5.15.* When sufficient quantities of soluble fiber cannot be obtained

Table 5.13
Steps for Calculating a High-Carbohydrate, High-Fiber Maintenance (HTM) Diet for Hyperlipidemic Individuals

Step	Guidelines
1. Estimate energy requirements	Approximate energy needs: • weight maintenance (sedentary) 10–12 calories/lb actual body weight • weight maintenance (active) 13–15 calories/lb actual body weight • weight reduction (gradual) 5–8 calories/lb actual body weight
2. Distribute calories	Multiply calorie level by: • carbohydrate 55% • protein 20% • fat 25%
3. Convert calories to grams	Divide: • carbohydrate by 4 calories/g • protein by 4 calories/g • fat by 9 calories/g
4. Translate grams into HCF exchanges	Begin with essential exchanges • multiply the exchanges for each group by exchange-group nutrient values for carbohydrate, protein, fat, fiber, and calories • try to stay within ± 3 g for nutrients and within 30 calories
5. Distribute exchanges into meals and snacks	Individualize according to diet history

Reprinted with permission from Anderson JW, Deakins DA, Floore TL, et al. Dietary fiber and coronary heart disease. *Crit Rev Food Sci Nutr.* 1990;29:95. Copyright CRC Press, Inc, Boca Raton, FL.

from food sources, fiber supplementation can be initiated using psyllium hydrophilic mucilloid. A regimen of 3.4 g of psyllium three times per day has been found to be well tolerated.[73]

Most people can increase their fiber intake with little difficulty if they do so gradually (5- to 10-g increments) while also increasing their fluid intake.[76] Some persons report flatulence with increased fiber intake. However, as the body adapts to increased fiber intake, the flatulence will decrease or cease.

Well-balanced high-fiber, high-carbohydrate diets have been found to be safe for long-term use.[77] High-fiber diets do not cause nutrient deficiencies in Western-type populations.[78] However, as a precautionary measure, a low-dose multivitamin-mineral preparation may be prescribed.[67]

DIETARY MANAGEMENT OF HYPERTRIGLYCERIDEMIA*

Restriction of calories. Most patients with hypertriglyceridemia are overweight. The secretion of VLDL by the liver is greatly stimulated by a calorie intake in excess of requirements for basal and physical activity. Therefore, the total caloric intake should be reduced. With weight loss, plasma triglyceride levels decline. After weight maintenance or when ideal body weight is achieved, plasma triglyceride levels stabilize.

Role of carbohydrates. Isocaloric substitution of carbohydrates for saturated fatty acids lowers the plasma total-cholesterol level; however, plasma triglyceride levels may increase because more substrate is available for endogenous triglyceride synthesis.[79] The increase in triglyceride levels is usually transient. Replacing dietary starch or glucose with sucrose usually elevates plasma triglyceride levels and occasionally increases the plasma total-cholesterol level.[79]

Most calories, therefore, should be derived from unrefined carbohydrates. Refined sugar and fruit juices should be limited as much as possible. Consumption of large quantities of whole fruits may also elevate the plasma triglyceride level in a small percentage of the population.

Restriction of fat. Total fat is usually restricted to less than 30% of calories when the triglyceride level is greater than 240 mg/dL. A combination of monounsaturated and polyunsaturated fatty acids should replace saturated fatty acids. Saturated fatty acids should be limited to less than 7% of total calories.[80]

In severe lipemia or acute pancreatitis, fat is usually restricted or avoided until the triglyceride level falls below the danger level (<1,000 mg/dL). Elimination of fat leads to a rapid decrease in chylomicron triglyceride levels (and hence, plasma triglyceride levels).

Fat intake for patients with primary chylomicronemia should be restricted to less than 10 to 20 g per day because of the underlying defect in lipolysis. Five grams should be from vegetable oil such as safflower oil to provide essential fatty acids.[80] One tablespoon of cod liver oil is recommended for two reasons: (1) it is rich in omega-3 fatty acids and will lower triglyceride levels, and (2) it provides fat-soluble vitamins.

*By Raksha Shah

Table 5.14
Sample 1,800-Calorie, High-Carbohydrate, High-Fiber Maintenance (HCF) Menu

Breakfast	
Oatmeal	½ cup
Peach slices, raspberries, almonds	½ cup
Whole-wheat toast	4 slices
Corn-oil margarine	2 tsp
Spice tea	1 cup
Mineral-vitamin supplement	1
Lunch	
Tuna salad in pita pocket	2 halves
Tomato slices and sprouts	½ cup
Fresh orange quarters	1 small
Pumpkin-oat bran muffin	1
Skim milk	1 cup
Dinner	
Spinach salad	½ cup
Light Italian dressing	1 tbsp
Rye crackers	6 small
Kidney-bean lasagna	8 oz
Steamed broccoli	2 stalks
Whole-wheat bread stick	1
Corn-oil margarine	1 tsp
Snack	
Bran flakes	⅔ cup
Skim milk	1 cup

Reprinted with permission from Anderson JW, Deakins DA, Floore TL, et al. Dietary fiber and coronary heart disease. *Crit Rev Food Sci Nutr.* 1990;29:95. Copyright CRC Press, Inc, Boca Raton, FL.

Table 5.15
Tips for Adding Fiber to Meals

Choose fresh fruits over canned fruits or juices.
Choose whole-grain breads.
Leave the peels on fruits such as apples, pears, and peaches.
Leave the peels on vegetables such as potatoes, squash, and carrots.
Have a salad every day.
When mashing potatoes, leave the skin on.
Use brown rice rather than white rice.
Use oats as a filler in casseroles, meat loaf, or salmon patties.
Use whole-grain flours for baking.
Use oats or oat bran as a thickening agent for sauces.
Use high-fiber breakfast cereals.
Have a high-fiber cereal daily.
Choose raw vegetables and fresh fruits for snacks.
Use whole-wheat pasta.
Eat beans and peas often.
Have a serving of dried beans or peas daily.
Blenderize oats and use in cooking and baking.
Eat foods in their most naturally occurring state.

Reprinted with permission from Anderson JW. *The HCF Guide Book.* HCF Nutrition Research Foundation, Inc, PO Box 22124, Lexington, KY 40522; 1987.

Medium-chain triglyceride (MCT) oil can be used to increase the palatability of the diet. Its fatty acids are transported to the liver in portal-vein blood rather than plasma chylomicrons.[80]

Alcohol. Ingestion of alcohol is a common cause of secondary hyperlipidemia, probably due to overproduction of endogenous VLDL. Some people with familial endogenous hypertriglyceridemia are particularly sensitive to alcohol. Abstinence may normalize triglyceride levels.

There is little evidence that soluble fiber significantly lowers plasma triglycerides. The nutritional goal in treating people with hypertriglyceridemia who are symptomatic (ie, abdominal pain and pancreatitis) is to alleviate these symptoms and prevent their recurrence. The initial treatment of hypertriglyceridemia always consists of changes in diet and life style. The patient should decrease caloric intake and reduce weight to ideal body weight. Alcohol should be avoided and the consumption of refined sugar should be limited. Complex carbohydrates should be emphasized and should provide the majority of calories. A summary of the dietary treatments for hypertriglyceridemia is presented in *Table 5.16.*

DIETARY TREATMENT OF HYPERTENSION*

There are many nonpharmacological therapies for the prevention and control of hypertension. Unless the blood pressure is especially high (systolic blood pressure $\geq$200; diastolic blood pressure $\geq$115) consistently, life-style modifications should be initiated for at least three to six months before drug therapy is advised.[82] Nonpharmacological measures such as dietary modification may lower blood pressure in hypertensive persons and should be used either alone, if control can be established, or as a useful adjunct to drug therapy. In addition, dietary changes may prevent the development of hypertension in healthy persons who may be considered high risk because of family history.

Weight Reduction. The goal weight for hypertensive patients should be within 15% of their desirable weight. However, modest weight reduction through caloric restriction with or without a reduction in sodium intake may cause a decrease in blood pressure in overweight people. Health professionals should stress weight control and maintenance for everyone, but especially for those who are at risk because of genetic predisposition.

Alcohol. Since excess alcohol intake may increase blood pressure or affect the adherence or efficacy of drug treatment, hypertensive patients should drink no more than 1 oz of ethanol daily—the amount in 2 oz of liquor, 8 oz of wine, or 24 oz of beer.

Sodium. High sodium intakes have been linked to high blood pressure in some hypertensive persons, but the individual response to sodium restriction is variable. Additionally, trial and error seems to be the only way at present to identify sodium-sensitive or sodium-resistant people. Patients most likely to have the greatest response are older, black, and have a high initial blood pressure reading or have a family history of hypertension. Genetic markers may soon be available to identify those who would benefit most from sodium restriction. At the present time, a modest reduction in intake (of 4 to 6 g sodium chloride daily) is recommended initially to lower blood pressure. The reduction can be used either alone or as an adjunct to drug therapy. This approach seems to be effective for many hypertensive persons.

*By Patricia Volz-Clarke

Table 5.16
Dietary Treatment of Primary Hypertriglyceridemia*

Type	Fat	Carbohydrate	Calories	Alcohol	Protein/Other
I. Familial hyperchylomicronemia Treatment entirely dietary	10% or less of total calories (15–30 g/day) Because the defect involves lipolysis, both saturated and polyunsaturated fats must be curtailed. Medium-chain triglyceride (MCT) oil may be added to increase palatability At least 5 g of total fat should be from vegetable oil like safflower for essential fatty acids	60%–65% total calories or higher Because fat is restricted, simple carbohydrates should be avoided	Not limited	Not recommended	Protein not limited Fat-soluble vitamins recommended
IV. Familial endogenous hypertriglyceridemia Primary mode of treatment is dietary	Total fat severely restricted (if acute pancreatitis or epigastric pain present) for a short term or until symptoms subside. For long-term management: 20% or less of total calories	60%–65% of total calories or higher if fat is severely restricted. Simple carbohydrates should be avoided	Restricted. If patient is overweight, maintenance of ideal body weight recommended	Not recommended	Not limited other than to achieve and maintain ideal weight
V. Fixed hyperlipidemic	20% or less of total calories. If severe lipemia is present, fat is totally restricted until triglyceride levels fall to acceptable range	60%–65% of total calories	Restricted to maintain ideal body weight	Not recommended	20% of total calories to maintain ideal weight

* For patients with borderline hypertriglyceridemia, very-low-fat, high-carbohydrate diets may not be advised.[6]

Adapted with permission from Connor WE, Connor SL. The dietary treatment of hyperlipidemia, rationale, technique and efficacy. *Med Clin North Am.* 1982;66:685.

Potassium and Calcium. Research has suggested that a high potassium intake (>80 mEq or 3 to 4 g/day) may cause a modest reduction in blood pressure in hypertensive individuals. However, supplementation does not appear to have any effect on blood pressure in normotensive people. Potassium supplements should be restricted only in patients who have normal renal function and who are not taking potassium-sparing diuretics or angiotensin-converting inhibitors.

Although a high calcium intake may lower blood pressure in some hypertensives, its effects are much smaller than sodium restriction and, as with sodium, variable. Additionally, an increase in dietary calcium may lead to the development of renal calculi in a small number of susceptible persons.

Dietary fats. Although some studies have indicated that limiting saturated-fatty-acid intake and increasing omega-6 fatty-acid intake may be associated with lowered arterial pressure, more of the research is inconclusive. However, as discussed in previous sections, dietary modification may be useful in lowering the plasma cholesterol level. Additionally, although nutritionists recommend consuming more fish for many reasons, there is little evidence that fish oil lowers blood pressure, and fish-oil supplements are not recommended.

References

1. Hoeg J, Gregg RE, Brewer HB Jr. Special communication: an approach to the management of hyperlipoproteinemia. *JAMA.* 1986;225:512.
2. Carroll MD, Abraham CS, Dresser CM. *Dietary Intake Source Data: United States, 1976-80.* Washington, DC: US Govt Printing Office; March 1983. US Dept of Health and Human Services publication PHS 83-1681. Vital and Health Statistics series 11-231.
3. Rosenthal MD, Barnard RJ, Rose DP, et al. Effects of a high complex carbohydrate, low fat cholesterol diet on levels of serum lipids and estradiol. *Am J Med.* 1985;78:23.
4. Hennekens CH. Alcohol. In: Kaplan NM, Stamler JS, eds. *Prevention of Coronary Heart Disease.* Philadelphia, Pa: WB Saunders Co; 1983:130.
5. Committee on Diet and Health, Food and Nutrition Board, and Commission on Life Sciences, National Research Council. *Diet and Health: Implication for Reducing Chronic Disease Risk.* Washington, DC: National Academy Press; 1989.
6. National Cholesterol Education Program Expert Panel. Report on detection, evaluation, and treatment of high blood cholesterol in adults. *Arch Intern Med.* 1988;148:36.
7. Connor SL, Connor WE. *The New American Diet.* New York, NY: Simon & Schuster Inc; 1986.
8. American Heart Association. *Dietary Treatment of Hypercholesterolemia: A Handbook for Counselors.* Dallas, Tex: American Heart Association; 1988.
9. Grundy SM. Comparison of monounsaturated fatty acids and carbohydrates for lowering plasma cholesterol. *N Engl J Med.* 1986;314:745.
10. Grundy SM, Nix D, Whelan MF, et al. Comparison of three cholesterol-lowering diets in normolipemic men. *JAMA.* 1986;256:2351.
11. Mensink RP, Katan MB. Effects of monounsaturated fatty acids versus complex carbohydrates on high density lipoproteins in healthy men and women. *Lancet.* 1987;1:122.
12. Mattson FH. A changing role for dietary monounsaturated fatty acids. *J Am Diet Assoc.* 1989;89:387.
13. Pritikin N. *The Pritikin Program for Diet and Exercise.* New York, NY: Grosset & Dunlap; 1982.
14. Ornish D. *Stress, Diet and Your Heart.* New York, NY: Holt, Rinehart & Winston; 1982.
15. McDougall M. *The McDougall Plan for Super Health and Life-Long Weight Loss.* Piscataway, NJ: New Century; 1983.
16. Kenney J. *The LA Diet.* Chicago, Ill: Contemporary Books; 1988.

17. American Dietetic Association. Position of the ADA: vegetarian diets—technical support paper. *J Am Diet Assoc.* 1988;88:352.
18. Oster G, Epstein AM. Cost effectiveness of antihyperlipidemic therapy in the prevention of coronary heart disease. *JAMA.* 1987;258:2381.
19. Connor WE, Cerqueira MT, Connor RW, et al. The plasma lipids, lipoproteins, and the diet of the Tarahumara Indians of Mexico. *Am J Clin Nutr.* 1978;31:1131.
20. Sacks F, Ornish D, Rosner B, et al. Plasma lipoprotein levels in vegetarians. *JAMA.* 1985;254:1337.
21. Kenney JJ, Hall JA, Inkeles S, et al. Lipid lowering and nutritional adequacy with long-term use of a high fiber, high complex carbohydrate diet. American Dietetic Association 71st Annual Meeting; October 3-7, 1988; San Francisco, Calif. Abstract.
22. Manilow M. Atherosclerosis: regression in non-human primates. *Circ Res.* 1980;46:311.
23. Clarkson TB, Bond MG, Bullock BC, et al. A study of atherosclerosis in regression in macca mulatta. *Exp Mol Pathol.* 1984;41:96.
24. Barnard RJ, Guzy PM, Rosenberg JM, et al. Effects of an intensive exercise and nutrition program on patients with coronary artery disease: five-year follow-up. *J Cardiac Rehab.* 1983;3:183.
25. Ornish D, Brown S, Scherwitz LW, et al. Can lifestyle changes reverse coronary heart disease? *Lancet.* 1990;336:129.
26. Ornish D, Scherwitz B, Brown SE, et al. Adhering to lifestyle changes and reversal of coronary atherosclerosis. *Circulation.* 1989;80(suppl):0239. Abstract.
27. Blankenhorn DH, Johnson RL, Mach WJ, et al. The influence of diet on the appearance of new lesions in human coronary arteries. *JAMA.* 1990;263:1646.
28. Anderson JW, Ferguson SK, Karounos D, et al. Mineral and vitamin status on high-fiber diets: long-term studies on diabetic patients. *Diabetes Care.* 1980;3:38.
29. Garg A, Bonanome A, Grundy S, et al. Comparison of a high carbohydrate diet with a high monounsaturated fat diet in patients with non-insulin dependent diabetes mellitus. *N Engl J Med.* 1988;319:829.
30. Zavaroni I, Bonora E, Pagliara M, et al. Risk factors for coronary artery disease in healthy persons with hyperinsulinemia and normal glucose tolerance. *N Engl J Med.* 1989;320:702.
31. Garg A, Grundy S. *N Engl J Med.* 1989;320:536. Letter.
32. Rock C, Coulston A. Review of the LA Diet. *Nutr MD.* 1988;14:8.
33. Kimura N. A farming and fishing village in Japan: Tanusimaru and Ushibuka. *Acta Med Scand.* 1967;460(suppl):231.
34. Sinhett PF, Whyte HM. Epidemiological studies in a total highland population, Tukisenta, New Guinea. *J Chronic Dis.* 1973;26:265.
35. Lacey H. Bulimia: factors associated with its etiology and maintenance. *Int J Eat Dis.* 1986;5:475.
36. Dreon DM, Frey-Hewitt B, Ellsworth N, et al. Dietary fat: carbohydrate ratio and obesity in middle-aged men. *Am J Clin Nutr.* 1988;47:995.
37. Romieu I, Willet WC, Stampfer MJ, et al. Energy intake and other determinants of relative weight. *Am J Clin Nutr.* 1988;47:406.
38. Reaven G. Dietary therapy for non-insulin-dependent diabetes mellitus. *N Eng J Med.* 1988;319:862.
39. Lissner L, Levitsky DA, Strupp BJ, et al. Dietary fat and the regulation of energy intake in human subjects. *Am J Clin Nutr.* 1987;46:886.
40. Odea K, Trainedes K, Ireland P, et al. The effect of diets differing in fat, carbohydrate, and fiber on carbohydrate and lipid metabolism in type II diabetics. *J Am Diet Assoc.* 1989;89:1076.
41. Duncan K. The effects of high and low energy density diets on satiety, energy intake, and eating time of obese and nonobese subjects. *Am J Clin Nutr.* 1983;37:763.
42. Danforth E. Diet and obesity. *Am J Clin Nutr.* 1985;41:1132.
43. Flatt J. Dietary fat, carbohydrate balance, and weight maintenance: effects of exercise. *Am J Clin Nutr.* 1987;45:296.
44. Bray G. Obesity: a disease of nutrient and energy balance? *Nutr Rev.* 1987;45:33.
45. Friedman M, Ramirez I. Relationship of fat metabolism to food intake. *Am J Clin Nutr.* 1985;42:1093.
46. Pan X. Comparison of plasma lipoproteins and apoproteins in Chinese and American non-insulin-dependent diabetic subjects and controls. *Diabetes Care.* 1986;9:395.

47. Kenney J, Rosenthal M, Inkeles S, et al. High monounsaturated fat diet for non-insulin-dependent diabetes mellitus. *N Engl J Med.* 1989;320:537. Letter.
48. Thusen L. One-year experience with a low-fat, low-cholesterol diet in patients with coronary heart disease. *Am J Clin Nutr.* 1986;44:212.
49. Meinertz H, Nilausen K, Faergeman O, et al. Soy protein and casein in cholesterol enriched diets: effects on plasma lipoproteins in normolipemic subjects. *Am J Clin Nutr.* 1989;50:786.
50. Jenkins DJA, Wolever TMS, Vuksan V, et al. Nibbling versus gorging: metabolic advantages of increased meal frequency. *N Engl J Med.* 1989;321:929.
51. Anderson JW, Chen WL. Plant, fiber, carbohydrate and lipid metabolism. *Am J Clin Nutr.* 1979;32:346.
52. Stevens J. Does dietary fiber affect food intake and body weight? *J Am Diet Assoc.* 1988;88:939.
53. Carroll K, Braden LM, Bell JA, et al. Fat and cancer. *Cancer.* 1986;58:1818.
54. Connor WE, Connor SL. Dietary treatment of familial hypercholesterolemia. *Arteriosclerosis.* 1989;9(suppl 1):1-91-1-105.
55. Anderson JW, Tietyen-Clark J. Dietary fiber: hyperlipidemia, hypertension and coronary heart diseases. *Am J Gastroenterol.* 1986;81:907.
56. Pilch SM. *Physiologic Effects and Health Consequences of Dietary Fiber.* Bethesda, Md: Federation of American Societies of Experimental Biology Life Sciences Research Office; 1987:36.
57. Anderson JW. Physiological and metabolic effects of dietary fiber. *Fed Proc.* 1985;44:2902.
58. Anderson JW, Bridges SR. Dietary fiber content of selected foods. *Am J Clin Nutr.* 1988;47:440.
59. Anderson JW. Physiological and metabolic effects of dietary fiber. *Fed Proc.* 1985;44:2902.
60. Anderson JW, Story L, Sieling B, et al. Hypercholesterolemic effects of oat-bran or bran intake for hypercholesterolemic men. *Am J Clin Nutr.* 1984;40:1146.
61. Anderson JW, Bridges SR, Tietyen J, et al. Dietary fiber content of a simulated American diet and selected research diets. *Am J Clin Nutr.* 1989;49:352.
62. US Dept of Health and Human Services. *The Surgeon General's Report on Nutrition and Health.* Washington, DC: US Govt Printing Office; 1988.
63. American Heart Association Nutrition Committee. Dietary guidelines for healthy American adults: a statement for physicians and health professionals. *Circulation.* 1988;721A.
64. Butrum RR, Clifford CK, Lanza E. NCI dietary guidelines rationale. *Am J Clin Nutr.* 1988;48:440.
65. Nutrition guidelines for health education in Britain. *Nutr Today.* 1986;21:21.
66. Nutritional recommendations and principles for individuals with diabetes mellitus. *Diabetes Care.* 1987;10:126.
67. Anderson JW. About fiber. In: *The HCF Nutrition Program: The HCF Guidebook.* Lexington, Ky: HCF Diabetes Foundation; 1987:11.
68. Anderson JW, Gustafson NJ. Alternative lipid-lowering diets. *Practical Cardiol.* 1988;14:84.
69. Anderson JW, Story L, Sieling B, et al. Hypercholesterolemic effects of high-fiber diets rich in water-soluble plant fibers: long-term studies with oat-bran and bean supplemented diets for hypercholesterolemic men. *Am J Clin Nutr.* 1984;40:1140.
70. Anderson JW, Chen WJL, Sieling B. Hypolipidemic effects of high-carbohydrate, high-fiber diets. *Metabolism.* 1980;29:551.
71. Anderson JW, Ward K. High-carbohydrate, high-fiber diets, for insulin treated men with diabetes mellitus. *Am J Clin Nutr.* 1979;32:2312.
72. Anderson JW, Story L, Sieling B, et al. Hypocholesterolemic effects of oat-bran or bean intake for hypercholesterolemic men. *Am J Clin Nutr.* 1984;40:1140.
73. Anderson JW, Zettwoch N, Feldman T, et al. Cholesterol-lowering effects of psyllium hydrophilic mucilloid for hypocholesterolemic men. *Arch Intern Med.* 1988;148:292.
74. Anderson JW. *The HCF Exchanges: The High Carbohydrate–High Fiber (HCF) Nutrition Plan.* Lexington, Ky: HCF Diabetes Foundation; 1987.
75. Anderson JW, Deakins DA, Floore TL, et al. Dietary fiber and coronary heart disease. *Crit Rev Food Sci Nutr.* 1990;29:95.
76. Floch MH, Maryniuk MD, Bryant C, et al. Practical aspects of implementing increased dietary fiber intake. *Nutr Today.* 1986;21:27.

77. Anderson JW, Ferguson SK, Karounos D, et al. Mineral and vitamin status on high-fiber diets: long-term studies of diabetic patients. *Diabetes Care.* 1980;3:74.
78. Rattan J, Levin N, Graff E, et al. A high-fiber diet does not cause mineral and nutrient deficiencies. *J Clin Gastroenterol.* 1981;3:389.
79. Story JA. Dietary carbohydrate and atherosclerosis. *Fed Proc.* 1982;41:2799.
80. Kane JP, Malloy MJ. Disorders of lipoprotein metabolism. In: *Basic and Clinical Endocrinology.* Los Angeles, Calif: Appleton-Lane; 1988:557.
81. Connor WE, Connor SL. The dietary treatment of hyperlipidemia, rationale, technique and efficacy. *Med Clin North Am.* 1982;66:685.
82. National Kidney Foundation. *Education Program on Nonpharmacologic Management of Hypertension.* National Kidney Foundation Inc; 1988.

6. NUTRITION MANAGEMENT OF HEART-TRANSPLANTATION AND CORONARY-BYPASS SURGERY PATIENTS

NUTRITION MANAGEMENT OF THE HEART-TRANSPLANT PATIENT*

As a result of cyclosporine therapy, which has helped to reduce the incidence of organ rejection, cardiac transplantation now offers many patients with end-stage heart disease additional productive years. Heart transplantation is no longer considered an experimental procedure but, rather, an effective therapy for the end-stage heart disease patient.

According to the Registry of the International Society for Heart Transplantation,[1] 3,623 heart transplants were performed from 1981 to 1986. Survival rates have improved significantly because of refinements in immunosuppressive therapy and patient selection, as well as better methods for diagnosing rejection and treating infection. For patients treated with the immunosuppressive drug cyclosporine, one-year actuarial survival has increased to 80.6%, and five-year actuarial survival has increased to 78.3%.[1] Nevertheless, infection and rejection remain the primary causes of death following heart transplantation.[1]

The nutritional status of heart-transplant patients can significantly affect the surgical outcome, length of hospitalization, and mortality. End-stage heart disease is often associated with multiorgan failure and significant loss of lean body and adipose tissue. Liver enlargement and accompanying ascites may result in edema. Serum albumin, iron stores, and total lymphocyte count levels may also be low, suggesting compromised visceral protein status.

Patients with heart failure are also at risk of becoming malnourished due to anorexia, hypermetabolism, increased nutrient loss through urine and stool, and impaired delivery of nutrients to tissues and removal of their toxic waste products.[2] Nausea and vomiting may result in anorexia. Hypermetabolism may increase energy needs by 20% to 30% because of greater cardiac and pulmonary energy metabolism.[3] Malabsorption can also occur as the intestinal tract becomes engorged with fluid associated with edema, leading to reduced absorption of essential nutrients.[2]

When all other treatments for cardiac failure have been unsuccessful, heart transplantation may be recommended. Preoperative and postoperative nutrition support can help reduce operative complications, including major sepsis and respiratory failure.[3] Because nutrition management has become an important factor in total care of the surgical patient, many organ-transplant centers are now incorporating nutrition into their multidisciplinary care programs.

Few reports have addressed the nutrition needs of heart-transplant recipients. To evaluate the current status of nutrition support programs for these patients, a national survey of the major transplant centers was conducted.

In December 1988, nutrition-program surveys were mailed to 23 Medicare-approved heart-transplant centers. Three additional hospitals where a relatively large number of heart transplants are performed each year were also

*By Carolyn Moore and Zakera Chowdhury

included in the study. Of the 26 hospitals asked to participate in the survey, 20 centers (76.9%) completed the questionnaire and provided samples of educational materials used in their nutrition programs.

Characteristics of Hospitals Surveyed

Hospitals participating in the survey were affiliated with medical schools (63.6%) or were private (not-for-profit) institutions (31.8%). The number of hospital beds varied widely among the hospitals surveyed, ranging from 250 to 500 beds to 1,000 to 1,500 beds.

The majority of the hospitals surveyed (95%) employed special heart-transplant teams that were either headed by a cardiologist (24%) or surgeon (67%). Clinical dietitians functioned as a member of the heart-transplant team at most of the hospitals surveyed (80%).

Patient Characteristics

Selection of recipients for cardiac transplantation may be the most important factor in determining long-term outcome. A number of causes may result in end-stage heart disease. Cardiomyopathy (58%) and coronary artery disease (36.9%) were the primary indications for cardiac transplant surgery[1] from 1967 to 1986. Other indications included congenital heart disease (1.9%), allograft rejection (1.1%) and valvular heart disease (2.0%).

During the same period, the average age of patients undergoing heart transplantation was 42 years, ranging from newborn to 66 years.[3] Typically, heart-transplant recipients have also been men, with only 15% of the recipients being women. The survey of patient characteristics was similar to those reported by the International Society of Heart Transplantation Registry for 1967 to 1986.

Teaching Conferences Prior to Transplantation

The nutritional status of potential candidates for heart transplantation is often evaluated prior to surgery.[4–6] The likelihood of dietary compliance after transplantation may be assessed by dietitians, influencing decisions regarding acceptance of a patient as a transplant candidate. Furthermore, knowledge of the patient's food preferences prior to surgery can be useful during the postoperative period and can increase dietary compliance.[6]

Of the hospitals surveyed, 95% require heart-transplant candidates or family members to attend pretransplant teaching conferences. Members from the different transplant services discussed prospective plans and procedures during the preoperative and postoperative periods; however, dietitians participated in the pretransplant conferences at only one half of the hospitals surveyed.

When included in the conferences, the dietitians reviewed pretransplant and posttransplant dietary restrictions that typically included modifying sodium and fat intake. In addition, during the pretransplant teaching conference dietitians usually discussed the patient's nutritional status, nutrition care plans, and possible drug-nutrient interactions.

Nutrition Assessment

Nutrition-assessment of heart-transplant patients often includes a review of a detailed diet history, noting food preferences and weight changes.[4–6] Anthropometric measurements may be included in an evaluation of nutritional status to assess somatic protein stores.[4–6] A review of laboratory parameters reflecting nutritional status and an analysis of food records by computer to determine nutrient intake can also provide useful information.

At most of the hospitals surveyed, the nutritional status of heart-transplant patients was assessed on a routine basis following transplantation, but not always prior to the procedure. After transplantation, nutrition assessments were usually performed every seven to ten days until the patient was discharged.

Nutrition-assessment parameters that the surveyed hospitals usually used are summarized in *Table 6.1*. A few parameters were included only occasionally for research purposes and were not considered to be part of the routine assessment (eg, creatinine-height index, 24-hour urinary nitrogen excretion, and plasma vitamin levels).

Table 6.1
Nutrition-Assessment Parameters Used by Hospitals When Evaluating Patients for Heart Transplant

Percentage of Hospitals Surveyed	Parameters
100	Past medical history, medications, and weight changes
90	Usual dietary intake and drug-nutrient interactions
60	Total lymphocyte count (TLC)
55	Physical examination for signs of nutritional deficiencies
40	Anthropometrics and serum transferrin
20	Call-mediated immunity
15	24-hour urinary nitrogen excretion
5	Creatinine-height index, thyroxine-binding prealbumin, retinol-binding protein, and plasma vitamin levels

In general, the energy needs of heart-transplant patients were estimated using the Harris-Benedict Equation[7] and the appropriate stress and injury factors. To a lesser extent, caloric factors expressed per unit of body weight were used to estimate caloric needs (eg, 30 calories per kilogram of body weight). Indirect calorimetry was rarely used to measure resting energy expenditure.

Whereas compromised preoperative nutritional status may not preclude acceptance into a heart-transplant program, assessing the patient's status can indicate whether nutrition support prior to surgery is advisable. Frazier and coworkers[4] evaluated 52 heart-transplant patients before and after surgery. Ten patients were severely compromised prior to surgery and were given commercial liquid supplements. Of these ten patients, five died, whereas six of 29 (21%) patients whose nutritional status was considered adequate died.

Another similar study[5] showed that somatic and visceral protein stores improved following heart transplantation. Body weight generally increased and returned to usual levels, which often exceeded ideal body weight.

Drug-Nutrient Interactions

Heart recipients adhere to complex immunosuppressive drug regimens following transplantation. Nutritional status may be influenced by the maintenance dosages of cyclosporine, prednisone, and azathioprine that are used to suppress rejection.[5,6]

Side effects associated with cyclosporine include hypertension and kidney and liver dysfunction as well as an increased susceptibility to viral infections and malignancy.

Prednisone, a corticosteroid, affects protein, carbohydrate, and lipid metabolism. Prednisone may cause sodium and fluid retention, loss of muscle mass, steroid-induced diabetes mellitus, redistribution of fat, increased appetite, increased infection, and mood swings. Side effects associated with azathioprine include gastrointestinal problems such as nausea and vomiting. Therefore, dietary management needs to be individualized to minimize the potential side effects of immunosuppressive therapy.

Nutrition Management and Counseling

Immediately following heart transplantation, patients are in a catabolic state, and, as with other postsurgical patients, nutritional requirements are increased. The goal of nutrition management has been to provide heart-transplant patients with a high intake of calories (1.5% to 1.75% basal energy expenditure) and protein (1.2 to 1.5 g per kg body weight).[4,8]

Over a 48-hour period following transplant, patients typically receive clear liquids, full liquids, and then a general or therapeutic diet.[2] During this transition period, oral intake is low, and colder, softer foods or liquids are often preferred.[6] As the patients recuperate, they are given meals incorporating their food preferences. Occasionally commercial supplements are used to help patients satisfy their increased calorie and protein needs.[4,8]

Once the patients are in anabolic state, long-term nutrition goals are developed.[4,8] Maintaining ideal body weight and moderately restricting sodium and fat are often important objectives. Patients may be advised to take a vitamin or mineral supplement or both after the dietitian has reviewed drug-nutrient interactions.

The diets that were routinely prescribed for pretransplant and posttransplant patients at the hospitals surveyed are shown in *Table 6.2*. Prior to transplantation, sodium intake was generally restricted, with or without a reduction of dietary fat and cholesterol.

Following transplantation, sodium intake was again limited. Immediately after the operation, patients were frequently placed on high-protein and high-calorie diets to prevent weight loss and negative nitrogen balance. In addition, one hospital placed patients on a low-purine diet after transplantation[4] because purines are believed to decrease the effectiveness of immunosuppressive drug therapy, thereby increasing the risk of infection.

During the two to four weeks following heart transplantation, the most common diets prescribed were low-fat, low-cholesterol diets that typically limited sodium intake. Dietary guidelines proposed by the NCEP[9] were generally followed to help lower blood cholesterol levels, which often increase after heart transplantation.

Table 6.2
Diets Routinely Prescribed for Heart-Transplant Patients

Type of Diet	Percentage of Diets Pretransplant	Percentage of Diets Immediately Following Transplant	Percentage of Diets Postransplant (>2–4 Weeks)
General	3.9	7.1	2.3
2 g sodium	31.4	19.0	14.0
4 g sodium, high-protein, high-calorie	15.7	26.2	9.3
Low cholesterol	15.7	23.8	11.6
2-4 g sodium, low-fat, low-cholesterol	21.6	19.0	30.2
Step One AHA*	7.8	2.4	11.6
Step Two AHA†	3.9	0	16.3
Low-purine	0	2.4	0
Weight loss	0	0	4.7
Total	**100%**	**99.9%**	**100%**

*The American Heart Association Step One Diet.
†The American Heart Association Step Two Diet.

The average hospital stay for heart-transplant recipients in the institutions surveyed was 25 days. Most heart-transplant centers (68%) continued to provide nutrition care to patients after discharge. The nutritional status of patients was monitored during periodic clinical visits and yearly evaluations. Diet instructions were given primarily on an individual basis (72%) rather than in a group setting (28%).

Heart-transplant patients are often readmitted to the hospital during episodes of infection, rejection, and pneumonia. Anorexia occasionally associated with the antibiotic therapy used to treat these conditions may place the heart recipient at risk of malnutrition. Thus, reassessing nutritional status and developing appropriate care plans following discharge are important components of any comprehensive heart-transplant program.

Dietary Concerns

One dietary concern that is unique to patients undergoing organ transplantation is the use of fresh fruits and vegetables. While the patient receives large dosages of immunosuppressive drugs (eg, cyclosporine, prednisone, and azathioprine) the risk of bacterial infection increases. Therefore, several of the hospitals surveyed (30%) restricted patients from eating fresh fruits and vegetables to minimize the risk. This restriction was applied from three weeks to three to four months following surgery. This practice, however, is controversial.

Heart-transplant patients often initially receive 200 to 400 mg of cyclosporine per day to maintain plasma levels between 200 and 350 ng/mL. Oral cyclosporine dissolves in an olive oil base. Experience indicates that tolerance to cyclosporine is increased when the medication is mixed with certain fluids. At the hospitals included in the study, most patients preferred mixing cyclosporine with chocolate milk or fruit juices.

Nutrition Support

Most heart-transplant patients (65%) did not receive liquid nutrition supplements as between meal nourishments among the hospitals surveyed. Commercial supplements or milkshakes were generally ordered on the basis of need rather than as standard practice. Likewise, enteral feedings were generally used only to prevent sustained weight loss.

Total parenteral nutrition (TPN) was only employed when heart-transplant patients were unable to tolerate oral and enteral feedings. TPN was instituted if the following conditions were present: renal failure, severe rejection, gastrointestinal complications, intubation, malnutrition, and cardiac cachexia. However, the possibility of the development of sepsis secondary to infection at the catheter site was the major concern that influenced decisions rather than the use of TPN itself.

HYPERLIPIDEMIA FOLLOWING HEART TRANSPLANTATION*

Graft atherosclerosis has been an important problem following heart transplantation, but the causes are not known. Some researchers[10–12] believe that hyperlipidemia may be an important factor and that a chronic form of graft rejection may possibly accelerate the process. Immunologic injuries associated with rejection might damage the arterial endothelium and expose the surface to thrombogenic processes, which eventually result in infiltration of plasma lipids and formation of atheromatous plaque.

Elevated blood cholesterol and triglyceride levels are frequently associated with weight gain after transplantation.[5,10] Factors that may contribute to weight gain include resumption of adequate caloric intake, improved gastrointestinal absorption with reversal of cardiac cachexia, and the use of corticosteroids and cyclosporine.[10] Weight gain associated with prednisone administration seems to correlate most closely with hyperlipidemia.

The mechanism by which cyclosporine elevates plasma lipid levels is unknown. Altered hepatic synthesis of lipoproteins or reduced peripheral catabolism may explain the elevation of blood lipids reported in both renal and cardiac transplant patients undergoing cyclosporine therapy. Recently, lovastatin was used successfully in two cardiac transplant patients receiving cyclosporine to lower serum total-cholesterol levels, without changing cyclosporine dosage levels or producing adverse side effects.[12] Thus, in the future, immunosuppressive drug therapy may be combined with medication to prevent hyperlipidemia following heart transplantation.

Summary

Cardiac transplantation now provides effective therapy for the end-stage heart disease patient. Research has shown that assessing the nutritional status of heart recipients may significantly reduce operative complications, length of hospitalization, and mortality. Eighty percent of the hospitals surveyed have recognized the importance of nutrition support and now include a dietitian as a member of the heart-transplant team.

Nutrition assessment has become an important component of the comprehensive health care provided to heart-transplant patients. In addition to the parameters that are typically evaluated, nutrition assessment should include consideration of the complex immunosuppressive drug regimes used to prevent

*By Carolyn Moore and Zakera Chowdhury

organ rejection. Finally, with continued research, nutrition support of the heart-transplant patient will become more refined as our understanding of the drug-nutrient interactions increases and the methods of assessing nutritional status improve.

NUTRITION MANAGEMENT OF THE CORONARY ARTERY BYPASS SURGERY PATIENT*

Coronary artery bypass (CAB) surgery is commonly used for treating symptoms and preventing death caused by cardiovascular disease (CVD). In 1987, approximately 284,000 CAB procedures were performed in the United States, more than double the number performed in 1980.[13] Improved survival with surgical rather than medical treatment has been demonstrated for patients with left main disease and for patients with certain types of three-vessel coronary disease.[14] In addition, CAB surgery has been shown to decrease anginal symptoms and improve the quality of life for patients who have been unresponsive to medical therapy.[15]

The appropriateness of performing CAB surgery has been recently evaluated.[16] In this study, 56% of the surgeries were performed for appropriate reasons, 30% were performed for equivocal reasons, and another 14% for inappropriate reasons. Nationwide, the number of CAB and coronary angiography procedures continues to increase. Another recent study[17] indicated that rates of CAB surgery and coronary angiography in persons ranging in age from 45 to 64 years are lowest in the northeast. Overall, rates were highest in the west, with the exception of slightly higher rates in the midwest for 45- to 64-year-olds.

The role of nutrition in the care of CAB patients is important. Coronary patients have special needs during their hospitalization, and often must make long-term changes in their eating habits to prevent the further build-up of atherosclerotic plaque and the need for additional surgery.

Effects of Malnutrition on Cardiac Function

One of the most important goals of nutrition support of CAB patients is the prevention of malnutrition, which has an independent effect on cardiac function. In the classic starvation studies of Keys, significant loss of weight in normal, healthy subjects resulted in bradycardia, mild hypotension, reduced venous pressure, decreased cardiac output and stroke volume, and decreased oxygen consumption.[18] As the subjects resumed normal eating, their cardiac function slowly returned to normal. Although usual body weight had been achieved by the 20th week, cardiac function remained at 10% below normal levels.

Previously, the heart was thought to be spared the adverse effects of malnutrition until the end stages of the disease. However, cardiac function has been shown to be affected early during the development of nutritional deficiencies. In fact, impaired cardiac function may be a fairly sensitive indicator of malnutrition.[19] Furthermore, patients with impaired cardiac function often do not eat enough calories. Without nutrition intervention, the patient's medical status may deteriorate rapidly.

*By Carolyn Moore

Nutrition Management

Nutrition management of CAB patients can be divided into two broad categories. The first group includes CAB patients who typically require nutrition support during the period immediately following surgery, especially when the recovery phase is prolonged. The second group includes patients who may have been well nourished prior to surgery, but who suffer from postoperative complications that are associated with an inability to resume normal eating. These patients are at risk of developing cardiac cachexia. Moreover, if a patient with preexisting cardiac cachexia undergoes CAB surgery, the risk of complications is greatly increased.

The nutritional requirements of a CAB patient without cardiac cachexia are similar to those of any other surgical patient during the postoperative period. Initially, the CAB patient is catabolic and requires a high intake of calories and protein to promote wound healing. Oral intake is preferred as long as the gut is functioning.

In contrast, the CAB patient with cardiac cachexia is at an increased risk of protein-calorie malnutrition. Classically, cardiac cachexia is associated with moderate to severe cardiac failure and a specific form of protein-calorie malnutrition that has multifunctional causes. Most of these patients develop sepsis and respiratory failure, spend more days in the intensive care unit, and incur higher medical bills than nonmalnourished patients.[20]

Four mechanisms have been used to describe the protein-calorie malnutrition associated with cardiac cachexia: anorexia, malabsorption caused by increased nutrient losses in urine and stool, a relatively hypermetabolic state, and impaired delivery of nutrients and oxygen to tissues.[20] Heymsfield and coworkers[2] have suggested that decreased cardiac output deprives tissues of nutrients and may further compound the problem of anorexia. Gastrointestinal hypomotility associated with edema, liver enlargement and ascites or hypokalemia also may be associated with anorexia and fat malabsorption.[21]

Preoperative nutrition support for one to two weeks has been recommended for CAB patients with cardiac cachexia.[20] Postoperatively, patients are introduced to oral feedings as soon as possible. However, if patients with cardiac cachexia remain on mechanical ventilation for more than 24 hours or develop an early complication associated with poor nutritional intake, tube feedings generally are initiated. When tolerance to enteral feedings is poor, TPN is administered.[8]

Nutrition Assessment

A physical examination and medical history are important components of the nutrition assessment of CAB patients. Indications of nutrient deficiencies may be noted during a physical examination. Knowledge of the patient's usual weight and dietary intake as well as the rate of any weight loss will help to evaluate the presence and the degree of any malnutrition.

Particular attention should be given to drugs often administered to CAB patients. Diuretics may deplete potassium and zinc stores, leading to hypomotility of the gastrointestinal tract and decreased taste acuity, respectively. In addition, digitalis intoxication may cause nausea, vomiting, and anorexia. Likewise, quinidine may decrease gastrointestinal tolerance to food.

Nutrition assessment of the CAB patient requires consideration of physiological changes that often accompany heart disease. One of the most important factors is the presence of abnormally large amounts of extracellular fluid. This fluid may artificially increase body weight, giving the false impression of good nutritional status.[2] Significant wasting of body mass may be obscured by an increase in extracellular fluid, resulting in little change in body weight. Therefore, edematous patients may appear to have adequate subcutaneous fat and muscle stores. However, measurements of an edema-free upper extremity can be used to assess somatic protein stores. Subclavicular and temporal wasting are also indicative of muscle wasting.

Visceral protein markers such as serum albumin, retinol-binding protein, and transferrin may be low because of the dilutional effects of excessive extracellular fluid. In addition, serum albumin and transferrin levels may be decreased by proteinuria or iron-deficiency anemia rather than malnutrition per se. Therefore, it may be necessary to rely on other biochemical parameters when assessing nutritional status. Creatinine-height index is generally a reliable indicator of protein stores in patients with cardiac failure.[21] The ratio of serum urea nitrogen to serum creatinine may also be used as an accurate measure of protein intake in stable patients.[21]

Biochemical assessment often reveals decreased levels of potassium, calcium, and sodium in CAB patients. Electrolyte abnormalities can result from retention of excess fluid and diuretic medications. Calcium can also be chelated by fat molecules; thus, fat malabsorption may contribute to calcium depletion. In addition, laboratory tests may indicate folate, iron, magnesium, thiamin, and zinc deficiencies.[22] Thus, nutrient requirements of CAB patients (*Table 6.3*) may exceed the RDAs[23] for adults.

Table 6.3
Nutrient Requirements of Coronary Artery Bypass Patients

Nutrient	Requirement
Water	0.5–1.0 mL/calorie
Calories	Basal energy expenditure × 1.3–1.5
Protein	0.75–1.0 g/kg or calorie-nitrogen ratio of 150:1
Sodium	1.5–2.4 g/day
Potassium	≥2–6 g/day
Magnesium	≥280–350 mg/day
Calcium	≥800 mg/day
Iron	≥10–15 mg/day
Water-soluble vitamins	RDA
Fat-soluble vitamins	RDA

Adapted from "Recommended Dietary Allowances", 1989, with permission from the National Academy Press, Washington, DC.

Estimates of the caloric needs of CAB patients should allow for the hypermetabolism that follows surgery. Energy needs can be calculated by determining basal energy expenditure (BEE) and adding 30% to 50%. Caloric needs may be further increased by preexisting malnutrition, fat malabsorption, or proteinuria.

An excess intake of calories, however, can lead to hyperglycemia, which is also a concern in the CAB patient. The incidence of diabetes among CAB patients is relatively high, and excess calories may contribute to the glucose intolerance that often accompanies the stress of surgery.

Protein needs of well-nourished CAB patients range between 0.8 to 1.0 g per kg of body weight postsurgically. However, protein requirements may be increased by the stress of surgery and possible postoperative complications. In addition, cardiac cachexia and loss of protein in the urine as a result of proteinuria or in the feces as a result of impaired digestion and absorption may increase protein needs. A calorie-nitrogen ratio of 100:1 can be used to estimate protein requirements for stressed patients. Generally, nitrogen balance studies to determine actual protein needs are reserved for research purposes.

Nutrition Support

Nutrition support to the CAB patient can be divided into acute and long-term needs. Immediately following surgery, patients typically receive clear liquids, followed by full liquids, and then a general or therapeutic diet. As the patient recuperates, meals that incorporate food preferences are provided.

Many factors, however, can interfere with the ability of the CAB patient to consume an adequate amount of calories in the postoperative period. Pain, medications, and restrictive diets may have an adverse effect on appetite. Thus, the dietitian often needs to work closely with a patient whose appetite is depressed. Easing some of the dietary restrictions and encouraging between-meal nourishments can often improve dietary intake.

Some patients may require nutrition supplements during the postoperative period. Most commercial supplements are equivalent to a 2-g sodium diet and provide 1 calorie per milliliter. Generally, these supplements are about 75% free water. When fluid intake needs to be further restricted, however, high-calorie supplements providing 1.5 to 2.0 calories per milliliter can be used. In addition, modular supplements can be used to increase the intake of protein, carbohydrates, or fat if patients require a more severe sodium restriction of less than 2 g. For example, 1,000 mL Magnacal plus 5 tbsp ProMix RDP at 4 mL per hour provides 2,000 calories, 85 g protein, and 1,000 mg sodium.

Enteral nutrition may be indicated if the CAB patient cannot eat enough food to satisfy caloric and protein needs. However, although the gastrointestinal tract may appear to be functioning normally, as evidenced by the presence of bowel sounds, problems may still exist. Gastrointestinal hypermotility may be associated with electrolyte abnormalities. Cardioreactive drugs such as digitalis and vasopressors may also compromise gastrointestinal function.

If enteral nutrition is required, the following considerations are important. Placement of enteral gastric tubes occasionally increases vagal tone, causing transient cardiac decompensation.[21] Soft, small-bore enteral tubes should be used, especially if an endotracheal or tracheostomy tube is in place.[22] Tracheoesophageal fistulas can occur if a soft enteral tube is used with a tracheal balloon as a result of pressure ischemia of the surrounding tissue. The risk of aspiration will be reduced if the tube is placed beyond the pylorus.

Often, tube feeding formulas equivalent to 2 g sodium per total volume and 1.5 to 2.0 calories per milliliter are necessary when fluid intake is of concern. Ideally, enteral feedings should begin with an iso-osmolar solution at a rate of 25 to 30 mL per hour, and the rate should be advanced slowly. However, if calorie-dense formulas are chosen, dilution will initially be necessary to prevent osmotic diarrhea. Gastric residuals, glucose and fluid control, and diarrhea should be monitored.

Elemental formulas may be more appropriate for patients with fat malabsorption or protein-losing enteropathies. Modular formulas may also be useful when sodium and fluid intake needs to be restricted.

Indication for instituting parenteral nutrition support of the CAB patient is the presence of conditions that can cause the gut to malfunction, such as prolonged ileus. Renal failure, prolonged ventilatory support, or poor wound healing are other indications.[22] Likewise, when tube feedings are not well tolerated, or aspiration is of concern, parenteral nutrition may be the best course of therapy.

The major difference between parenteral therapy for CAB patients and traditional parenteral nutrition is the need to restrict sodium and fluid intake. TPN solutions often contain 40% dextrose instead of 20% to 25% to provide calories in a small volume. However, these dextrose concentrations may pose a problem. Glucose intolerance occurs fairly often because CAB patients frequently have diabetes. Therefore, infusion rates should be initiated slowly (eg, 30 to 50 mL per hour), and insulin may need to be added directly to TPN bags.

Glucose should be monitored every four to six hours. When glucose levels range between 200 and 300 mg/dL, a sliding scale should be used to administer insulin.[22] If levels are over 300 mg/dL, a separate, continuous infusion of insulin is usually recommended.

When renal and hepatic function are normal, fluid intake rarely needs to be restricted to less than 1,500 mL/day. Adjustment of diuretic therapy can allow high volumes of TPN to be administered as long as renal function is not compromised. However, marked water losses with diuretics can lead to sodium, potassium, and magnesium depletion. Thus, replacing minerals in parenteral solutions may become necessary.

Intravenous fat emulsions contain a concentrated source of calories, which may be beneficial for patients in whom fluid intake must be limited. In the past, some problems were associated with fat-emulsion administration, but they were found to be dose related.[24] Most patients can tolerate the administration of 20% fat emulsions at rates lower than 1 mL/min. Nevertheless, plasma triglycerides should be monitored periodically to assess lipid clearance.

Long-term Nutrition Management

As the CAB patient recovers from surgery, nutrition-education programs should be initiated to facilitate long-term dietary management. Hypercholesterolemia is an important factor that may accelerate atherosclerosis in both vein grafts and native vessels following CAB surgery. Because of this, the NCEP dietary guidelines are recommended for dietary management of CAB patients.[9] If necessary, drug therapy should be initiated.

Blood cholesterol and triglyceride levels, however, may be influenced by the stress of surgery. Therefore, decisions regarding the dietary and medical treatment of hyperlipidemia should not be based on measurements obtained during the first few weeks following CAB surgery.

Most CAB patients should follow the Step One Diet upon discharge. Total plasma-cholesterol levels should be determined four to six weeks and three months after surgery, and adherence to the Step One Diet should be assessed.[9] If the desired reduction of plasma total cholesterol has not been achieved, the patient should be placed on the Step Two Diet. A minimum of six months of intensive dietary therapy and counseling should be employed before initiating drug therapy.

Omega-3 Fatty Acids

Manipulating the dietary of fatty acids may have a special role in the dietary treatment of CAB patients. Omega-3 fatty acids reportedly reduce the rate of early restenosis after coronary angioplasty.[25] Administering 3.2 g of eicosapentaenoic acid for one week prior and for six months after coronary angioplasty significantly reduced restenosis in 82 men. The incidence of early vessel restenosis was 36% in the control group and 16% in the treatment group. These findings suggest that frequent inclusion of fish in the diet may be beneficial to the CAB patient and may reduce the need for future coronary angioplasty and possible surgery.

In another study, the dietary supplementation of diets with omega-3 fatty acids for 12 weeks in men significantly reduced blood triglyceride levels and lowered heart rate, blood pressure, and systolic arterial pressure in response to exercise.[26] Despite the beneficial biochemical and hemodynamic effects, short-term dietary supplementation did not appear to alter subjective or objective parameters of myocardial ischemia.

Drug Therapy

Drug therapy should be considered for the CAB patient when LDL-cholesterol levels greater than 190 mg/dL do not respond to intensive dietary therapy after six months.[9] However, when LDL cholesterol is greater than 225 mg/dL, shorter periods of intensive dietary therapy can be considered before instituting drug therapy. The drugs commonly used for the treatment of hypercholesterolemia are described in chapter 11.

In the past, drugs of first choice were the bile-acid sequestrants (cholestyramine, colestipol) and nicotinic acid. Nicotinic acid has been the drug of choice when triglyceride levels are also elevated.

Inhibitors of hydroxymethylglutaryl coenzyme-A (HMG-CoA) such as lovastatin are very effective in lowering LDL cholesterol levels and now may be considered to be the drug of first choice for CAB patients. In a recent multicenter study, lovastatin was found to be more effective and better tolerated than cholestyramine for the treatment of hypercholesterolemia.[26] After 12 weeks of treatment with 80 mg/day of lovastatin, LDL-cholesterol levels were reduced 34% compared to only 17% when 12 g/day of cholestyramine was prescribed for the same period of time. Adverse effects for both treatment groups primarily included gastrointestinal-tract symptoms such as constipation and dyspepsia.

Treatment of Hypertension

For CAB patients with hypertension, the step-by-step approach using diet therapy and antihypertensive drugs (*Table 6.4*) is recommended.[27] Reducing blood pressure with drugs has been clearly shown to decrease cardiovascular mortality and morbidity when diastolic blood pressure is greater than 104 mm Hg.[27] If, after a one to three month interval, the response to therapy is inadequate, three options are available: the first drug dosage can be increased if it is below the maximum; an agent from another class can be added; or the initial drug can be discontinued and a drug from a different class can be substituted.

Table 6.4
Stepped-care Therapy for Hypertension

Step	Treatment
1.	Nonpharmacologic approaches: sodium and alcohol restriction; weight control; exercise
2.	Add first drug: diuretic, beta-blocker, calcium antagonist or angiotensin-converting enzyme inhibitor
3.	Add second drug of a different class: increase dose of first drug or substitute another drug
4.	Add third drug of a different class or substitute second drug
5.	Further evaluation and/or referral; or add third or fourth drug

Adapted from 1988 Joint National Committee. Report on detection, evaluation, and treatment of high blood pressure. *Arch Intern Med.* 1988;148:1023.

Summary

Coronary artery bypass surgery has proved useful to treat symptoms and to prevent deaths caused by CVD. Moreover, nutrition has been shown to play an important role in the comprehensive medical care of the CAB patient. Preventing malnutrition is a major goal of nutrition support following surgery. Nutritional status can significantly affect surgical outcome, length of hospitalization, and mortality.

Nutrition support of the CAB patient can be divided into acute and long-term phases. Immediately following surgery the patient is in a catabolic state. Nutrition supplements, tube feedings, or total parenteral nutrition may be indicated to satisfy increased protein and energy needs during the postoperative period.

In contrast, long-term dietary management employs a progressive approach to lower blood pressure and elevated cholesterol levels. Dietary therapy usually requires the CAB patient to make changes in lifetime eating habits to prevent the formation of atherosclerotic plaque and the need for additional surgery. Plasma total-cholesterol levels and dietary adherence should be monitored periodically. Finally, incorporating appropriate behavioral strategies is crucial for successful dietary change and long-term adherence.

References

1. Kaye MP. The Registry of the International Society for Heart Transplantation: fourth official report—1987. *J Heart Transplantation.* 1987;6:63.
2. Heymsfield SB, Smith J, Reed, et al. Nutritional support in cardiac failure. *Surg Clin North Am.* 1981;61:635.
3. Mullen JL, Gordon PB, Matthews P, et al. Reduction of operative morbidity and mortality by combined preoperative and postoperative nutritional support. *Ann Surg.* 1980;192:604.
4. Frazier OH, Van Buren CT, Poindexter S, et al. Nutritional management of the heart transplant recipient. *Heart Transplant.* 1985;4:450.
5. Grady KL, Herold LS. Comparison of nutritional status in patients before and after heart transplantation. *J Heart Transplantation.* 1988;7:123.
6. Rogsdale D. Nutritional program for heart transplantation. *J Heart Transplantation.* 1987;6:228.
7. Blackburn GL, Bistrain BR, Maini BS, et al. Nutritional and metabolic assessment of the hospitalized patient. *J Parenteral Enteral Nutr.* 1977;1:11.
8. Kumar MR, Coulston AM. Nutritional management of the cardiac patient. *J Am Diet Assoc.* 1983;83:463.

9. National Cholesterol Education Program Expert Panel. Report on detection, evaluation, and treatment of high blood cholesterol in adults. *Arch Intern Med.* 1988;148:36.
10. Kaegh A, Simons L, Spratt P, et al. Hyperlipidemia after heart transplantation. *J Heart Transplantation.* 1988;7:171.
11. Hess ML, Hastillo A, Thompson JA, et al. Lipid mediators in organ transplantation: does cyclosporine accelerate coronary atherosclerosis? *Transplantation Proc.* 1987;19:71.
12. Ballantyne CM, Jones PH, et al. Hyperlipidemia following heart transplantation: natural history and intervention with mevinolin (lovastatin). *Transplantation Proc.* 1987;19(supplement 5):60.
13. American Heart Association. *Heart Facts.* Dallas, Tex: American Heart Association;1988.
14. European Coronary Surgery Study Group. Long term results of prospective randomized study of coronary artery bypass surgery in stable angina pectoris. *Lancet.* 1982;2:1173.
15. Peduzzi P, Hultgren HN. Effect of medical versus surgical treatment of symptoms in stable angina pectoris: the Veterans Administration Cooperative Study for Coronary Arterial Occlusive Disease. *Circulation.* 1979;60:888.
16. Winslow CM, Kosecoff JB, Chassin M, et al. The appropriateness of performing coronary artery bypass surgery. *JAMA.* 1988;260:505.
17. Gillum RF. Coronary artery bypass surgery and coronary angiography in the United States. *Am Heart J.* 1987;113:1255.
18. Keys A, Brozek J, Henschel A, et al. *The Biology of Human Starvation.* Minneapolis, Minn: University of Minnesota Press; 1950.
19. Abel RM, Grimes JB, Alanso D, et al. Adverse hemodynamic and ultrastructural changes in dog hearts subjected to protein-calorie malnutrition. *Am Heart J.* 1979;97:733.
20. Abel RM. Nutritional support and the patient. In: Rombeau JL, Caldwell MD, eds. *Parenteral Nutrition.* Philadelphia, Pa: WB Saunders Co; 1986:575.
21. Bernard MA, Jacobs DO, Rombeau J. *Nutritional and Metabolic Support of Hospitalized Patients.* Philadelphia Pa: WB Saunders Co; 1986:129.
22. Talamini MA. The cardiac patient. In: Lang CE, ed. *Nutritional Support in Critical Care.* Rockville, Md: Aspen Publishers Inc; 1987:149.
23. *Recommended Dietary Allowances.* Washington, DC: National Academy of Sciences; 1989.
24. Abel RM, Fisch D, Grossman ML. Hemodynamic effects of intravenous 20% soy oil emulsion following coronary artery bypass surgery. *J Parenteral Enteral Nutr.* 1983;7:534.
25. Dehmer GJ, Popma JJ, Egerton KV, et al. Reduction in the rate of early restenosis after coronary angioplasty by a diet supplemental with n-3 fatty acids. *N Engl J Med.* 1988;319:733.
26. The Lovastatin Study Group III. A multicenter comparison of lovastatin and cholestyramine therapy for severe primary hypercholesterolemia. *JAMA.* 1988;260:359.
27. 1988 Joint National Committee. Report on detection, evaluation, and treatment of high blood pressure. *Arch Intern Med.* 1988;148:1023.

7. PEDIATRIC PREVENTION AND TREATMENT OF HYPERCHOLESTEROLEMIA

EPIDEMIOLOGIC BACKGROUND*

Preventive medicine, by its very nature, must be initiated early for optimal results. Although children are typically not at risk of coronary mortality during childhood, they may begin the atherosclerotic process in their preschool years. Pathologic precursors of coronary heart disease (CHD) such as fatty streaks have been observed in children as young as age 4.[1] Epidemiologic evidence indicates that children with lipid and lipoprotein levels in the upper 95th percentile of the age- and sex-specific population means are potentially at the highest risk for subsequent CHD morbidity.[1-4] In the Bogalusa Heart Study, aortic fatty streaks were strongly related to both antemortem levels of plasma total- and LDL- cholesterol levels in 35 subjects (mean age of death, 18 years).

In countries with significantly lower CHD incidence, the distributions of serum cholesterol in pediatric populations plot at lower values when compared with those of North American children and children from countries with higher CHD rates.[5,6] *Table 7.1* illustrates normal lipid and lipoprotein levels by age and sex for males and females during the first two decades of life in the United States, as determined by the Lipid Research Clinics (LRC).[7] Umbilical cord blood cholesterol levels are similar cross-culturally with means in the range of 65 to 75 mg/dL, but differences are noted after the first year of life.[7]

No group of children has yet been followed for several decades to examine the diet-lipid relationship over time as it ultimately relates to CHD. Data from the Bogalusa Heart Study (a prospective study among biracial—64% white, 36% black—infants and children from a semirural area in Louisiana) demonstrated that the lowest levels of serum total cholesterol accompanied the lowest total dietary fat intake.[8]

Data from other major prospective studies among children (including the Muscatine Study in Iowa and the Beaver County Study in Pennsylvania, as well as Bogalusa) reported that children in the upper quintile of serum total cholesterol maintain the same relative position in the cholesterol distribution curve over time.[9-11] Studies tracking plasma total cholesterol, triglycerides, LDL cholesterol, and HDL cholesterol in children illustrate that the top deciles of the distribution have the highest correlations between childhood and adult cholesterol levels.[4] These relationships persist despite the influence of regression toward the mean.

An increased propensity for the development of coronary artery disease occurs among families of children with persistently elevated cholesterol levels.[12,13] The tracking of dietary components such as total and saturated fat and cholesterol and their correlations with risk for CHD have also been reported by the Bogalusa Study.[8] Since only 0.2% to 1.0% of all children in the United States are estimated to have genetically induced familial hypercholesterolemia, the majority of hypercholesterolemia in pediatric populations is likely due to environmental influences such as obesity, smoking, and diet.[13] Other factors that are known to influence lipid-lipoprotein levels in the first two decades of life include age, sex, and hormones.[14] To achieve maximum benefit,

*By Linda V. Van Horn and Gail C. Frank

it is particularly appropriate to initiate family-oriented intervention to reduce the serum cholesterol level of all family members and to strengthen environmental support for the child.

Table 7.1
Normal Plasma Lipid Concentrations in the First Two Decades of Life

Age (yr) and Sex	No.	Cholesterol (mg/dL)			Triglyceride (mg/dL)			No.	Cholesterol (mg/dL): High-Density Lipoprotein			No.	Low-Density Lipoprotein			No.	Very-Low-Density Lipoprotein		
		5th	Mean	95th	5th	Mean	95th		5th	Mean	95th		5th	Mean	95th		5th	Mean	95th
0-4																			
M	238	114	155	203	29	56	99												
F	186	112	156	200	34	64	112												
5-9																			
M	1,253	121	160	203	30	56	101	145	38	56	75	132	63	93	129	132	0	8	18
F	1,118	126	164	205	32	60	105	127	36	53	73	114	68	100	140	113	1	10	24
10-14																			
M	2,278	119	158	202	32	66	125	298	37	55	74	288	64	97	133	288	1	10	22
F	2,087	124	160	201	37	75	131	248	37	52	70	245	68	97	136	245	2	11	23
15-19																			
M	1,980	113	150	197	37	78	148	300	30	46	63	298	62	94	130	297	2	13	26
F	2,079	120	158	203	39	75	132	297	35	52	74	295	59	96	137	295	2	12	24

Data given are from the Lipid Research Clinic Data Book. Lipids were determined on plasma from 11,219 fasting, white subjects (5,749 boys, 5,470 girls) who were studied in seven North American Lipid Research Clinics, using common protocols and laboratory methodology.

Data are from the Lipid Research Clinic Data Book. Lipoproteins were determined on plasma from 1,415 fasting, white subjects (743 boys, 672 girls) who were studied in seven North American Lipid Research Clinics, using common protocols and laboratory methodology.

Adapted from Lipid Research Clinics.[7]

DIETARY PATTERNS OF CHILDREN*

Dietary studies of four cross-sectional surveys of 10-year-old children in Bogalusa reported that an excessive energy and protein intake— ie, above the RDA range—resulted in nutrient intakes well above the RDA *(Table 7.2)*.[15,16] More than 80% of children exceeded the RDA for protein. Boys averaged 7 calories per kilogram of body weight more than girls. Two thirds of dietary protein came from animal sources and one third came from vegetable sources. Total carbohydrate consisted of two thirds simple sugars and one third starch. Approximately 40% of the children consumed more than 300 mg of cholesterol per day, and fat intake averaged 38% of total calories. Significant increases in omega-6 fatty acids were reported in later cross-sectional surveys, but only 5% of the children had polyunsaturated to saturated-fatty-acid (P/S) ratios greater than 1.0. These dietary patterns reflected health-risk eating behaviors among healthy children; however, consistent significant correlations between diet components and the serum total-cholesterol levels were not observed.[8,16,17]

*By Linda V. Van Horn and Gail C. Frank

Table 7.2
Mean Nutrient Intake of Four Surveys of 10-year-olds, Bogalusa Heart Study, 1973–1982

	Group 1 1973–1974 (n = 185)		Group 2 1976–1977 (n = 158)		Group 3 1978–1979 (n = 224)		Group 4 1981–1982 (n = 304)	
Dietary Component	**x**	**2 SD**	**x**	**2 SD**	**x**	**2 SD**	**x**	**2 SD**
Energy, kcal	2,141	± 1,691	2,316[a]	± 1,747	2,145	± 1,877	2,054[b]	± 1,562
kcal/kg	65.5[a]	± 57.1	67.2[a]	± 57.5	62.1[a]	± 54.4	57.4[b]	± 48.6
Protein, g	69.1[b]	± 60.2	79.8[a]	± 86.5	72.1[b]	± 79.0	67.4[b]	± 62.2
g/1,000 kcal	32.5	± 17.0	33.9	± 17.0	33.3	± 19.6	32.7	± 15.6
g/kg	2.10	± 1.92	2.32[a]	± 2.72	2.09	± 2.37	1.90[b]	± 1.93
Fat, g	93.1	± 93.0	100.5	± 100.0	96.1	± 122.6	87.3[b]	± 88.7
g/1,000 kcal	42.7	± 17.5	42.5	± 16.7	42.8	± 19.1	41.5	± 16.1
g/kg	2.83[a]	± 2.91	2.92[a]	± 3.25	2.77[a]	± 3.41	2.44[b]	± 190.5
Carbohydrate, g	261.5	± 216.7	280.5[a]	± 198.4	253.1[b]	± 191.6	255.6[b]	± 190.5
g/1,000 kcal	123.6	± 47.5	123.9	± 46.0	123.0	± 52.1	127.1	± 46.8
g/kg	8.06[a]	± 7.57	8.11[a]	± 6.32	7.35	± 5.82	7.13[b]	± 5.77

a > b, $p < 0.05$

Reprinted with permission from Frank GC, Farris RP, Cresanta JL, et al. Dietary intake as a determinant of cardiovascular risk factor variables: observations in a pediatric population. In: Berenson GS, ed. *Causation of Cardiovascular Risk Factors in Children: Perspectives in Causation of Cardiovascular Risk in Early Life.* New York, NY: Raven Press; 1986:254.

Limitations in dietary assessment methodology in studies of adults as well as children have contributed to the difficulties in obtaining significant correlations between dietary factors and serum lipid levels.[8,18] Wide variability in dietary intake within and between individuals and cultures further confounds meaningful interpretations.[19] However, findings from dietary intervention studies of adults and children using different assessment methods continue to demonstrate cholesterol-lowering benefits from fat-modified dietary patterns.[20,21]

RESPONSE TO DIETARY INTERVENTION AT VARIOUS AGES*

Children with high plasma total-cholesterol levels have been shown to be responsive to dietary intervention (ie, reducing saturated fat and cholesterol.[14,22,23] Studies that compared the plasma total-cholesterol levels in infants fed different commercial formulas with those of infants fed human milk showed plasma lipid level differences due to diet.[24–26] Currently, most infant formulas have a P/S ratio of around 0.4, which is similar to the P/S ratio of human milk.[14] A clinical study of children who were fed a diet low in cholesterol (<200 mg/day) with a P/S ratio of 1.0 from birth demonstrated significantly lower plasma total-cholesterol levels (145 mg/dL) at 3 years than children following a typical American diet (154 mg/dL).[27] Studies of healthy adolescents who reduced their daily intake of saturated fatty acids and cholesterol (to 10% of calories and 300 mg/day, respectively) showed a significant reduction in serum total-cholesterol levels (a 15% reduction, compared with controls).[28] These values returned to baseline levels when previous dietary patterns were resumed. Other school-based intervention studies (such as the American Health Foundation's Know Your Body Program[29] and the Child and

*By Linda V. Van Horn and Gail C. Frank

Adolescent Trial on Cardiovascular Health [CATCH], a prospective intervention study in progress) are beginning to accumulate data on the efficacy and feasibility of school-based nutrition intervention for blood cholesterol-lowering.[30]

Community intervention studies in Finland have shown a reduction in plasma cholesterol of about 10% among teenage children who reduced total fat from 37% to 32% of calories over two years.[31] Although the response to dietary intervention is variable in children, just as it is in adults, children with the highest baseline total-cholesterol levels generally experience a response to dietary intervention that is more dramatic than in children with lower baseline levels.[25,26] Kwiterovich et al[22] have reported that on the average, plasma total-cholesterol and LDL-cholesterol levels of children with heterozygous familial hypercholesterolemia can be reduced by approximately 10% to 15% by dietary intervention alone.

SAFETY OF MODIFIED DIETS FOR CHILDREN*

Optimal growth and development are dependent on adequate nutrient intake. Various members of the pediatric community have expressed concern that the consumption of fat-modified diets (eg, low in cholesterol, total fat, and saturated fatty acids) by children might pose a threat to the adequate intake of calories, protein, and certain trace minerals such as iron and zinc.[32,33] Data from studies among vegetarian children whose dietary intake of animal fat and protein is reduced (compared with that of omnivorous children) did not show deficiencies in essential vitamins and minerals.[34] The increased intake of complex carbohydrates in these children was associated with the improved intake of certain nutrients compared with nonvegetarian children.[34] Subsequent work by the same investigator, however, demonstrated compromised growth curves in vegetarian (0.5 to 1.0 kg and 1 to 2 cm lower) versus age- and gender-matched nonvegetarian children.[35] Data regarding the efficacy, safety, and feasibility of dietary intervention in hyperlipidemic children have yet to be conclusively established. The Dietary Intervention Study in Children (DISC), sponsored by the National Heart, Lung and Blood Institute (NHLBI) of the NIH, will investigate these issues in preadolescent children.

Theoretically, there is no reason why a decrease in saturated fatty acids and dietary cholesterol to levels commonly recommended should be deleterious to growing children as long as other nutrient and caloric needs are met.[14] There is no dietary requirement for saturated fatty acids or dietary cholesterol, due to endogenous synthesis of these nutrients. Limited cross-cultural data illustrate no significant growth differences, based on height, between American and Israeli adolescents, despite significantly lower intakes of saturated fatty acids and dietary cholesterol among the latter.[36] In Mediterranean and Far Eastern countries, childhood diets that are rich in fish, fruits, vegetables, grains, and legumes and lower in animal products, fats, and sugar are consumed with safety.[14] Definitive results about the safety of fat-modified diets among a sample of US children are forthcoming from DISC in 1993.

RECOMMENDATIONS FOR CHILDREN*

The American Heart Association's Nutrition Committee has issued dietary recommendations for healthy children older than 2 years.[37] These recommendations and their practical implications as interpreted by Kwiterovich[14] are presented in *Table 7.3.* These recommendations are consistent with the Surgeon General's Report on Nutrition,[38] the report of the National Academy of Sciences,[39] and the earlier report of the Senate Select Committee on Nutrition and Human Needs.[40]

*By Linda V. Van Horn and Gail C. Frank

Table 7.3
Dietary Recommendations for Healthy Children Older Than 2 Years of Age

Recommendations	Practical Implications
1. Nutritionally adequate diet consisting of a variety of foods	1. Satisfies RDA of the Food and Nutrition Board of the National Research Council for protein, vitamins, and minerals
2. Calorie intake based on growth rate and activity level	2. Maintain growth curve and weight appropriate for height
3. Decrease total fat intake to approximately 30% of calories and saturated fat to 10% of calories	3. Emphasize consumption of lean meat, fish, and poultry and decrease use of fatty meats; substitute vitamin D–fortified skim milk or lowfat milk for whole milk; broil or bake rather than fry foods
4. Moderate use of polyunsaturated fats (not more than 10% of calories)	4. Use soft margarine rather than solid margarine or butter; use vegetable oils such as safflower or corn oil rather than lard for cooking or salads
5. Lower cholesterol intake to <300 mg/day	5. Limit eggs to 2 to 3 per week; items 3 and 4 above
6. Maintain protein at about 15% to 20% of calories	6. Protein of both animal and vegetable sources will provide all essential amino acids
7. Increase percentage of calories from carbohydrates to about 50% to 55%, derived primarily from complex carbohydrates, and increase fiber	7. Increase consumption of whole-grain or enriched breads and whole-grain, enriched, and fortified cereals; increase consumption of fruits and vegetables; decrease consumption of desserts, snack foods, candy bars, sweets

Reproduced by permission of *Pediatrics* vol 78 page 349 copyright 1986.

In 1985, the Consensus Conference on Lowering Blood Cholesterol to Prevent Heart Disease[41] made several recommendations both for adults and for children older than age 2 (*Table 7.4*). From this report, as well as extensive animal, laboratory, clinical, and epidemiological evidence, the NCEP was launched.[42] The NCEP has convened several panels to address the issues of treatment and prevention of high blood cholesterol levels.[43] At the time of this writing, the reports of the Adult Treatment Panel, the Laboratory Standardization Panel, and the Panel on Population Strategies for Lowering Blood Cholesterol have been written. The Panel on Blood Cholesterol in Children and Adolescents is expected to release its report by early 1991. Representatives from the pediatric and dietetic communities have been appointed to this panel; they will weigh the existing epidemiologic, intervention, and nutrition data on children to develop their recommendations for the evaluation, detection, and treatment of high cholesterol levels.

The American Academy of Pediatrics' Committee on Nutrition, in its statement on "Prudent Lifestyle for Children: Dietary Fat and Cholesterol,"[33] listed seven dietary recommendations (*Table 7.5*). One recommendation is that the "current dietary trends in the U.S. toward a decreased consumption of saturated fats, cholesterol, and salt and an increased intake of polyunsaturated fats should be followed with moderation." A further precaution was that "diets that avoid extremes are safe for children." Some parents have been overly zealous in their application of the dietary recommendations and severely restrict fat and energy in their very young children. A number of cases of failure to thrive have been reported.[44] The recommendations for reduced fat intake are directed at children over the age of 2 years; they imply that a moderate reduction in saturated and total fat among children currently eating high-fat diets can have beneficial health effects.

Table 7.4
Special Guidelines by Consensus Conference for Management of Children

1. It is desirable to begin prevention in childhood because patterns of life-style are developed in childhood. The moderate-fat and moderate-cholesterol diets recommended for the population at large in this report should be suitable for all family members, including healthy children older than 2 years. For children, the diets should provide all nutrients in quantities adequate for growth and development and meet energy requirements. Excessive gain in weight should be avoided.
2. Children at "high-risk" should be identified primarily by carefully obtained family histories rather than routine screening. The history should include parents, grandparents, and all first-degree relatives. A family history of hypercholesterolemia or premature CHD should alert the physician to obtain at least two blood cholesterol determinations.
3. If the blood cholesterol level in such "high-risk" children is above the 75th percentile (approximately 170 mg/dL for children aged 2 to 19 years), total and HDL-cholesterol measurements should be obtained. Those children with blood cholesterol levels between the 75th and 90th percentile (170 to 185 mg/dL) should be counseled regarding diet and other cardiovascular risk factors and then followed up at one-year intervals. Those with levels above the 90th percentile ($>$185 mg/dL) require special dietary instruction and close supervision with evaluation of other risk factors. A child with a blood cholesterol level above the 95th percentile ($>$200 mg/dL) on two occasions is in a special category and may have one of the hereditary hypercholesterolemias. Strict dietary intervention is indicated and will be sufficient for many children. Nonresponders should be considered for treatment with a lipid-lowering agent, eg, a bile-acid sequestrant (such as cholestyramine). All family members should be screened.
4. Dietary management of children with elevated blood cholesterol levels should be part of total management that includes regular exercise programs, maintenance of ideal weight, avoidance of excess salt, and avoidance of cigarette smoking.

From NIH Consensus Conference. Lowering blood cholesterol to prevent heart disease. *JAMA.* 1985;253:2080.

THE ROLE OF THE REGISTERED DIETITIAN: BEHAVIOR ISSUES*

To apply the concept of preventive medicine successfully to coronary risk reduction among children, a blueprint for eating behavior must be established. Drawing from their experiences with the pitfalls that limit adult eating-behavior change, registered dietitians must actively counsel both the adults who may be promoting an unhealthy eating environment at home or at school, as well as the children themselves.

The pediatrician, pediatric cardiologist, or family practitioner is responsible for the medical management of the child who presents with either a clinically defined hyperlipidemia or a strong family history of CHD. The registered dietitian who works directly with the family and the physician implements a "high-risk model" to manage the hyperlipidemia.[45] The registered dietitian with training in behavioral counseling can skillfully interpret scientific data

*By Linda V. Van Horn and Gail C. Frank

into practical life-style recommendations.[46] The registered dietitian who becomes knowledgeable about the child-nutrition program in the schools can add an important dimension to the preventive effort by creating a "population model" to manage hyperlipidemia.[47] The five major objectives of a lipid-lowering program that involves both the home and the school are outlined in *Table 7.6.*

Table 7.5
Committee on Nutrition, American Academy of Pediatrics: Recommendations for Feeding Children

1. When breast-feeding is unsuccessful, inappropriate, or stopped early, infant formulas provide the best alternative for meeting nutritional needs during the first six months of life. During the second six months of life, whole cow's milk may be introduced for infants who are consuming one third of their calories as supplemental foods consisting of a balanced mixture of cereal, vegetables, fruits, and other foods. Supplementary foods are recommended beginning at four to six months of age. Dietary fat should probably not be restricted in this age group.
2. After 1 year of age, infants should receive a varied diet including each of the major food groups. This provides the best assurance of nutritional adequacy; the key is balance from variety.
3. Detection of obesity by measuring height and weight and detection of hypertension by measuring blood pressure according to the schedules published by the Academy will permit the early recognition and treatment of obesity and hypertension.
4. Counseling on the maintenance of ideal body weight and a regular exercise program and, in teenagers, counseling concerning the dangers of smoking should be a routine part of all health visits.
5. Family history for each patient should include information about family members who have had a premature (before 60 years of age) heart attack or stroke, hypertension, obesity, diabetes mellitus, and/or hyperlipidemia.
6. Screening of children more than 2 years old who are at risk because of family history should consist of at least two serum cholesterol measurements. HDL-cholesterol level should be measured in those who consistently have levels above the 95th percentile for age and sex. If HDL-cholesterol is not the cause of the hypercholesterolemia, the child should be treated with an appropriate diet and/or medication.
7. Currently dietary trends in the U.S.—decreased consumption of saturated fats, cholesterol, and salt and an increased intake of polyunsaturated fats—should be followed with moderation. The optimal total fat intake cannot be determined, but 30% to 40% of calories seems sensible for adequate growth and development. Diets that avoid extremes are safe for children for whom there is no evidence of special vulnerability. Any recommendations for changing toward a more restrictive dietary pattern during the first two decades of life should await demonstration that such dietary restrictions are needed and, in addition, that such restrictions would support adequate growth and development for children and adolescents.

Reproduced by permission of *Pediatrics* vol 71 page 78 copyright 1983.

Table 7.6
Major Objectives of the Registered Dietitian When Planning a Program to Lower Plasma Lipid Levels

1. Identify eating behaviors that influence a child's risk for CVD.
2. Target eating behaviors that are modifiable.
3. Structure modifications of a child's eating behavior considering a complementary home and school environment.
4. Plan a progressive sequence of eating-behavior-change activities.
5. Incorporate others in the child's home and school to aid and support the change process.

The registered dietitian's challenge is to design an appropriate eating-behavior program that is practical for the family on a daily basis and that also initiates the changes needed to establish a new, healthier eating environment. The recommended composition of a healthy eating pattern is outlined in Table 7.3. To target, structure, and plan a program to achieve this pattern, the registered dietitian may find it productive to focus activities on the home or on the school.

The home environment is the most important site for teaching and practicing sound eating behaviors. The child should not have sole responsibility to make all behavioral changes. Children receive environmental imprints. Mothers, who are the gatekeepers of their children's diets, tend to plan meals in response to their husbands' food likes.[48] Children react to the media.[49] Parents imprint children via the foods they bring into the home and the restaurants they select when dining out. Conversely, children direct their parents' food choices.[50] These subtle activities may assist or negate the child's attempt to make positive, healthy behavioral changes.

Table 7.7
Timeline for Introducing Selected Dietary Components for Management of Hyperlipidemia in a Private Physician's Office

Activity/Instruction	**Monthly Consultation Visit**								
	Phase I (Months)			**Phase II (Months)**			**Phase III (Months)**		
	1	**2**	**3**	**4**	**5**	**6**	**7**	**8**	**9**
Assessment*									
Anthropometric	X	X	X	X	X	X	X	X	X
Record of food intake	X	X			X		X		
Computerized analysis of food intake			X			X		X	
Lipid/lipoprotein determination				X			X		X
Instructions									
Energy reduction	X		X		X			X	X
Fat modification									
Fat quantity	X	X		X			X		
Fat quality		X		X			X		X
Cholesterol		X					X		X
Alcohol			X	X		X			
Complex carbohydrate			X	X			X		
Fiber			X					X	

*Initial visit after evaluation of serum lipids/lipoproteins.

Reprinted with permission from the American College of Cardiology (*Journal of the American College of Cardiology*, vol 12, 1988, page 1090).

Parental encouragement to eat, the frequency of food prompts, and the use of food as a reward are significant contributors to a child's relative weight.[51] Parental modeling, positive reinforcement, food contacts, and discipline motivate the food preferences and food choices of children.[52] Social learning theory (SLT) provides a framework for organizing an eating-behavior-change program.[53] SLT integrates cognitive and behavioral change strategies within the family dynamics. The application of SLT has been shown to be effective not only with short-term behavior change but also when one is promoting a new life style.[54]

The registered dietitian who is involved in lipid-lowering should begin a series of family-nutrition consultation sessions within the private pediatrician's office, medical clinics, and health agencies in the community. Over a 6- to 12-month period, contact with the family may need to be as frequent as once every three to four weeks within a minimum of one to one and one-half hours assigned to each session. *Table 7.7* outlines a flow sequence for private consultation.[45] Activities can be planned within the sessions to integrate the tenets of SLT, eg, record keeping, pledging, and modeling.

A food record that focuses on the health-risk eating behaviors of children is an efficient way to identify and modify unhealthy eating habits. A one-week period is an appropriate time frame for recording food intake. After family members record their foods and beverages, the registered dietitian can evaluate whether the foods are high, medium, or low in fat, saturated fat, or fiber. During nutrition consultations, the registered dietitian reviews the checklists and provides criteria (such as a fat-counter booklet) for evaluating the content of foods.[55] This activity gradually teaches the family to identify healthful foods.

Each family member can select activities that create health-risk situations and can agree to become actively involved as "change agents."[55] Individual commitment may take the form of a behavioral pledge—a personal commitment to change or to modify a habit.[56] Adding one piece of fruit to the daily diet might be the skill that is targeted at one session. Each family member must become involved with individual complementary tasks. For example, the child may pledge to eat a banana instead of cookies after school; the parent may pledge to make more of the child's favorite fruits available and accessible. Siblings may pledge to eat more fruit or drink more juice as well.[57,58]

Pledging can be directed toward fat intake, fiber intake, total energy intake, meal time, eating out, snacks, or a variety of other behaviors. The skilled registered dietitian addresses only one or two complementary pledges at each consultation with the family. Pledges become small steps that accumulate to form a critical mass of positive behavior change. It is the magnitude of change and the persistence of the new habit patterns that will allow eating behavior change to occur.[59]

Self-responsibility and self-management are other basic constructs of SLT. Teaching the child and family to identify their own behaviors and to modify behaviors that are related to unhealthy eating habits strengthens self-efficacy and empowers the child with the ability to feel in control of his or her health.[60] The children and families who believe they can make changes and who experience successful change are, in fact, successful with change.

Modeling is another important SLT tenet; it aligns learning with observations of what others do. Peer and sibling influence as well as parental influence cannot be controlled, but they can be directed toward healthy eating behavior. Family skills and tasks that support environmental change are outlined in *Table 7.8*.

To modify school lunches successfully, efforts must occur at the local, state, and national levels.[47,61] Making an effort in a single cafeteria to assure that a high-risk child has proper food choices is worthwhile and needed, but medical and dietetic professionals must wage efforts to create broad-based change. Creating a healthy eating environment in schools is essential, since 27 million children are fed school lunches and 3 million eat breakfast at school.

If a student with hyperlipidemia has been identified by his or her pediatrician and the child's school has no formal program to assure a lowfat lunch, the registered dietitian can meet with school-lunch personnel at the county or school level to outline the specific needs of the child. The goals are to become aware of existing efforts within the school and to plan for lower-fat versions of foods without causing the child to feel different. Using a "population strategy" that assures a lower fat intake for all children is the preferred format.[62-64]

Table 7.8
Assignment of Meal-Related Tasks To Help Families Create Healthy Life Styles

Skill/Task	Family Member
General	
• Select family recipes for change	Mom
• Alter eating times for total family participation	Mom and Dad
• Make meals a separate event away from TV	Each member
• Avoid eating on the run	Each member
• Keep family problems away from meals	Each member
• Define times for watching TV	Dad
• Select family physical activities	Each member
Specific	
• Purchase measuring spoons and nested cups	Dad
• Purchase a functional food scale	Dad
• Use healthy recipes	The cook
• Make salad dressings with preferred oils	Mom
• Use herbs and spices in cooking	The cook
• Remove the saltshaker from the table	Dad
• Measure total margarine allowance at the beginning of the day	Mom
• Replace baked desserts with fresh fruits	The cook
• Replace fried foods with fresh vegetables	The cook

In the United States, the basic goals of the child nutrition program are: (1) to meet one third of the child's RDA with acceptable, low-cost meals; and (2) to serve as a laboratory for health and nutrition education, where students have an opportunity to practice food behaviors consistent with classroom instruction.[65] Children learn from and within their school environments. When the classroom imparts sound nutrition information that is reinforced by the cafeteria's serving foods lower in saturated fat, salt, and sugar and higher in fiber, children are given the stimuli for responding positively when selecting foods in school.[66]

A fat-modified school-lunch program along with classroom programs and physical-education programs can enhance students' behavioral changes within a learning environment.[62] These instructive settings provide the knowledge base for students, and they complement home activities. Registered dietitians are not usually skilled in coordinating programs of this nature. To identify elements in the school environment that support a lipid-lowering effort, the "precede model" can be used to aid program planning.[67] The precede model identifies variables for effective intervention strategies in schools (*Figure 7.1*). It groups factors that influence health-related behaviors into three categories: predisposing, enabling, or reinforcing. Most of the predisposing factors (eg, demographic and population norms) are beyond the scope of a school education program. However, when these factors are positively affected, often outside the school environment, they motivate students to make preventive behavior changes that influence peer behaviors. For example, a shift in dietary behaviors to lower saturated fat and energy intakes may establish a new preferred peer norm.

The attitudes and behaviors of peers, school personnel, and the media are a reinforcing factor—they either support or discourage behavioral change. Daily physical-education classes indirectly support nutritional well-being.

Physical activity can be therapeutic for weight loss (besides providing improved muscle tone and cardiovascular conditioning). Beginning in first grade, the nature of cafeteria food interacts with the classroom curriculum and physical activities to further reinforce positive attitudes and enhance children's behavioral changes. Using this planning tool, the registered dietitian can organize and present a strategy for food change in schools.

Fig. 7.1
Cardiovascular health promotion for school-age children. Reproduced with permission from Green LW, Kreuter NW, Deeds SG, et al.* Health Education Planning: A Diagnostic Approach. *Palo Alto, Calif: Mayfield; 1980:142.

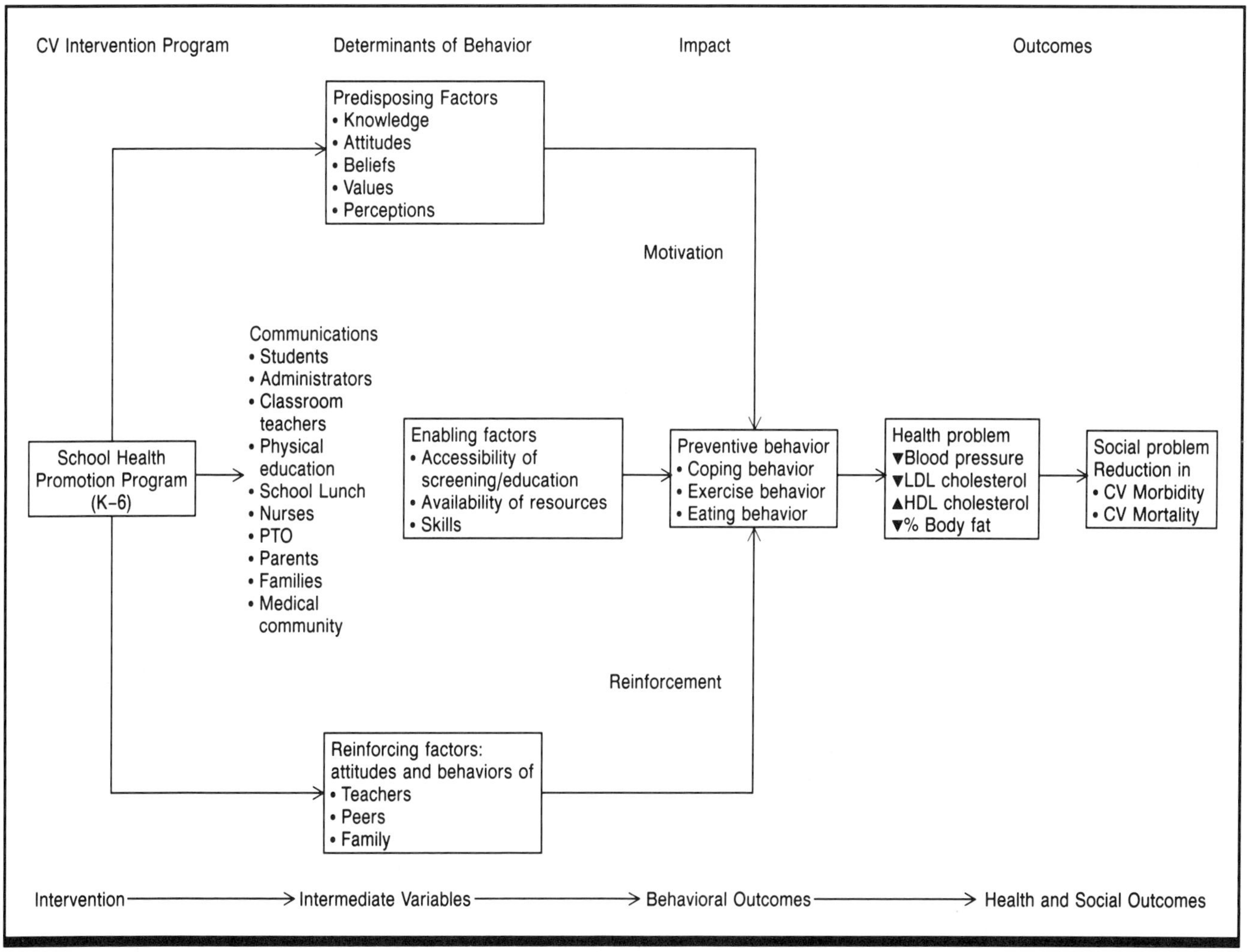

The American School Food Service Association and state education agencies have made a national commitment to promote the decreased use of salt, sugar, and fat. Training programs and modified recipes are offered to teach food-service personnel how to adjust ingredient levels to be consistent with the prudent-diet recommendations. By 1990, 50% of school-cafeteria employees and managers should be promoting USDA and US Dept of Health and Human Services Dietary Guidelines, and all states should have nutrition education as part of their required comprehensive school health education programs at the elementary and secondary levels.[68] A growing number of registered dietitians teach classes for foodservice staff and school faculty. They also plan school menus and design programs for the classroom to meet these requirements.[63,64]

One major concern of parents and professionals has been the content of the USDA commodities, which contribute 20% of the foods used for lunches. An average of 55 different commodities are used during a school year. Specifications have continually reduced the fat and salt content in these foods to make them healthier, and there is a continuing effort to encourage the use of foods lower in salt, sugar, and fat. Current commodities include unsalted peanuts, meats canned with less salt, lowfat cheeses, vegetable oils (excluding palm, palm kernel, or coconut oils), and fruits and juices canned in light syrup.

A second concern is that students are required to take only three of the five lunch components: milk, vegetables, protein-rich foods, fruit, and bread. Although children are encouraged to take one of all five items, the "offer versus serve" format may create an imbalance of nutrients and violate the one-third RDA requirement. Creative programs such as the School Nutrition Action Project (SNAP) bring positive, healthy changes to school-lunch menus and to nutrition education by opening communication between schools and parents through newsletters and interactive parent-child fact sheets.[69]

A third concern involves the sale of snacks to students either during the school day or as fund raisers. Four criteria have been established to evaluate food selected for sale in schools:

1. Nutrient density—A single food should contain
   a. a minimum of three nutrients in a nutrient to energy ratio that is at least equal, or
   b. two nutrients with a double nutrient to energy ratio.
2. Sugar content—Sugar concentration should be less than 20% of weight, with less than 20 mg carbohydrate retained after five minutes, or sugar concentration should be less than 10%, with retentiveness less than 10 mg.
3. Salt content—A single snack food should not exceed 400 mg of sodium per item.
4. Food additives—Additives are acceptable if they return the original nutritive value to a processed food, keep the food palatable, and extend the shelf-life for packaged goods.[70]

The local school administration is responsible for enforcing these criteria.

IMPLICATIONS AND FUTURE DIRECTIONS*

Unhealthful eating behavior is common among American children. Epidemiologic data strongly suggest that these behaviors are linked to higher lipid levels that can ultimately increase a child's risk for CHD. The challenge for the 1990s is to add a new dimension to the word prevention—a dynamic eating behavior—to guide parents, children, and schools toward establishing healthy eating environments.

Registered dietitians are the facilitators of eating-behavior changes. They work in tandem with the pediatrician, family, school, and child. Based on evidence from social learning theory, the registered dietitian's counseling methods can build positive interdependence, which provides support and encourages

*By Linda V. Van Horn and Gail C. Frank

eating-behavior change. Setting small, realistic goals and identifying specific skills and tasks for each family member strengthens the process. The home provides the foundation for change. The pediatrician's office becomes a magnet for change. The school cafeteria becomes a laboratory for experimenting with change. All three settings link health with healthy behaviors, optimize nutritional status, and promote a lifestyle that reduces each child's risk of CHD.

SCHOOL-BASED HEART-HEALTHY PROGRAMS*

Special Program in Nutrition. An innovative nutrition-education guide for third- and fourth-grade elementary-school students and their families, the Special Program in Nutrition (SPIN) was designed and developed by the Gladstone Foundation Laboratories, San Francisco, Calif, and piloted and validated in the Millbrae, Calif, Elementary School District. The program comes in three volumes: (1) introductory material, in-service for teachers, and parent program; (2) 27 lessons for third-grade students and seven follow-up lessons for fourth-grade students, each complete with background information for teachers, worksheet/activities, homework, flash cards, posters, etc; and (3) a cookbook of heart-healthy, low fat, and low-cholesterol recipes.†

Know Your Body Disease Prevention Program. Available through the American Health Foundation,‡ the Know Your Body Disease Prevention Program promotes healthy life styles to lower the incidence of cancer, heart disease, and stroke. The program contains workshop materials, a teacher's manual, screening materials, classroom activities, and resource materials.

The Heart Treasure Chest. This 1984 program is directed to young children. The curriculum has three modules: the work of the heart, physical activity and rest, and heart-healthy foods. Each module contains key concepts, background information for teachers, planning activities, and directions for activities, as well as a promotional kit. The Heart Treasure Chest is an American Heart Association program.§

Putting your Heart Into the Curriculum. This 1982 American Heart Association program is divided into grade levels K through 2, 3 through 5, 6 through 8, and 9 through 12. Each level contains three to six modules, and the material may be duplicated for classroom use.§

Heart Health Education of the Young. A resource guide for teachers of kindergarten through 12th-grade students, Heart Health Education of the Young was prepared by the Pennsylvania affiliate of the American Heart Association in 1983. The breakdown of grade levels is K through 3, 4 through 6, 7 through 9, and 10 through 12.||

*By Anne H. Snyder and Laura Walsh

†The complete set is $35, or $10 for the cookbook, and $30 for the curriculum. To place an order or to request further information, contact Anne H. Snyder, RD, Gladstone Foundation Laboratories, 2550 23rd St, PO Box 40608, San Francisco, CA 94140, 415/826-7500.

‡The American Health Foundation, 1370 Avenue of the Americas, New York, NY 10019, 212/489-8700.

§American Heart Association, National Center, 7320 Greenville Avenue, Dallas, TX 75231, 214/373-6300.

||American Heart Association, Pennsylvania Affiliate, 3700 Vartan Way, Harrisburg, PA 17110, 717/657-3383.

References

1. Newman WP, Freedman DS, Voors AW, et al. Serum lipoproteins and systolic blood pressure are related to atherosclerosis in early life: the Bogalusa Heart Study. *N Engl J Med.* 1986;314:138.
2. Schrott H, Clarke W, Wiebe D. Increased coronary mortality in relatives in hypercholesterolemic school children: the Muscatine Study. *Circulation.* 1979;59:320.
3. Strong W. Distribution of plasma lipid concentrations in infancy and childhood. *Proceedings from the Primary Prevention of Atherosclerosis in Childhood: The Role of Lipids*; March 28, 1985; New York, NY.
4. Laskarzewski P, Morrison J, DeGroot I, et al. Lipid and lipoprotein tracking in 108 children over four-year period. *Pediatrics.* 1979;64:584.
5. Knuiman JT, Hermus RJJ, Hautvast JGAJ. Serum total and high density lipoprotein (HDL) cholesterol concentrations in rural and urban boys from 16 countries. *Atherosclerosis.* 1980;36:529.
6. Blackburn H. Conference on the health effects of blood lipids: optimal distributions for populations. *Prev Med.* 1979;8:612.
7. Lipid Research Clinics. *Population Studies Data Book, I: The Prevalence Study.* 1980. US Dept of Health and Human Services NIH publication 80-1527.
8. Frank G, Berenson G, Webber L. Dietary studies and the relationship of diet to cardiovascular risk factor variables in 10-year old children: the Bogalusa Heart Study. *Am J Clin Nutr.* 1978;131:328.
9. Clarke W, Schrott H, Leaverton P. Tracking of blood lipids and blood pressures in school-age children: the Muscatine Study. *Circulation.* 1978;58:626.
10. Frerichs R, Srinivasan S, Webber L, et al. Serum lipids and lipoproteins at birth in a biracial population: the Bogalusa Heart Study. *Pediatr Res.* 1978;12:858.
11. Orchard TJ. Cholesterol screening in childhood: does it predict adult hypercholesterolemia? The Beaver County experience. *J Pediatr.* 1983;103:687.
12. Conference on Blood Lipids in Children. Optimal levels for early prevention of coronary artery disease. *Prev Med.* 1983;12:725.
13. Glueck CJ, Laskarzewski P, Rao D, et al. Familial aggregation of coronary risk factors. In: Connor W, Bristow JD, eds. *Coronary Heart Disease.* Philadelphia, Pa: JB Lippincott Co; 1984:173.
14. Kwiterovich P. Biochemical clinical, epidemiologic, genetic, and pathologic data in the pediatric age group relevant to the cholesterol hypothesis. *Pediatrics.* 1986;78:349.
15. Frank GC, Webber LS, Farris RP, et al. *Dietary Databook: Quantifying Dietary Intakes of Children and Adolescents—The Bogalusa Heart Study, 1973–1983.* New Orleans, La: Louisiana State University Printing Office; 1986.
16. Frank GC, Berenson GS, Webber LS. Dietary studies of infants and children. In: Coates T, Petersen A, Perry C, eds. *Promoting Adolescent Health: A Dialogue on Research and Practice.* New York, NY: Academic Press; 1982:329.
17. Frank GC, Farris RP, Cresanta JL, et al. Dietary intake as a determinant of cardiovascular risk factor variables: observations in a pediatric population. In: Berenson GS, ed. *Causation of Cardiovascular Risk Factors in Children: Perspectives in Causation of Cardiovascular Risk in Early Life.* New York, NY: Raven Press; 1986:254.
18. Morrison JA, Larsen R, Glatfelter L, et al. Interrelationships between nutrient intake and plasma lipids and lipoproteins in school children aged 6 to 19: the Princeton School District Study. *Pediatrics.* 1980;65:727.
19. Beaton GH, Milner J, Corey P, et al. Sources of variance in 24-hour dietary recall data: implications for nutrition study design and interpretation. *Am J Clin Nutr.* 1979;32:2546.
20. Lipid Research Clinics Program. Relationship between reduction in coronary heart disease and in low density lipoprotein cholesterol in hypercholesterolemic men: the diet plus placebo group of the Lipid Research Clinics Primary Prevention Trial. *Clin Res.* 1984;33:520A. Abstract.
21. Lauer RM, Shekelle RB, eds. *Childhood Prevention of Atherosclerosis and Hypertension.* New York, NY: Raven Press; 1980.
22. Kwiterovich PO Jr, Bachorik PS, Franklin FA Jr, et al. Effect of dietary treatment on the plasma levels of lipids, lipoprotein cholesterol and LDL B protein in children with type II hyperlipoproteinemia: detection and treatment of lipid and lipoprotein disorders in childhood. *Prog Clin Biol Res.* 1985;188:123.

23. Stein EA. Changes in plasma lipid and lipoprotein fractions after alteration in dietary cholesterol, polyunsaturated, saturated, and total fat in free-living normal and hypercholesterolemic children. *Am J Clin Nutr.* 1982;35:1375.
24. Fomon SJ. *Infant Nutrition.* 2nd ed. Philadelphia, Pa: WB Saunders Co; 1974.
25. Carlson SE, DeVae PW, Barness LA. Effects of infant diets with different polyunsaturated to saturated fat ratios on circulating high density lipoproteins. *J Pediatr Gastroenterol Nutr.* 1982;1:303.
26. Farris RP, Frank GC, Webber LS, et al. Influence of milk source on serum lipids and lipoprotein during the first year of life: the Bogalusa Heart Study. *Am J Clin Nutr.* 1982;35:42.
27. Friedman G, Goldberg SJ. An evaluation of the safety of a low saturated fat, low cholesterol diet beginning in infancy. *Pediatrics.* 1976;58:655.
28. Ford CH, McGandy RB, Stone FJ. An institutional approach to the dietary regulation of blood cholesterol in adolescent males. *Prev Med.* 1972;1:426.
29. Walter H, Hofman A, Vaughn R, Wynder E. Modification of risk factors for coronary heart disease: five year results from a school based intervention trial. *N Engl J Med.* 1988;318:1093.
30. Stone E. School-based health research funded by the National Heart, Lung and Blood Institute. *J School Health.* 1985;55:168.
31. Puska P, Vartiainen E, Pallonen U, et al. The North Karelia Youth Project: evaluation of two years of intervention on health behavior and CVD risk factors among 13 to 15 year old children. *Prev Med.* 1982;11:550.
32. Mauer AM. A pediatrician attends the National Institutes of Health Consensus Conference on Lowering Blood Cholesterol. *Pediatrics.* 1985;76:125.
33. American Academy of Pediatrics Committee on Nutrition. Toward a prudent diet for children. *Pediatrics.* 1983;71:78.
34. Dwyer J. Diets for children and adolescents that meet the dietary goals. *AJDC.* 1980;134:1080.
35. Dwyer JT, Andrew E, Berkey C, et al. Growth in "new" vegetarian preschool children using the Jenss-Bayley curve fitting technique. *Am J Clin Nutr.* 1983;37:815.
36. Kaufmann NA, Friedlander Y, Halfon S, et al. Nutrient intake in Jerusalem—consumption in 17-year olds. *Isr J Med Sci.* 1982;18:1167.
37. Weidman W, Kwiterovich P Jr, Jesse MJ, et al. Diet in the healthy child: AHA Nutrition Committee Report. *Circulation.* 1983;67:1411A.
38. *The Surgeon General's Report on Nutrition and Health.* 1988. Dept of Health and Human Services publication 88-50210.
39. National Research Council, Committee on Diet and Health, Food and Nutrition Board. *Diet and Health: Implications for Reducing Chronic Diseases Risk.* Washington, DC: National Academy Press; 1989.
40. *Dietary Goals for the United States.* 2nd ed. Washington, DC: US Senate Select Committee on Nutrition and Human Needs; 1977.
41. Consensus Conference. Lowering blood cholesterol to prevent heart disease. *JAMA.* 1985;253:2080.
42. Lenfant C. New National Cholesterol Education Program. *Cardiovasc Med.* 1985;10:39.
43. National Cholesterol Education Program Expert Panel. Report on detection, evaluation, and treatment of high blood cholesterol in adults. *Arch Intern Med.* 1988;148:36.
44. Pugliese M, Weyman-Daum M, Moses N, et al. Parental health beliefs as a cause of non-organic failure to thrive. *Pediatrics.* 1987;80:175.
45. Frank GC. Nutritional therapy for hyperlipidemia and obesity: office treatment integrating the roles of the physician and the registered dietitian. *J Am Col Cardiol.* 1988;12:1090.
46. Snetselaar LG. *Nutrition Counseling Skills.* London, England: Aspen Publishers, 1983:275.
47. Frank GC, Vaden A, Martin J. School health promotion: child nutrition programs. *J School Health.* 1987;57:451.
48. Moore MC, Beasley CD, Moore M. Why the boys? *J Home Econ.* 1970;69:338.
49. Lesser H. *Television and the Preschool Child.* New York, NY: Academic Press; 1977.
50. Rodin J. Social and immediate environmental influences on food selection. *Int J Obesity.* 1980;4:364.
51. Klesges RC, Coates TJ, Brown G, et al. Parental influence on children's eating behavior and relative weight. *J Appl Behav Anal.* 1983;16:371.

52. Eppright E, Fox H, Fryer B, et al. Eating behavior of preschool children. *J Nutr Educ.* 1969;1:16.
53. Bandura A. *Social Learning Theory.* Englewood Cliffs, NJ: Prentice-Hall; 1977.
54. Mahoney MJ, Mahoney K. Treatment of obesity: a clinical exploration. In: Williams BJ, Martin S, Foreyt JP, eds. *Obesity: Behavioral Approaches to Dietary Management.* New York, NY: Brunner/Mazel; 1976.
55. Raab C, Tillotsen J, eds. *Heart to Heart: A Manual in Nutrition Counseling for Reduction of Cardiovascular Disease Risk Factors.* NIH publication 83-1528.
56. Ferguson JM. *Habits, Not Diets—The Real Way to Weight Control.* Palo Alto, Calif: Bull Publishing; 1976.
57. Erickson F. Gatekeeping and the meeting pot: interaction in counseling encounters. *Harvard Educ Rev.* 1975;45:44.
58. Kanfer F, Goldstein A, eds. *Helping People Change.* New York, NY: Pergamon; 1975, 1986.
59. Frank GC, Farris RP, Ditmarsen P, et al. An approach to primary preventive treatment for children with high blood pressure in a total community. *J Am Col Nutr.* 1982;1:357.
60. Bandura A. Self-efficacy: toward a unifying theory of behavior change. *Psychol Rev.* 1977;84:191.
61. Frank GC. Primary prevention in the school arena: a dietary approach. *Health Values.* 1983;7:14.
62. Butcher AH, Frank GC, Harsha DW, et al. Heart smart: a school health program meeting the 1990 objectives for the nation. *Health Educ Quar.* 1988;5:17.
63. Frank GC, Nicklas TA, Forcier JS, et al. Cardiovascular health promotion for school children, part 1: the "heart smart" nutrition intervention. *School Food Serv Res Rev.* 1989;13:130.
64. Frank GC, Nicklas TA, Forcier JS, et al. Cardiovascular health promotion for school children, part 2: observations on institutional food service change affecting student eating behavior. *School Food Serv Res Rev.* 1989;13:137.
65. Food and Nutrition Service. *Menu Planning Guide for School Food Service.* Washington, DC: December 1983. US Dept of Agriculture program aid 1260.
66. Frank GC, White M. Sodium-modified recipes in school lunch. *School Food Serv Res Rev.* 1983;7:2.
67. Green LW, Kreuter NW, Deeds SG, et al. *Health Education Planning: A Diagnostic Approach.* Palo Alto, Calif: Mayfield; 1980:142.
68. *Promoting Health/Preventing Disease: Objectives for the Nation.* Washington, DC: US Dept of Health and Human Services; 1980.
69. Blakely CK. SNAP project catches on in the Southwest. *Food Nutr.* 1985;15:9.
70. Oregon Public Health Association. *Guide for Selection of Snack Foods.* Nutrition Task Force Report. February 1980.

8. WEIGHT MANAGEMENT

People who are obese are at greater risk for CHD, hypertension, diabetes, and some forms of cancer.[1] The effects of overweight and obesity on CHD were thought to be mediated through coronary risk factors such as hyperlipidemia, hypertension, and impaired glucose tolerance.[2] However, the Framingham Heart Study[3] demonstrated that obesity is a significant independent predictor of CHD. Furthermore, the results indicated that weight gain in the young adult years was associated with an increased risk of CHD in both sexes that could not be attributed either to initial body weight or to other risk factors that might have resulted from weight gain. The authors concluded that "intervention in obesity, in addition to the well established risk factors, appears to be an advisable goal in the primary prevention of CHD."[3]

EFFECT OF BODY WEIGHT ON PLASMA LIPIDS*

Obesity is associated with a more atherogenic plasma lipid profile. Obesity (assessed by relative weight or body mass index) is positively correlated with plasma total-cholesterol, LDL-cholesterol, and triglyceride levels and negatively correlated with HDL cholesterol.[4–6] Kannel et al[7] estimated that for each percentage increase in relative weight there was a corresponding 1.1 mg/dL increase in the plasma cholesterol level in men and approximately half the increase for women gaining a similar amount of weight.

The relationship between body-fat distribution and plasma lipids and lipoproteins has been the focus of recent attention. Foster et al[8] showed that both men and women with a high waist-to-hip ratio reflective of android obesity (excess fat deposits located predominantly in the upper body) were more likely to have elevated plasma total-cholesterol, triglyceride, and apolipoprotein-B levels and lower HDL-cholesterol levels than those with gynoid (lower-body) obesity. Two recent population studies[9,10] have shown that waist-to-hip circumference and subscapular skinfold thickness were associated with a higher incidence of ischemic heart disease and coronary events.

Weight reduction has been recommended to reduce CHD risk.[11] Many studies have evaluated the influence of weight loss on plasma lipoprotein levels. Although results are inconsistent, the studies frequently show that weight loss favorably affects plasma lipid levels.

In a recent meta-analysis of a number of studies, Tran and Weltman[12] reported that weight loss from exercise and/or exercise plus caloric restriction was associated with lower plasma total-cholesterol, LDL-cholesterol, and triglyceride levels. Plasma total-cholesterol and LDL-cholesterol levels decreased 5% to 10% in response to weight loss. Clinically, a greater plasma total-cholesterol and LDL-cholesterol reduction can be achieved if initial plasma lipid levels are high, if weight loss is substantial, if diet composition changes in the direction of current recommendations, and if exercise is a component of the weight-reduction program. Some investigations, however, have not observed changes in plasma lipids during weight loss or during the postintervention follow-up period.[13,14] The reasons for the disparate findings include: the experimental design employed, the clinical characteristics of the study subjects, the rate of weight loss, the amount and composition of weight loss, the posttreatment body mass index, and the weight-stabilization period, among others.

*By Linda S. McDonald

BODY WEIGHT AND HYPERTENSION*

The incidence of hypertension is greater in overweight persons and those who have recently gained weight.[15-19] Weight loss reduces blood pressure, even when ideal body weight has not been achieved.[20]

Caloric restriction leading to weight loss is commonly associated with a fall in arterial pressure, independent of whether the patient restricts salt intake.[16-18,21,22] (In an uncontrolled setting, however, when calories are reduced, so too is sodium.) The mechanisms by which weight loss reduces blood pressure are not clear. Weight reduction is accompanied by a reduction in adrenergic activity, plasma renin activity, and aldosterone levels, and these changes are independent of sodium intake.[23]

FACTORS AFFECTING RESTING ENERGY NEEDS†

A variety of factors influence resting energy needs, including basal metabolic rate, the thermic effect of food, the thermic effect of exercise, and adaptive thermogenesis. These factors can significantly affect weight balance.

Resting metabolic rate (RMR) is the energy expended during rest in a comfortable environment several hours after eating or exercising. It is the energy required for basic body functions and homeostasis, and it is responsible for approximately 60% to 75% of caloric needs in the average male.[24]

The thermic effect of food (TEF) is the energy required to digest and completely metabolize ingested food. TEF also represents the stimulation of numerous chemical processes by the amino acids present in ingested food.[24,25] (TEF is also known as the specific dynamic action of protein.) TEF's contribution to total metabolic needs is dependent on several factors, including meal composition and nutritional status, but it averages approximately 10% of total caloric intake.[24]

The thermic effect of exercise (TEE) is the direct consequence of performing muscular work, and it varies directly with the amount and intensity of the work performed. In a moderately active male, TEE contributes approximately 30% of the daily caloric expenditure.[24]

Also known as "nonshivering thermogenesis," adaptive thermogenesis (AT) is the increase in RMR in response to homeostatic changes such as temperature and stress. AT is associated with brown adipose tissue, which is the site of rapid lipid oxidation and heat production. Although researched extensively in animals, AT is not well understood in humans.[24]

FOOD INTAKE STIMULI†

Humans respond to a variety of eating cues such as chemical and psychological stimuli in order to meet their energy needs. These cues either stimulate or inhibit the feeding and satiety centers of the hypothalamus, which, in turn, stimulate or inhibit the act of eating.[24,25]

Distention of the stomach stimulates inhibitory feedback to the brain, terminating food intake. Distention of other portions of the gastrointestinal tract elicits similar signals.[24,26]

A frequent complaint of people on calorie-restricted diets is that the rapid weight loss often observed at the onset of the diet later slows and even ceases for periods. Explanations for the development of plateaus include: (1) a decrease in

*By Linda S. McDonald
†By Monika Woolsey

lean tissue mass, and achieving caloric equilibrium with time,[27] and (2) a subsequent slow rate of fat loss after glycogen loss occurs within the first weeks of a caloric deficit. An average deficit of 3,500 calories is required to lose 1 lb of fat. Therefore, for those with a 500-calorie daily deficit, 1 lb weight loss (of fat) is expected weekly. Some obese people report that they consume diets already low in calories that do not permit a 500-calorie deficit per day (as some would then be consuming as little as 300 to 500 calories daily). Practitioners may want to suggest a nutritionally balanced diet that contains the low calorie level such a client reportedly consumes, and then monitor his or her weight. Weight reduction is likely to occur, especially when exercise is a component of the weight-loss program.

Hunger and succeeding food intake are stimulated by low blood glucose and amino acid levels (chemical stimuli). Plasma hormones also influence intake. Insulin, for example, stimulates hunger and intake, while glucagon and cholecystokinin cause a decrease in food intake.[25]

Aside from physiological factors, a number of external factors influence intake in the short run, including the time of day, location, availability of food, and tastiness of food (psychological stimuli). Emotions such as stress, anger, boredom, and fear can also induce eating.[26] However, there is no compelling evidence that any of these factors influences the development or maintenance of obesity.

ESSENTIAL COMPONENTS OF A SUCCESSFUL WEIGHT-LOSS PROGRAM*

Successful weight-control programs require a nutritionally adequate but reduced-calorie diet. A regular exercise program and behavior-modification therapy with psychological support should also be included.[28] Diet therapy for weight reduction should be based on a sound scientific rationale. It should be safe, nutritionally adequate, and practical, and it should promote long-term effectiveness. An exercise program for weight reduction should also be safe, and it should promote an increased energy expenditure, fat loss, maintenance of lean body mass, and lasting increases in physical activity throughout life. Behavior and psychological therapy are important in helping patients acquire the new eating habits that are needed for weight loss and maintenance. Treatment should focus on methods of acquiring new behaviors and on problems that arise with weight loss. A pretreatment psychosocial assessment is required. In addition, the following therapeutic modalities are the minimum required for a weight-loss program. Instruction is recommended on the following topics: (1) self-monitoring (record keeping), (2) stimulus control, (3) sensible diet, (4) cognitive restructuring, and (5) psychosocial intervention such as assertiveness training and supportive psychotherapy. Therapeutic modalities are also required for the maintenance of weight loss.

Caloric Restriction as a Weight-Loss Strategy

Early attempts to reduce weight focused on restricting energy intake. Caloric restriction alone (especially significant caloric restriction) is not the preferred method for weight reduction for most people, because it has been shown to cause a lowered metabolic rate, plateauing, poor nutrient intake, boredom with the weight-loss program, and chronic hunger.

While the goal of a weight-reduction program is to reduce fat tissue while maintaining lean tissue,[28,29] caloric restriction alone leads to significant lean-tissue[32] and bone-mass losses.[6-8] Moreover, fat-free mass (eg, muscle and bone)

*By Monika Woolsey

loss through dieting is not likely to be regained.[28] A reduction in muscle mass can significantly reduce calorie needs. In fact, dieting has been reported to reduce metabolic needs by as much as 15%.[25,26] In addition to decreasing the metabolic rate, dieting reduces the energy cost of physical activity.[27] It is not surprising that the success rate is bleak (5% to 20%) for weight loss and maintenance using low-calorie dieting alone.[30]

Caloric intake may not be the primary factor influencing weight. Several studies have demonstrated that obese people actually eat less than nonobese people, despite their excess weight.[27,30] This metabolic anomaly may be genetic, as children of obese parents also have been shown to have lower-than-normal basal metabolic rates.[27] If obesity is at least partially due to a defect in metabolism, it may not be appropriate to concentrate totally on diet therapy for weight control for such people. Instead, therapy should consist of modalities that do not further alter metabolism. It is interesting to note, however, that in a recent study, Prentice et al[31] measured energy expenditure in obese women and found that it was 25% to 35% higher than in lean women. The authors were unable to find evidence of energy-sparing mechanisms in the obese women studied. The results of this study, together with studies that suggest differences in metabolic efficiency in obese people, make it impossible to resolve this issue at the present time.

Exercise as a Weight-Reduction Strategy

Exercise has been shown to facilitate weight loss while maintaining lean body mass.[27] Proponents of exercise for losing and maintaining weight cite the following benefits: a decrease in body fat and a faster rate of weight loss when combined with a calorie-restricted diet, better maintenance of lean tissue and bone mass, an increased metabolic rate, decreased appetite, and better maintenance of long-term weight goals. A recent study reported by Wood et al[32] found that dieting and exercise produced comparable losses in fat mass, but lean tissue was also lost in dieters—a response not observed in subjects who exercised to lose weight. The effects of exercise on adipose tissue mass are the result of a decrease in adipocyte lipid content rather than any effect on adipocyte number.[26]

Weight-bearing exercise is important for maintenance of bone health.[28] In addition, exercise that causes muscle hypertrophy can reduce the loss of lean body mass during caloric restriction. Regular exercise (both aerobic and nonaerobic) increases lean body mass.[27,30]

Exercise-induced changes in the proportion of lean body mass to body fat increase the amount of metabolically active tissue, as lean tissue requires three times the calories that fat tissue requires. An exercise bout can increase resting caloric expenditure.[27] These changes, along with the actual energy cost of exercise, significantly increase daily caloric needs. A major benefit of increased caloric expenditure is that the decrease in metabolic rate experienced with caloric restriction can be offset,[28] resulting in a significant decrease in body fat not reported with the severe caloric (only) restriction.[33]

Exercise has been shown to increase, decrease, or have no effect on food intake.[34-36] In a recent study designed to examine the acute effects of exercise on appetite in young men, Thompson et al[27] reported that high-intensity exercise briefly suppressed hunger. The appetite suppression was of short duration and did not affect total calorie intake. While these results are not supportive of an exercise-induced appetite suppression leading to a caloric deficit, they nonetheless demonstrate that exercise did not stimulate appetite and increase food intake. Therefore, as a result of the caloric cost of the exercise, a negative calorie balance was achieved. In support of these findings, several studies[37-39] showed that caloric intake was unchanged in obese women and men in response to exercise. The caloric cost of exercise alone, however, led to a negative calorie balance in these subjects. In nonobese people, however, vigorous exercise does lead to an increase in caloric intake. Moreover, studies conducted by Wood and associates at Stanford University have shown that active, normal-weight people consume more calories than sedentary, overweight people (P. Wood, personal communication). These studies demonstrate the importance of physical activity in weight control. An effective program to promote initial weight loss and long-term weight maintenance requires both exercise and caloric restriction.[40]

While exercise is beneficial for long-term weight control, significant weight loss also requires an accompanying caloric restriction.[32] Exercise is thought to be an adjunct to reduced-calorie diets for weight loss. A combination of diet and exercise appears also to decrease plasma triglycerides and, specifically, VLDL triglycerides.[32] Thus, successful weight-loss and weight-control programs require changes in both energy intake and energy expenditure.

THE WEIGHT-REDUCTION DIET*

Moderate calorie restriction is recommended for the treatment of obesity. A calorie level that is ±10% of the measured or estimated resting metabolic rate is a good starting point.[41] For example, if a client's resting metabolic rate is 1,200 calories, then a calorie-restricted diet with 1,080 to 1,320 calories is appropriate. The calorie-restricted diet should lead to a slow, steady weight loss of 0.5 to 2 lb per week, depending on the client's level of physical activity. An average deficit of 3,500 calories is required to lose 1 lb of fat. Calorie-restricted diets should provide at least 1,000 to 1,200 calories daily to assure that nutrient needs are met. The American Dietetic Association recommends that weight-reduction diets for people whose body weights are greater than 20% of the ideal should provide at least 10 calories per pound of their present body weight. This particular recommendation does not apply to people with diabetes or people who are more than 30% heavier than ideal body weight.

A steady weight loss reduces weight loss from fat-free compartments and promotes adherence. Dietitians recommend a maximal weight loss of 2 lb per week. To achieve this, some clients may require a higher-calorie diet than typically prescribed for weight reduction. Both diet (reduced calorie intake) and exercise (increased physical activity) should contribute to the caloric deficit. There are no specific guidelines for the proportional contribution of each to the prescribed caloric deficit. (Specific aerobic exercise guidelines are described below.) Weight-reduction programs must be individualized and based on many factors (ie, physiological, psychological, social, economic).

The distribution of macronutrients (carbohydrate, protein, and fat) is generally not specified, although calorie-reduced diets should also meet the Step One Diet recommendations of the American Heart Association and the National Cholesterol Education Program (NCEP). Carbohydrate-restricted diets generally cause a greater initial weight loss,[42] but the total amount of fat lost at the end of the weight-reduction program is similar in response to isocaloric low- and high-carbohydrate diets.

Advocates of high-carbohydrate weight-reduction diets believe that since relatively large volumes of food are allowed, long-term compliance with the diet is easier. There has been a great deal of attention directed toward the recent

*By Monika Woolsey

work of Donato and Hegsted,[43] who report that the energy utilization from dietary fat was greater than the energy utilization from dietary carbohydrate during growth. Using Atwater values of 4 and 9 calories per gram for carbohydrate and fat, respectively, the energy from dietary fat was more efficiently utilized for body-fat deposition than was energy derived from carbohydrate. Specifically, fat provided approximately 11 calories per gram, whereas gross energy from sucrose was approximately 4 calories per gram. The efficiency of dietary fat utilization was 124% of that expected. Donato[43] notes that the direct conversion of dietary fat to body fat is a very energy-efficient process. She notes that dietary fat supplements increased body-fat deposition even when energy intake was restricted. The practical application of these findings await clarification. One expert in the field believes that the utilization of fat may be more efficient during positive energy balance (growth, weight gain, pregnancy), but not in a state of caloric equilibrium (T. Van Itallie, personal communication). Clearly, more work is needed in this area. The role of dietary fat in promoting weight gain, loss, and maintenance needs to be established.

Recent evidence suggests that self-selected diets high in carbohydrates promote weight loss, while self-selected diets higher in fat do not. Lissner et al[44] measured spontaneous food consumption of people whose diets contained 15% to 20%, 30% to 35%, or 45% to 50% calories from fat. Relative to the diet with a moderate level of fat (30% to 35% of calories), subjects on the high-carbohydrate diet spontaneously consumed 11% fewer calories, whereas subjects on the diet higher in fat consumed 15% more calories. These results agree with previous studies and indicate that decreasing the caloric density of the diet causes spontaneous caloric deficits. Based on this, it appears that reducing fat intake in weight-reduction diets is promising because it imposes fewer food restrictions. For long-term weight control, high-carbohydrate diets may be more effective than diets higher in fat. In support of this hypothesis, Dreon et al[45] found in a cross-sectional study of middle-aged men that body fat increased as total fat intake increased.

There also is evidence to suggest that high-carbohydrate diets may not be more effective in promoting weight loss.[46,47] In two different studies, weight loss was not greater in the group on the high-carbohydrate diet compared with controls. It should be pointed out, however, that there were problems with compliance to the diets. At this time it is evident that more studies are necessary to establish the ideal macronutrient composition for long-term compliance for weight control.

In a recent review of the effect of dietary fiber on food intake and body weight, Stevens[48] reported that supplementation (other than wheat bran) may decrease energy intake slightly (approximately 100 to 200 calories) and increase weight loss. The author cautions, however, that because of the associated side effects, fiber supplements are not an instant cure for obesity. Moreover, the actual reduction in energy intake is relatively small and the duration of the effect is unknown.[48]

Calorie Awareness

Calorie awareness is essential in a weight-loss program. One of the most popular and patient-acceptable calorie-counting systems is the exchange system developed by the American Diabetes Association and The American Dietetic Association.[49] Food groups are recognizable by most, and knowledge of a few food groups rather than a few hundred foods allows for a reasonable estimate of daily intake. The nutritional basis for the exchange system is presented in *Table 8.1*. Calorie-counting books, available in most bookstores, can be used with or instead of the exchange system. A reduced-calorie diet should provide a variety of foods and should not include extreme calorie restrictions (not less than 1,000 to 1,200 calories per day) in order to promote nutritional adequacy, palatability, and adherence.[28,29]

Table 8.1
Nutrient Values per Serving from Exchange Lists

Exchange List	Carbohydrate, g	Protein, g	Fat, g	Calories
Starch/bread	15	3	trace	80
Meat				
Lean	—	7	3	55
Medium-fat	—	7	5	75
High-fat	—	7	8	100
Vegetable	5	2	—	25
Fruit	15	—	—	60
Milk				
Skim	12	8	trace	90
Low-fat	12	8	5	120
Whole	12	8	8	150
Fat	—	—	5	45

The Exchange Lists are the basis of a meal planning system designed by a committee of the American Diabetes Association and The American Dietetic Association. While designed primarily for people with diabetes and others who must follow special diets, the Exchange Lists are based on principles of good nutrition that apply to everyone.

AEROBIC-EXERCISE GUIDELINES*

The American College of Sports Medicine has established guidelines for obtaining the maximum benefit from aerobic exercise: The exercise should be performed three to five days per week, it should be performed at an intensity of 60% to 85% of maximum heart rate (220 minus one's age), and it should last for at least 30 minutes. Any aerobic activity that uses large muscle groups and that can be maintained continuously is recommended.[50] In addition, participation in exercise should represent a permanent life-style change, since the loss of any training effect can occur once regular exercise has ceased.[28,29] Recommended aerobic exercises include but are not limited to: running, swimming, bicycling, cross-country skiing, aerobic dancing, rowing, and brisk walking.

BEHAVIOR-MODIFICATION THERAPY*

Weight loss and maintenance are a struggle for many people. Behavior-modification therapy is essential for short- and long-term success with weight control.[28]

Most behavior-modification programs employ a problem-solving approach; that is, behaviors problematic to the client are identified, specific strategies to change these behaviors are developed, success in changing the behaviors is periodically assessed, and strategies are altered if necessary.[51] A sample behavior-modification approach to weight control is provided in *Table 8.2*. Several parameters have been identified as crucial components of behavior-modification therapy: self-monitoring, control of external stimuli, reinforcement of positive change, allowance for special occasions, assertiveness training, follow-up, and spousal support.[28,52]

*By Monika Woolsey

Table 8.2
Behavior Modification in Weight Control

Step 1.	Keep a food record for several days. In addition to the items eaten, record when, where, and how much was eaten, the mood when food was eaten, and the duration of feeding.
Step 2.	Identify overeating patterns.
Step 3.	Set strategies that alter these behaviors.
Step 4.	Decide how often the behavior must be changed in order to be successful. Insisting on 100% change might be unrealistic, whereas successful change might be enlisting a new behavior 75% of the time when the problem situation arises.
Step 5.	Decide on a nonfood reward for successful behavior. Examples include: • a night out at the movies • peace and quiet • a long-distance phone call • sleeping late • a relaxing bath or shower
Step 6.	Periodically evaluate success. For example: • Did the old behavior replace the new behavior? • How often? • If not, why not? Was the strategy unrealistic? Did the strategy induce other undesirable behaviors? • Should the strategy be completely changed? Or does the behavior need to be introduced more gradually? In the beginning, behavior changes should be monitored fairly frequently, even weekly, for motivational purposes. As time passes, self-evaluation can be performed less frequently, but should take place at least once per month.
Step 7.	Provide the reward for successful behavior.

Reprinted with permission from DeBakey ME, Gotto AM Jr, Scott LW, et al. *The Living Heart Diet.* New York, NY: Raven Press; 1984.

Record keeping (self-monitoring) is essential, as it serves to make clients aware of eating problems.[53] Without data to document that there are inappropriate eating behaviors, succeeding steps in behavior modification are not possible.

Conscious control of nonphysiological feeding stimuli (control of external stimuli) is of the utmost importance. Sample strategies for this technique are provided in *Table 8.3*. An important consideration in designing alternative behaviors is to avoid overwhelming the client with too many changes to make in too short a period. Most people can remain challenged with one or two behaviors to change at once. These changes may take two weeks or two months. Unrealistic goals should be discouraged.

While weight loss represents a positive change, a weight-loss program can nonetheless cause many negative feelings. An overall weight loss of 20 lb may easily be forgotten with one "cheating" incident. Negative feelings, if allowed to cultivate, can result in food binges, a return to former eating habits, and weight gain.[28] Therefore, it is important to reinforce positive behavior. Rewarding positive behaviors helps prevent and/or reduce negative feelings about occasional deviations from the weight-control program.

Assertiveness training is important for teaching clients about responding to internal feeding cues. Instruction in maintaining behavior changes in a variety of social situations allows clients to take charge of their own eating behaviors rather than permitting others to dictate what and when they eat.

Table 8.3
Common Problem Eating Behaviors and Strategies to Change Them

Behavior	Strategy
Eating in front of the television	Limit eating to one room only.
Eating midnight snacks	Choose an alternative, hand-consuming activity such as letter writing or knitting.
Eating too fast	Lay eating utensils down between bites. Take a sip of water between each bite.
Eating multiple portions	Eat more slowly. Place a regular portion of food on a smaller plate.
Eating while cooking	Chew gum while cooking. Brush teeth before cooking.
Constant snacking	Keep problem foods stored out of sight. Schedule alternative activities at usual snack times.
Eating in response to emotion	Engage in other activities (exercise, housework, etc).
Poor food choices in restaurants	Plan choices ahead of time. Avoid fatty foods.
Overeating in social situations	Eat before attending the event. Position oneself away from food.

Allowance for Special Occasions

Special occasions should be viewed as enjoyable and not unmanageable events. It is important to reinforce overall positive changes in behavior and in weight, and to allow for an occasional treat.[28] Anticipating and planning for, rather than avoiding, special occasions can help the client approach these events with a positive outlook and be motivated to follow the prescribed diet plan.

Follow-up and Weight Maintenance

Follow-up is an important component of a weight-control program.[54] Obviously, change is not likely with just one visit with a dietitian. Although no standard protocol exists for frequency of visits, Weisner et al[28] recommend a minimum of four months of weekly treatment, with monthly follow-ups for at least six months after the weight goal has been achieved. Many clients will benefit from more intensive follow-up for longer periods. Practitioners will be required to work intensively with some to prevent and deal with lapse and relapse.

Spouse Involvement

The involvement of the spouse (or significant other) is an important adjunct to any therapy.[52,54,55] Since the spouse can control available food, provide external stimuli, influence behavior, and dictate time commitments, it is essential that he or she pledge support for success. Support can take many forms: attending counseling sessions, participating in an exercise program with the client, modifying food preparation, helping eliminate external cues in the home, or even signing a contract that pledges support.[54,55] Without this effort, it may be difficult or even impossible for the client to make the changes necessary for long-term weight control.

YO-YO DIETING*

Yo-yo dieting refers to a repeated cycle of weight loss followed by weight gain. The syndrome is psychologically damaging and physiologically defeating to long-term weight control. Brownell and colleagues[56] reported that weight cycling made obese rats metabolically efficient. Weight cycling made animals both lose weight less efficiently (eg, a larger calorie deficit was required to lose weight) and gain weight more efficiently (eg, fewer calories were required to gain weight) than control (non–weight-cycled) obese rats.

Brownell has noted a similar phenomenon in many patients he has studied (K. D. Brownell, personal communication). Some of his patients lost little weight while following a diet of 700 to 800 calories/day. These findings are intriguing, and they clearly emphasize the importance of preventing overweight and obesity as well as maintaining ideal body weight for a lifetime. Some investigations have not supported the findings of Brownell and coworkers[56] that yo-yo dieting leads to metabolic efficiency. More work is needed to either support or refute this hypothesis.

VERY-LOW-CALORIE DIETS†

Conventional weight-reduction diets can be ineffective in moderately and severely obese people. Alternative weight-loss diets include: very-low-calorie diets (VLCDs—less than 400 calories per day), low-calorie diets (LCDs—less than 800 calories per day), and protein-sparing modified fasts (PSMFs—less than 400 calories per day, in the form of protein). These methods may seem more attractive to the clinician or patient because they result in rapid weight loss. In fact, Stuart et al[57] found that next to fasting, VLCDs produced the greatest weight losses in the shortest time. With these findings, more rigorous treatments for obesity have gained the interest of clinicians and the public.

Despite their many complications, VLCDs cause rapid weight loss. Medical risks and psychological side effects have been attractively modified.[58] These benefits, however, do not warrant the use of these diets and special products for all overweight people. Garrow's classification of obese patients (listed in *Table 8.4*) determines a management strategy based on body index.[59]

Table 8.4
Garrow's Management Strategies for Obesity

Body Mass Index	Management Strategy
20–24.9	Patient "normal"; assess basis for anxiety
25–29.9	Community-based group therapy
30–40	Individual attention, detailed management
> 40	Special measures, ie, surgery

Reprinted with permission from Garrow JS. *Treat Obesity Seriously.* Edinburgh, Scotland: Churchill-Livingston; 1981.

Conventional forms of weight-loss management are more realistically used for mild obesity. Severely obese people benefit more from rigorous treatment, ie, VLCDs (or surgery).[59] Patients selected to use rapid weight-loss methods should always be evaluated for emotional stability, medical complications, and degree of overweight.[60]

*By the Editors
†By Alison Murray

Very-low-calorie diets appear to be very effective in promoting rapid weight loss without compromising health.[60–62] When obese patients are treated with a calorie-restricted diet, behavior modifications, and anorectic drugs, mean weight loss is less than 7 kg.[63] Patients treated with VLCDs, however, have a mean weight loss of at least 20 kg in 12 weeks of treatment.[60] A treatment period of 19 to 24 weeks leads to losses of 31 to 41 kg.[64,65]

Maintenance of weight loss continues to be a significant problem with VLCDs. Even when patients continually receive behavior therapy and nutrition education, maintenance of weight loss has been poor. Genuth and associates[66] found that 56% of the patients enrolled in their study had regained 50% of their lost weight at 22 months. Similarly, Anderson et al[67] found that only 3% of over 2,000 clients maintained their weight loss (ie, they did not regain at least one half of the weight initially lost) after five years.[67] On the other hand, Wadden et al[68] found that initial weight losses of 20.5 kg were essentially maintained.[69] More research is needed to evaluate the long-term efficacy of VLCDs.

Various guidelines for VLCDs and protein-sparing, modified-fast protocols have been proposed. Some begin the program with an initial calorie restriction of 1,000 to 1,200 calories per day in order to predict adherence to the diet. Other protocols immediately subject the client to the VLCD. Some introduce the VLCD in a formula divided into three to five feedings daily. Others combine formula with animal protein, or use animal protein alone, in three to four meals daily.[60]

Behavior-modification therapy is important when clients are following a VLCD. Behavior therapy focuses on the maintenance of weight loss, cognitive restructuring, relapse-prevention training, avoidance of excessive dietary restraint, and preventing and dealing with weight gain.[68]

The most successful programs have been those that combine diet and behavior therapy. Behavior therapy teaches the patient better control over eating, decreases attrition and psychological complications, and improves maintenance of weight loss. VLCDs used alone have not produced the same positive results.[68]

In its position paper on VLCDs, The American Dietetic Association acknowledges that these diets can produce a large and rapid weight loss safely when administered properly. It cautions, however, that there are limitations and risks associated with the diets. Although they may be effective for certain persons, they should be undertaken only with the supervision of a multidisciplinary health team that includes monitoring by a physician and nutrition counseling by a registered dietitian. In addition, programs should be limited to predetermined periods, and the amount and composition of the weight loss should be monitored. The criteria for selecting candidates for VLCD therapy are described in the ADA position paper.[69]

FAD DIETS*

A variety of weight-loss diets are introduced on the market each year. Since many overweight people find it difficult to follow diets long enough to achieve their desirable body weight,[70] they seek "effortless" and "miracle" cures. It has been estimated that tens of billions of dollars are spent each year on these diet approaches.[71] Unfortunately, the effectiveness of these diets is often based on nothing more than testimonies.

*By Alison Murray

It is usually easy to recognize a fad diet. Fad diets make elaborate promises of success, understate the rigors of adherence, try to place the decision for dietary restriction in the hands of the dieter, and provide someone with substantial financial profits.[72] Fad diets have three characteristics[70]: They tell you it is easy to lose weight,[71] they promise quick, dramatic, miraculous cures,[72] and they use anecdotes and testimonials to support their claims.[73]

While the registered dietitian can easily identify a fad diet, the layperson often believes the claims that quacks make. Some of the claims are cleverly twisted theories from scientific studies.

Since new quack diets are published almost daily, it is not possible to be familiar with each one. Guthrie[74] lists criteria for assessing the soundness of weight-reducing diets (*Table 8.5*). These criteria will be of benefit to both practitioners and the general public in evaluating existing and new weight-loss diets that are introduced so frequently. Any weight-reduction diet that does not meet all of these criteria is not recommended.

Table 8.5
Criteria for Assessing Weight-Reducing Diets

- Must be deficient in kilocalories
- Must have adequate amounts of all other nutrients
- Must have sufficient fat or bulk to provide satiety
- Must be able to be adapted from family meals or when eating out
- Must be reasonable in cost
- Must be a diet that can be adhered to for a sufficient time to lose weight
- Must retrain the individual in a new set of eating habits

Reproduced by permission from Guthrie, Helen A.: *Introductory nutrition*, ed. 7, St. Louis, 1989, Times Mirror/Mosby College Publishing.

References

1. Simopoulos AP. The health implications of overweight and obesity. *Nutr Rev*. In press.
2. Simopoulos AP. Dietary control of hypertension and obesity and body weight standards. *J Am Diet Assoc*. 1985;85:4.
3. Hubert HB, Feinleib M, McNamara PM. Obesity as an independent risk factor for cardiovascular disease: a 26-year follow-up of participants in the Framingham Heart Study. *Circulation*. 1983;67:968.
4. Glueck CJ, Taylor HL, Jabcobs D, et al. Plasma high-density lipoprotein cholesterol: association with measurements of body mass. *Circulation*. 1980;62(suppl IV):62.
5. Little JA, Graves K, Suchindran CM, et al. Customary diet, anthropometry and dyslipoproteinemia in selected North American populations. The Lipid Research Clinics Program Prevalence Study. *Circulation*. 1986;73:I-80.
6. Brennan PJ, Simpson J, Blacket RB, et al. Effects of body-weight on serum cholesterol, serum triglycerides, serum urate, and systolic blood pressure. *Aust NZ J Med*. 1980;10:15.
7. Kannel WB, Gordon T, Castelli WP. Obesity, lipids and glucose intolerance: the Framingham Study. *Am J Clin Nutr*. 1979;32:1238.
8. Foster CJ, Weinseir RL, Birch R, et al. Obesity and serum lipids: an evaluation of the relative contribution of body fat and fat distribution to lipid levels. *Int J Obesity*. 1987;11:151.
9. Donahue RP, Abbott RD, Bloom E, et al. Central obesity and coronary heart disease in men. *Lancet*. 1987;1:821.

10. Lapidus L, Bengstsson C, Larrson B. Distribution of adipose tissue and risk of cardovascular disease and death: a 12 year follow up of participants in the population study of women in Gothenburg, Sweden. *Br Med J.* 1984;289:1257.
11. Kannel WB, Gordon T. Physiological and medical concomitants of obesity: the Framingham Study. In: Bray GA, ed. *Obesity in America.* 1979. US Dept of Health, Education, and Welfare NIH publication 79-359.
12. Tran ZV, Weltman A. Differential effects of exercise on serum lipid and lipoprotein levels seen with changes in body weight. *JAMA.* 1985;254:919.
13. Vaswani AN. Effect of weight reduction on circulating lipids: an integration of possible mechanisms. *J Am Col Nutr.* 1983;2:123.
14. Wolf RN, Grundy SM. Influence of weight reduction on plasma lipoprotein in obese patients. *Arteriosclerosis.* 1983;3:160.
15. Tyroler HA, Heyden S, Hames CG. Weight and hypertension: Evans County studies of blacks and whites. In: Paul O, ed. *Epidemiology and Control of Hypertension.* New York, NY: Stratton Intercontinental; 1975.
16. Genuth SM, Castro JH, Vertes V. Weight reduction in obesity by outpatient semistarvation. *JAMA.* 1974;230:987.
17. Reisin E, Abel R, Modan, et al. Effect of weight loss without salt restriction on the reduction of blood pressure in overweight hypertensive patients. *N Engl J Med.* 1978;298:1.
18. Johnson AL, Cornoni JC, Cassel JC, et al. Influence of race, sex and weight on blood pressure behavior in young adults. *Am J Cardiol.* 1975;35:523.
19. Stamler R, Stamler J, Riedlinger WF, et al. Weight and blood pressure: findings in hypertension screening of 1 million Americans. *JAMA.* 1978;240:1607.
20. Dyer A, et al. Alcohol consumption, cardiovascular risk factors, and mortality in two Chicago epidemiologic studies. *Circulation.* 1977;56:1067.
21. Haskell WL, et al. The effect of cessation and resumption of moderate alcohol intake on serum density lipoprotein subfractions: a controlled study. *N Engl J Med.* 1984;310:805.
22. Kannel WB. Prevalence and natural history of electrocardiographic left ventricular hypertrophy. *Am J Med.* 1983;75(suppl 3A):4-11.
23. Kaplan N. Use of non-drug therapy in treating hypertension. *Am J Med.* 1984;3:273.
24. Horton ES. Introduction: an overview of the assessment and regulation of energy balance in humans. *Am J Clin Nutr.* 1983;38:972.
25. Guyton AC. *Textbook of Medical Physiology.* Philadelphia, Pa: WB Saunders Co; 1976.
26. Van Itallie TB, Kissileff HR. Physiology of energy intake. *Am J Clin Nutr.* 1985;42:914.
27. Thompson JK, Jarvie GJ, Lahey BB, et al. Exercise and obesity: etiology, physiology and intervention. *Psychol Bull.* 1982;91:55.
28. Weisner RL, Wadden TA, Ritenbaugh C, et al. Recommended therapeutic guidelines for professional weight control programs. *Am J Clin Nutr.* 1984;40:865.
29. American College of Sports Medicine. Position statement on proper and improper weight loss programs. *Med Sci Sports Exer.* 1982;15:IX.
30. Franklin BA, Rubenfine M. Losing weight through exercise. *JAMA.* 1980;244:377.
31. Prentice AM, Lucas A, Vasquez-Velasquez L, et al. Are current dietary guidelines for young children a prescription for overfeeding? *Lancet.* 1988;2:1066.
32. Wood PD. Changes in plasma lipids and lipoproteins in overweight men during weight loss through dieting as compared to exercise. *N Engl J Med.* 1988;319:1173.
33. Hagan RD, Upton SJ, Wont L, et al. The effects of aerobic conditioning and/or caloric restriction in overweight men and women. *Med Sci Sports Exer.* 1986;18:87.
34. Stunkard AJ, Pennick BS. Behavior modification in the treatment of obesity. *Arch Gen Psychiatry.* 1979;36:801.
35. Bray GA. The myth of diet in the management of obesity. *Am J Clin Nutr.* 1970;23:1141.
36. Garrow JS. *Energy Balance and Obesity in Man.* 2nd ed. Amsterdam, the Netherlands: Elsevier; 1978.
37. Wooley SC, Wooley OW, Dyrenforth SR. Theoretical, practical and social issues in behavioral treatment of obesity. *J Appl Behav Anal.* 1979;12:3.
38. Wing RR, Jeffrey RJ. Outpatient treatments of obesity: a comparison of methodology and results. *Int J Obesity.* 1979;3:261.

39. Dempsey JA. Anthropometrical observations on obese and nonobese young men undergoing a program of vigorous physical exercise. *Res Quar.* 1964;35:275.
40. Brownell KD, Stunkard AJ. Exercise in the development and control of obesity. In: Stunkard AJ, ed. *Obesity.* Philadelphia, Pa: WB Saunders Co; 1980.
41. Mayo Clinic Committee on Dietetics. *Mayo Clinic Diet Manual.* 4th ed. Philadelphia, Pa: WB Saunders Co; 1971.
42. Rabast V, Vornberger KH, Ehl M. Loss of weight, sodium and water in obese persons consuming a high or low-carbohydrate diet. *Ann Nutr Med.* 1981;251:341.
43. Donato K, Hegsted DM. Efficiency of various sources of energy for growth. *Proc Natl Acad Sci.* 1985;82:4866.
44. Lissner L, Levitsky DA, Strupp BJ, et al. Dietary fat and the regulation of energy intake in human subjects. *Am J Clin Nutr.* 1987;46:866.
45. Dreon DM, Frey-Hewitt B, Ellsworth N, et al. Dietary fat: carbohydrate ratio and obesity in middle-aged men. *Am J Clin Nutr.* 1988;47:995.
46. Russ CS, Atkinson RL. Use of high fiber diets for the out-patient treatment of obesity. *Nutr Rep Int.* 1985;32:193.
47. Baron JA, Schori A, Crow B, et al. A randomized controlled trial of low carbohydrate and low fat/high fiber diets for weight loss. *Am J Public Health.* 1986;76:1293.
48. Stevens J. Does dietary fiber affect food intake and body weight? *J Am Diet Assoc.* 1988;88:939.
49. American Diabetes Association, American Dietetic Association. *Exchange Lists for Meal Planning.* Chicago, Ill: American Dietetic Association; 1986.
50. Pollock ML. The recommended quantity and quality of exercise for developing and maintaining fitness in healthy adults. *Med Sci Sports Exer.* 1978;10:8.
51. DeBakey ME, Gotto AM Jr, Scott LW, et al. *The Living Heart Diet.* New York, NY: Raven Press; 1984.
52. Frankle RT. Obesity: a family matter. *J Am Diet Assoc.* 1985;85:597.
53. Munro JF, Douglas JG. The management of obesity. *Hum Nutr Clin Nutr.* 1983;37C:1.
54. Jeffery RW, Bjornson-Benson WM, Rosenthal BS, et al. Correlates of weight loss and its maintenance over two years of follow-up among middle-aged men. *Prev Med.* 1984;13:155.
55. Black DR, Lantz CE. Spouse involvement and a possible long-term follow-up trap in weight loss. *Behav Res Ther.* 1984;22:557.
56. Brownell KD, Greenwood MRC, Stellor E, et al. The effects of repeated cycles of weight loss and regain in rats. *Physiol Behav.* 1986;38:459.
57. Stuart RB, Mitchell C, Jensen JA. In: Prokop CK, Bradley LA, eds. *Medical Psychology: Contributions to Behavioral Medicine.* New York, NY: Academic Press; 1980.
58. James WPT. Treatment of obesity: the constraints on success. In: James WPT, ed. *Clinics in Endocrinology and Metabolism.* London, England: WB Saunders Co; 1984.
59. Garrow JS. *Treat Obesity Seriously.* Edinburgh, Scotland: Churchill-Livingston; 1981.
60. Wadden TA, Stunkard AJ, Brownell KD. Very low calorie diets: their efficacy, safety, and future. *Ann Intern Med.* 1983;99:675.
61. Felig P. Very low calorie protein diets. *N Engl J Med.* 1984;310:589. Editorial.
62. Lockwood DH, Amatruda JM. Very low calorie diets in the management of obesity. *Ann Rev Med.* 1984;35:373.
63. Wing RR, Jeffrey RW. Outpatient treatments in obesity: a comparison of methodology and clinical results. *Int J Obesity.* 1979;3:261.
64. Genuth SM, Castro JH, Vertes V. Weight reduction in obesity by outpatient semistarvation. *JAMA.* 1974;230:987.
65. Vertes V, Genuth SM, Hazelton IM. Supplemented fasting as a large scale outpatient program. *JAMA.* 1977;238:2151.
66. Genuth SM, Vertes V, Hazelton J. Supplemented fasting in the treatment of obesity. In: Bray G, ed. *Recent Advances in Obesity Research.* London, England: Newman; 1978.
67. Anderson T, Stokholm H, Baker OG, et al. Long-term (5 year) results after either horizontal gastroplasty or very-low-calorie diet for morbid obesity. *Int J Obesity.* 1988;12:277.

68. Wadden JA, Stunkard AJ, Brownell KD, et al. Treatment of obesity by behavior therapy and a very low calorie diet: a pilot investigation. *J Con Clin Psy.* 1984;52:692.
69. The American Dietetic Association. Position of The American Dietetic Association: very low calorie weight loss diets. *J Am Diet Assoc.* 1990;90:722.
70. Friedman RB. Fad diets: evaluation of five common types. *Postgrad Med.* 1986;79:249.
71. Clydesdale FM. Fad diets and weight reduction. *Nutr MD.* 1984;10:1.
72. Consumer Union's Report, eds. *Health Quackery.* New York, NY: Holt, Rinehart & Winston; 1980.
73. Herbert V, Barrett S. *Vitamins and "Health" Foods.* Philadelphia, Pa: George F Stickly Co; 1982.
74. Guthrie HA. *Introductory Nutrition.* 7th ed. St Louis, Mo: Mosby Co; 1989:214.

PART 3
TREATMENT APPROACHES FOR CHD

9. EXERCISE INTERVENTION FOR CHD

LIPIDS AND LIPOPROTEINS*

People who participate in vigorous endurance-type exercise generally have plasma lipid and lipoprotein profiles consistent with lower risk for coronary heart disease (CHD). The major differences between people who exercise and matched, sedentary, control subjects appear to be lower triglyceride levels and higher HDL-cholesterol levels. Plasma total cholesterol and LDL cholesterol are less likely to differ from inactive controls. It appears more difficult to change the plasma lipoprotein concentration in young women with exercise training than in men; however, the evidence is limited. The modification of enzymes (either activity or enzyme protein mass) involved in triglyceride and cholesterol synthesis, transport, and catabolism likely mediate the exercise-induced changes in lipid and lipoprotein metabolism.[1] In addition, regular participation in exercise apparently has a positive effect on blood coagulation.[2,3] It has also been shown that exercise lowers platelet aggregation in men.[4,5] Since there is general agreement that platelets are involved in the atherosclerotic process and that thrombosis of coronary arteries acts as a mechanism of myocardial infraction, it appears that the effects of regular exercise on platelet aggregation could slow the development of atherosclerotic plaques and hence reduce the risk of CHD. A recent study[6] shows that a lower level of physical activity is associated with a higher risk of CHD in men, independent of conventional risk factors.

Plasma Total Cholesterol

Observational studies generally have demonstrated small changes in the plasma total cholesterol of endurance-trained athletes compared with less-active men or women of a similar age. Some studies with athletes[1,7,8] have not reported any effect of exercise on the plasma total cholesterol, while other studies with endurance-trained runners have reported either lower[1,9] or higher values.[1] Speed- or power-trained athletes have similar or higher plasma total-cholesterol levels compared with sedentary controls. Plasma total cholesterol also appears to be similar for active men (such as lumberjacks) in the general population, compared with their sedentary counterparts.[1]

Results from some longitudinal, endurance-training studies have shown that exercise reduces plasma total cholesterol[1,10–12]; however, most well-designed studies have not shown any change.[1,13] It has been speculated that an increase in the cholesterol content of one lipoprotein may be counterbalanced by a decrease in the cholesterol content of other lipoproteins with the result that total cholesterol is not changed.[1] Thus, the relationship between exercise and total cholesterol appears variable and inconclusive.[13]

Low-Density-Lipoprotein Cholesterol

The effect of exercise on LDL cholesterol generally has been small and highly variable in both cross-sectional comparisons of active and inactive subjects and in longitudinal training studies.[1,8,9] A number of training studies have found that LDL cholesterol is lower following training,[1,10,12,14] while others have shown no effect from either high- or low-intensity training.[1,15] The exercise intensity in studies reporting a decrease in LDL cholesterol has usually been moderate (60% to 85%), with exercise frequency ranging from daily to

*By Susan Bryant

three times weekly (30 to 60 minutes per session) and training duration ranging from 11 days (daily training) to 16 weeks. Reductions in LDL cholesterol have been more frequent when exercise caused weight loss, but decreases in LDL cholesterol have occurred in exercising subjects who did not lose weight. LDL cholesterol is more likely to decrease with exercise if it is elevated prior to training.[1]

High-Density-Lipoprotein Cholesterol

Physically active people[1,7,13] and endurance-trained athletes[1,16] consistently have higher plasma HDL cholesterol levels than the general public or sedentary controls. Elevations in HDL cholesterol have been reported for long-distance runners, cross-country skiers, speed skaters, soccer players, and tennis players.[1,7-9,17,18] In addition, HDL_2 cholesterol has been shown to account for most of the increase in HDL cholesterol noted in runners.[18]

Average HDL-cholesterol values are approximately 45 mg/dL for young men and 55 mg/dL for young women in the United States and Canada.[16] The difference between values for athletes and sedentary controls is 12 to 20 mg/dL or 20% to 35% of control values.[1,16] In contrast, HDL-cholesterol levels in trained weightlifters are similar to those of nonathletes.[19]

Men and women who are active on the job or during leisure time but are not endurance-trained athletes generally have higher concentrations of HDL cholesterol than their less-active counterparts. Although these differences are statistically significant, they are usually small and typically do not exceed 5 mg/dL.[1]

HDL cholesterol and exercise training. Prospective exercise studies have yielded conflicting results regarding the effect of exercise training on HDL cholesterol.[20] Approximately 50% of the endurance-training studies with clinically healthy men have reported significant or near-significant increases in HDL cholesterol,[1,10-12,14,21,22] whereas other studies have found no change or a decrease.[1,10,15,23] When HDL cholesterol is raised, the increase typically ranges from 5% to 16% or 3 to 8 mg/dL.[1,24]

Although physical conditioning consisting primarily of heavy resistance exercise has generally not increased HDL cholesterol,[1] body builders have been shown to have a higher HDL cholesterol than powerlifters,[13] and weight training has been shown to change lipid and lipoprotein levels favorably in previously sedentary men and women.[10]

The increase in HDL cholesterol in cross-sectional and longitudinal (training) studies is thought to largely be the result of increased HDL_2 cholesterol. Apolipoprotein A-I (but not A-II) also seems to increase concomitantly.[25]

Gender differences, exercise, and HDL cholesterol. The observation that exercise training increases HDL-cholesterol levels in men more frequently than in women suggests a gender-related difference in response to exercise.[10,26,27] Changes in endogenous testosterone and estrogens may account for the increase in HDL cholesterol in men.[26] However, HDL cholesterol has also been shown to increase in women running an average of 12 miles per week.[28] It has been suggested that sedentary women may need more frequent, more intensive, and longer training programs than men to increase HDL-cholesterol levels[23] and that higher initial levels of HDL cholesterol in women may be the result of a greater lipoprotein lipase (LPL) activity in women.[29]

Plasma Triglycerides

When exercise affects plasma triglycerides, VLDL triglyceride is the lipoprotein fraction that is changed.[1] Physically active people and endurance-trained athletes usually have lower concentrations of VLDL triglyceride and plasma triglyceride than inactive controls.[1,9,30] Compared with the general population, lower plasma triglyceride levels have been reported for long-distance runners, cross-country skiers, and tennis players,[1] but no difference from controls has also been reported.[8] Plasma triglyceride levels of athletes involved in power or speed-type training are similar to those observed in inactive people. Lower plasma triglyceride values have been reported for people who are more active on the job or during leisure time in selected populations, but not in others.[1,7] Little information has been published on the relationship between plasma triglyceride levels and habitual exercise status in the general population.[1,7] However, both acute and long-term increases in aerobic exercise have been shown to cause decreases in plasma triglycerides except in people who already have low normal levels.[1,18] This decrease is associated with an increase in the rate of triglyceride clearance.[31]

MECHANISMS BY WHICH EXERCISE AFFECTS PLASMA LIPIDS AND LIPOPROTEINS*

It is not clear what accounts for the variation in the lipoprotein (particularly HDL-cholesterol) and plasma lipid response to exercise training. It appears that changes in plasma lipoproteins are produced, in some way, by the large increase in energy expenditure required during exercise, by the higher caloric intake usually reported by very active people, and by body leanness. Exercise has been shown to alter the activities of LPL, hepatic lipase (HL), and lecithin-cholesterol acyltransferase (LCAT), all of which are of importance in cholesterol metabolism.[1]

The increase in LPL activity in the adipose tissue and skeletal muscle of highly trained athletes such as endurance runners (compared with sprinters and sedentary controls) suggests that hydrolysis of plasma triglycerides is increased. This may be the first step in a series of events that leads to elevations of HDL_2 *(Figure 9.1)*. Some of these differences may be due to an acute increase in LPL activity produced by vigorous exercise.[1,19,25]

Although LPL activity appears to increase with vigorous exercise, HL activity decreases. A significant negative correlation has been reported between HDL cholesterol and HL in highly trained runners, active military academy students, and middle-aged men before and after 15 weeks of exercise training. Since HL plays a role in the conversion of HDL_2 to HDL_3, the lower enzyme activity reported with exercise provides an explanation for the accompanying higher HDL_2 cholesterol levels (*Figure 9.2*).

LCAT catalyzes the transfer of fatty acids in plasma from lecithin to cholesterol during the production of HDL cholesterol. An increase in LCAT activity has been reported in endurance-trained athletes and with endurance training of young and middle-aged men. It is thought that this increase in LCAT might contribute to the increase in HDL-cholesterol concentrations (*Figure 9.3*).

*By Susan Bryant

Fig 9.1
Proposed mechanism by which high-density lipoprotein (HDL) increases in response to exercise via increased lipoprotein lipase (LPL) activity. During lipolysis, components of triglyceride-rich lipoproteins are transferred to and incorporated into HDL_3, leading to the formation of HDL_2. LDL indicates very-low-density lipoprotein; chylo, chylomicron. Reprinted with permission from Kris-Etherton PM. The effect of exercise on lipid and lipoprotein metabolism. **Am Chem Soc Symp Series.** ***1986;294:59.***

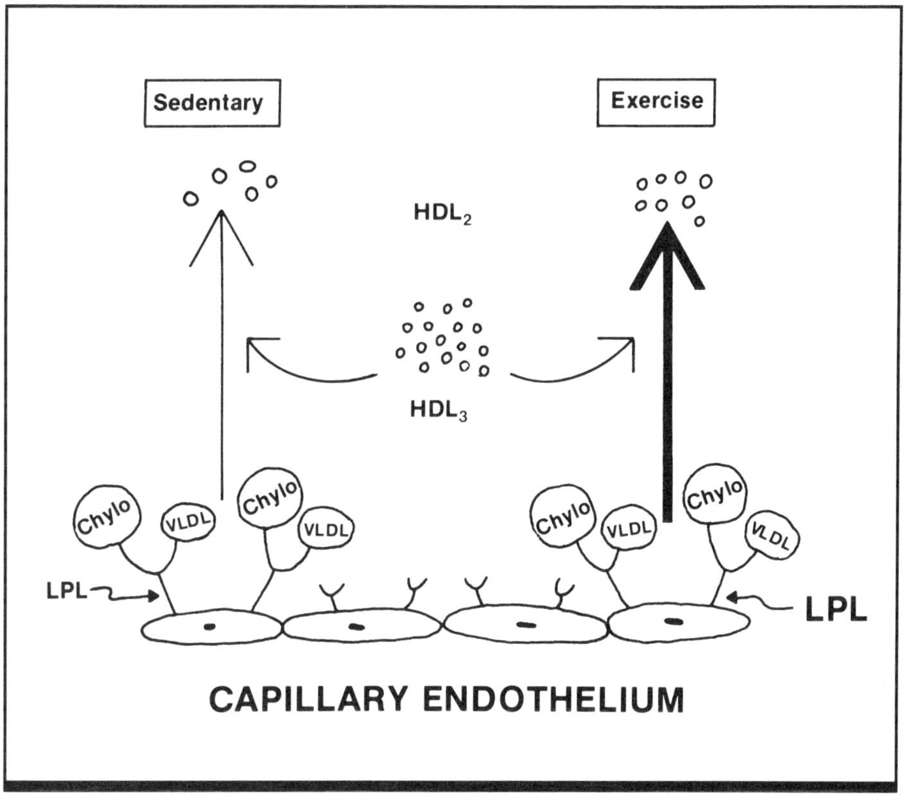

Fig 9.2
Proposed yet speculative mechanism by which high-density lipoprotein (HDL) increases in response to exercise via decreased hepatic lipase activity. LCAT indicates lecithin-cholesterol acyltransferase. Reprinted with permission from Kris-Etherton PM. The effect of exercise on lipid and lipoprotein metabolism. **Am Chem Soc Symp Series.** ***1986;294:59.***

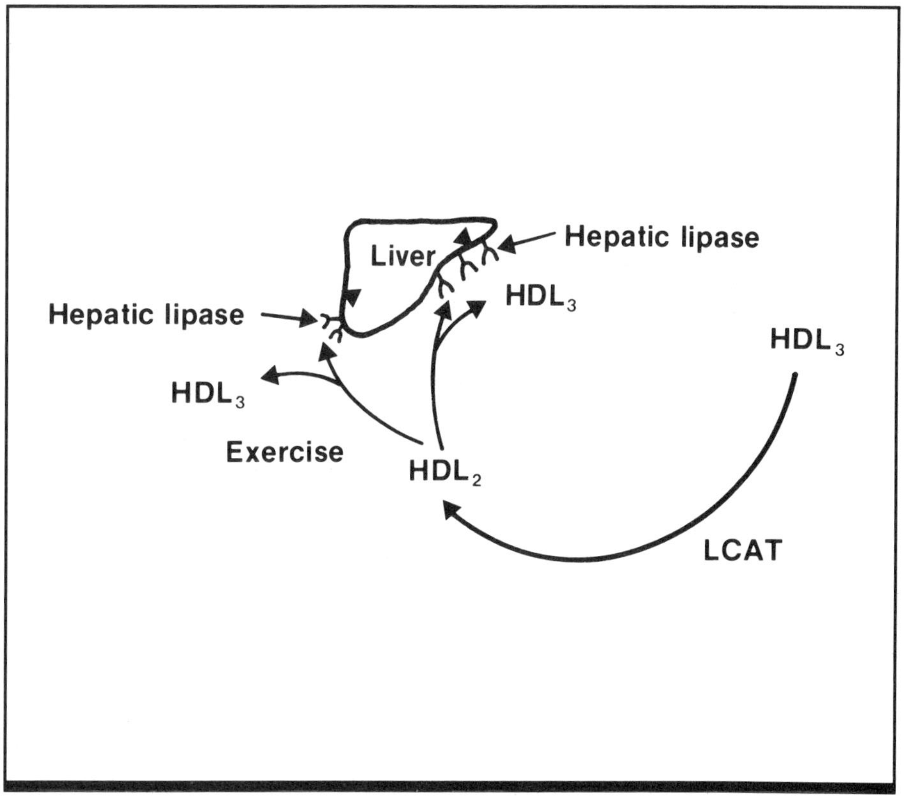

Fig 9.3
Proposed yet speculative mechanism by which high-density lipoprotein (HDL) increases in response to exercise via increased lecithin-cholesterol acyltransferase (LCAT) activity and/or increased apolipoprotein-A_1 concentration. Reprinted with permission from Kris-Etherton PM. The effect of exercise on lipid and lipoprotein metabolism. **Am Chem Soc Symp Series.** ***1986;294:59.***

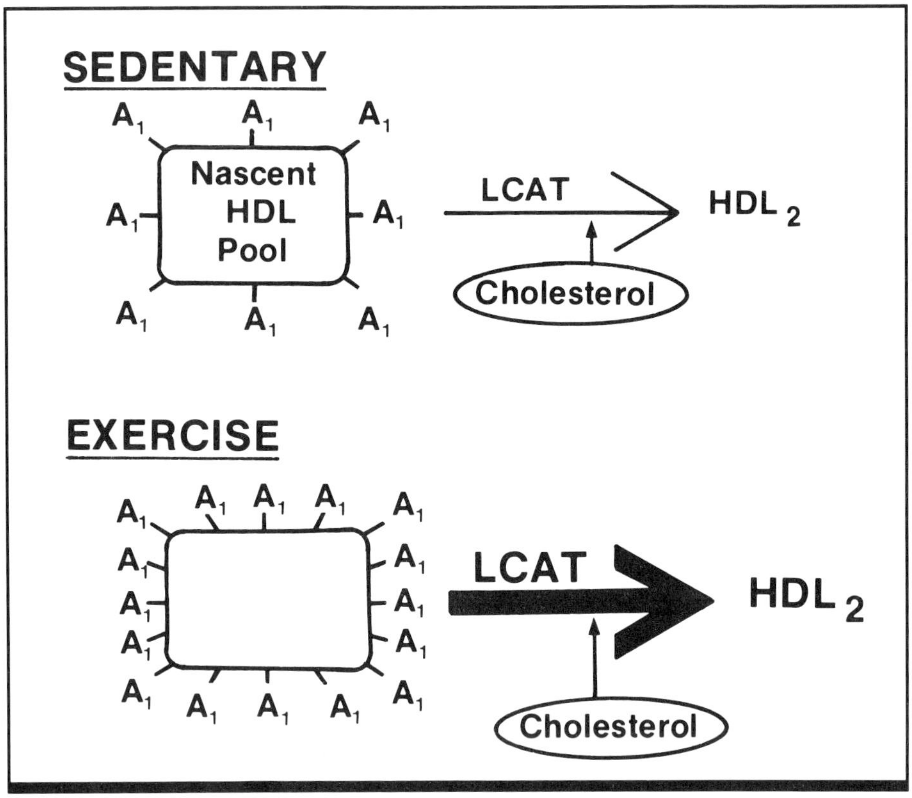

The effect of energy expenditure from exercise on HDL. A minimum beneficial threshold of 1,000 calories per week in energy expenditure has been recommended to increase HDL cholesterol.[1] In addition, it has been suggested that there is a dose-response relationship between the level of physical activity and HDL-cholesterol levels with increases in HDL cholesterol correlating with increases in energy expenditure up to about 4,500 calories per week.[1,13] However, this tissue is not resolved, and the greatest increase in HDL-cholesterol levels appears to occur when sedentary men become more active,[33] particularly if they have low HDL-cholesterol levels before training.[1,20] Running mileage and length of training have also been positively correlated with HDL cholesterol.[12,22]

The effect of exercise training, weight loss, and HDL cholesterol. A meta-analysis study of previous reviews was conducted to evaluate the relative contributions of fitness and weight reduction to lipoprotein levels.* This analysis showed that reductions in plasma total-cholesterol and HDL-cholesterol levels were greatest when exercise training was combined with reduction in body weight.[33]

EXERCISE AND GLUCOSE METABOLISM†

Physical training decreases insulin secretion[34] and improves glucose clearance by at least three separate mechanisms.

Evidence indicates that exercise training decreases plasma insulin concentrations both during fasting and after glucose ingestion in younger and

*Meta-analysis is a quantitative approach to research reviewing that uses a variety of statistical techniques for sorting, classifying, and summarizing information from the findings of many experimental studies.
†By Susan Bryant

middle-aged people and in older athletes.[13,20] A decrease in circulating insulin without any change in fasting blood glucose levels is indicative of an increase in tissue insulin sensitivity. Increased insulin binding to receptors (an increase in the number of available insulin receptors) due to physical activity is thought to be the mechanism for increased insulin sensitivity.[35] During muscle and liver glycogen repletion (24 to 48 hours after exercise), there is an improvement in glucose tolerance and diminished insulin requirements.[36]

Exercise has a potent insulinlike effect on glucose uptake by muscle. A residual effect of exercise on the permeability of the muscle cell to glucose could play a role in the rapid clearance of glucose, despite lower insulin levels in people who exercise regularly.[37] Although the mechanism by which exercise results in a marked increase in muscle glucose uptake has not been completely defined, insulin appears to play an important role since it has been shown that the exercise-enhanced muscle glucose uptake is inhibited in insulin-deficient states.[38]

Other factors thought to be responsible for exercise-dependent regulation of glucose uptake include a muscular activity factor, hypoxia, and an increase in intracellular calcium.[38,39] However, many investigators favor the hypothesis that increased glucose uptake during exercise is secondary to the increased availability of insulin and glucose to muscle cells as a result of increased blood flow.[38]

EXERCISE AND BLOOD PRESSURE*

The potential benefits of exercise on blood pressure modification are: (1) a reduction in systolic and diastolic blood pressure at rest, (2) a reduction in blood pressure at a given submaximal workload after exercise training, and (3) a reduction of circulating catecholamines at rest and during exercise.[34,39–41] These changes are thought to decrease the stress on the arterial wall, decrease the rate of atheroma formation,[34] and decrease myocardial oxygen demand.[13,33,42] The implications that exercise might benefit people with hypertension are of particular interest because elevated blood pressure has been identified as a primary risk factor for cardiovascular disease (CVD).[43,44]

Population studies have found an inverse correlation between physical activity and blood pressure.[32,45] Epidemiological studies have shown that men in physically active occupations[41] and people in developing countries where physical activity is greater[43] have lower systolic and diastolic blood pressures than those in sedentary occupations and those in developed countries where physical inactivity is greater. The resulting trend is an increased risk for the development of hypertension. The incidence of hypertension has also been associated with low levels of vigorous exercise in an epidemiologic study of Harvard alumni.[40]

Acute effects. The acute blood pressure response to exercise depends on the type, intensity, and duration of the activity. Two types of exercise with different blood pressure responses are dynamic (aerobic, isotonic)† exercise and static (isometric)‡ exercise.[45] A small proportion of people with hypertension who do not have excessively high blood pressure can manage their condition with a formal exercise program. The clinical efficacy of exercise training for the

*By Susan Bryant
†Strength training in which the muscle shortens as weight is moved against the force of gravity and the muscle lengthens as weight is moved in the direction of gravity.
‡Static muscle contraction in which the overall length of the muscle does not change during the application of force against a fixed resistance.

management of hypertension requires further study. Results of most acute studies of exercise training show a return of the hypertensive blood pressure patterns after three to six weeks of detraining.[46]

During dynamic exercise, the oxygen requirements of the exercising muscle increase, which requires an increase in minute ventilation, cardiac output, and exercising muscle blood flow. The vasodilating effect of an acute bout of exercise suggests the possibility that regular exercise could produce a chronic state of vasodilation and, therefore, a reduction in vascular resistance and blood pressure at rest.[45] Therefore, these changes are achieved, in part, by reduced peripheral resistance. During the exercise phase, systolic pressure rises while diastolic pressure usually remains unchanged or decreases. Mean arterial pressure also rises slightly.[45]

By contrast, static exercise increases both systolic and diastolic blood pressure. This, in turn, produces a greater increase in mean arterial pressure.[45] This acute cardiovascular strain could be harmful for people with hypertension or other forms of cardiovascular disease, for whom dynamic forms of moderate exercise would be more appropriate.[34]

In addition to the type of exertion, blood pressure response to exercise may vary depending on the amount of exercising muscle. As less muscle mass is used during dynamic exertion (as with arm ergometry), the hemodynamic response gradually begins to resemble the pattern reported with static exercise.[45]

Chronic effects. Although exercise acutely raises blood pressure, there is growing evidence that repeated physical exertion may reduce blood pressure in both normotensive and hypertensive persons.[45] A reduction in heart rate at rest following exercise training has been postulated as a means of reducing the blood pressure of hypertensive people who exhibit a hyperkinetic circulation (increased heart rate and cardiac output) at rest.[47] It has also been suggested that people with borderline hypertension who exhibit a hyperkinetic circulation may benefit more from exercise training than do people with established hypertension.

Early hypertension, characterized by hyperdynamic circulation with elevated heart rate and resulting in increased cardiac output, is probably due to increased sympathetic nervous system (SNS) activity. Lean borderline hypertensives show chemical evidence of heightened adrenergic activity by their elevated plasma norepinephrine levels. It is thought that exercise might exert its hypotensive effects directly through hemodynamic mechanisms or indirectly by promoting nutrition, metabolic, or behavioral changes (*Table 9.1*).

Exercise training has been shown to blunt the increase in plasma norepinephrine and cortisol that occurs during exhaustive exercise. Likewise, physical conditioning reduces sympathetic tone (decrease resting heart rate and cardiac output). Thus, borderline hypertensives may respond favorably to regular exercise. In addition, repeated dynamic exercise could conceivably produce chronic vasodilation and a resetting of baroreflexes, thereby reducing total peripheral resistance. As yet, there are few longitudinal data to support this concept.[45]

Positive changes in nutrition habits with increased physical activity may result from an awareness of life-style habits, a desire for improved eating habits, and the effects of exercise on body weight. These changes may result in a favorable blood pressure response.[45] Exercise has been shown to lower blood pressure modestly, independent of weight loss or a reduction in body fat.

Table 9.1
Postulated Mechanisms of Reduced Blood Pressure Associated with Repeated Physical Exercise

Hemodynamic	
	Decreased resting cardiac output
	Decreased sympathetic nervous system activity
	Decreased total peripheral resistance
Nutritional	
	Weight loss
	Reduced alcohol consumption
	Reduced sodium intake
	Changes in other dietary factors (fat, potassium, fiber, etc)
Endocrine-metabolic	
	Reduced plasma catecholamines
Behavioral	
	Relaxation techniques

Reprinted with permission from McMahan M, Palmer RM. Exercise and hypertension. *Med Clin North Am.* 1985;69:57.

A reduction in catecholamine levels has been suggested as a means by which blood pressure is reduced by exercise training. A decrease in norepinephrine in hyperadrenergic patients with mild essential hypertension has been demonstrated following exercise training. Similar findings of lower plasma and cardiac catecholamine levels after training suggest an alteration of sympathetic neural activity and a decrease in sympathetic tone.[40] Exercise may lead to positive behavior changes. Reduction of blood pressure via relaxation might also occur as a result of exercise training.[45]

In summary, while longitudinal studies have demonstrated decreases in systolic and diastolic blood pressure in response to endurance exercise, the change in blood pressure reported in most studies is modest. Regular exercise programs favorably influence other CHD risk factors independent of blood pressure.

EXERCISE PRESCRIPTION FOR HEALTHY PEOPLE*

It is well accepted that people of all ages who are physically active appear to be healthier and that regular exercise may be associated with these health benefits. If this is so, there must be some defined dose, or stimulus, of exercise required to get these responses. The question is frequently asked, "How much exercise is enough and what type is best for health?" Even though the consensus is that exercise is important for good health, an actual recommended level of exercise cannot be made at this time. The primary focus of this section is to discuss the characteristics of this level and to offer guidelines for designing a safe and effective lifetime physical activity plan. Questions such as, "What type, intensity, frequency, duration, and total energy output of exercise are required to produce the targeted health effects, and how do we guide people to maintain a program once they begin?" will be answered.

Assessing Readiness to Exercise

Before outlining specific characteristics for an exercise prescription, it is important to mention the need for preexercise screening. Most apparently

*By Barbara Frey-Hewitt

healthy people do not need a preexercise medical evaluation before starting an exercise program. However, three categories of people might benefit from a medical examination before a program:

1. Those who have a history of heart disease, high blood pressure, lung disease, or disease of the bones or joints that could be exacerbated by exercise
2. Those who are older than 35, are sedentary, and intend to plunge immediately into exercise that is more vigorous than brisk walking
3. Those who are interested in using their current fitness level as a measure of progress

Since preexercise screening is not within the scope of this chapter, the reader is referred to the references by the American College of Sports Medicine (ACSM), the American Heart Association (AHA), and the Young Men's (and Women's) Christian Association (YMCA) for more information.[44,48,49]

The Activity Prescription: Above All, Individualize

The first step in designing physical-activity programs is to discuss with the patients any medical concerns they may have regarding certain types of activities and to determine their fitness needs. It is important that all prescriptions be individualized. Gather information on the types of activities the patients enjoy (an activity enjoyed will be continued for the long term), their interests, daily schedules, capabilities, and their motivation to begin and maintain a physical-activity program. Effective prescriptions combine this information with more-specific elements such as the prescribed intensity, duration, frequency, and energy expenditure needed to attain fitness. The patient and practitioner should discuss the prescription as well as the short- and long-term goals and specific plans and activities. This section provides a brief discussion of these elements, as they specifically apply to fitness and health. For more detailed information the reader is referred to ACSM, AHA, and YMCA guidelines.[44,48,49]

Types of Activities for Physical Fitness and Health

The components that make up physical fitness are cardiovascular fitness, strength, and flexibility. Since most of the health benefits ascribed to physical activity are associated with cardiovascular fitness, the major activity prescriptions are the aerobic-type activities that use large muscle groups and are done continuously in a rhythmic, dynamic fashion. These activities cause a sustained increase in metabolic, cardiovascular, and respiratory functions. They are called *aerobic* or endurance exercises because the primary muscle fuel for the activity is derived from a continuous supply of oxygen delivered to the muscle from the blood (by the heart). The most common aerobic activities are brisk walking, jogging, swimming, stepping, cycling, rowing, and aerobic dancing. The safer forms of aerobic activities, in terms of injury risk, are walking, swimming, or stationary cycling. Patients should choose activities that are enjoyable, accessible (in terms of space and schedule), and within their capabilities. To keep the program interesting, two to three activities can be chosen (ie, alternative routes, seasonal options, and so forth).

Since all activity requires some degree of strength, a physical-activity program needs also to include some specific strength and flexibility exercises (particularly for the back and stomach). These exercises will improve activity performance and prevent injury as well as help patients perform everyday tasks such as lifting, carrying, and doing yard work.

Intensity of Activity

As recommended by the American College of Sports Medicine, exercising for 15 to 60 minutes three to five times per week at 65% to 90% of maximum heart rate is adequate to condition the muscles and cardiovascular system.[44] This level of exercise, which is related to exercise duration, is represented by a target zone (ie, the defined heart rate). If clients do not know their maximum heart rate (HR max) from a treadmill test, it can be determined by using an age-based average that is derived by the formula, 220 minus one's age. There is wide variability in this formula (SD = ± 10 beats per minute). The maximal attainable heart rates and target zones (60% to 85% HR max) for various age groups are shown in *Table 9.2.*[49] The same training effect can also be obtained by doing a lower-intensity task at 60% of HR max for a longer duration. This is important, since an overweight or very unfit person should begin with a low-intensity exercise, such as walking, and gradually work up to a duration of 40 to 60 minutes.

Table 9.2
Maximal Attainable Heart Rates (HR max) for Various Age Groups

Age	Predicted HR Max	Target Heart Rate 60%	70%	80%
20–29	200–191	120–114	140–134	160–153
30–39	190–181	114–109	133–127	152–145
40–49	180–171	108–103	126–120	144–137
50–59	170–161	102– 97	119–113	136–129

Duration and Frequency of Activity

The exercise session should consist of a 5- to 10-minute warm-up of slow walking and mild stretching, a cardiovascular conditioning period of 15 to 60 minutes depending on the intensity, a 5- to 10-minute cool-down period to slowly bring the heart rate down, and a 10- to 20-minute period for strength and flexibility work. The recommended frequency of activity ranges from a minimum of three days per week to a maximum of six, depending on the fitness level and the intensity of the activity. For example, a typical exercise schedule for a week may include 30 to 40 minutes of continuous swimming for three days and 20 minutes of brisk walking followed by strength and flexibility exercises for two days. It is important that clients recognize that duration and frequency of activity is flexible, with the general guideline being to maintain a three-day-per-week program of exercises in their target zone with at least a day in between to let their muscles recover.

Energy Expenditure

If the primary goal of a physical-activity program is weight loss, or if the instructions for intensity, duration, and frequency of exercise are too confusing to remember, then it is recommended that a required caloric output per week in physical activity be prescribed. This caloric output may be met by having clients exercise in their target zone as well as by having them lead a more active life style. Recent research by Paffenbarger et al[50] suggests that more walking and climbing stairs may be just as effective for maintaining health as a program that includes only vigorous physical activity. The caloric output suggested to achieve these benefits is approximately 2,000 kcal per week and can be achieved in split exercise bouts. The energy expenditure of various activities is presented in the appendix (see Table 14.35). To help clients determine the energy cost of their activities, an energy-expenditure table can be used (*Table 9.3*). An easier way to determine the energy cost of exercise, as used in the Stanford Weight Control Project, is to estimate a cost of approximately 10 calories per minute if the exercise was performed in the target zone.

Table 9.3
Examples of Daily Energy Expenditures of Mature Women and Men in Light Occupations*

		Man, 70 kg		Woman, 58 kg	
Activity Category	**Time, hr**	**Rate, kcal/min**	**Total kcal (kJ)**	**Rate, kcal/min**	**Total kcal (kJ)**
Sleeping, reclining	8	1.0–2	540 (2,270)	0.9–1.1	440 (1,850)
Very light seated and standing activities, painting trades, auto and truck driving, laboratory work, typing, playing musical instruments, sewing, ironing	12	up to 2.5	1,300 (5,460)	up to 2.0	900 (3,780)
Light walking on level, 2.5–3 mph, tailoring, pressing, garage work, electrical trades, carpentry, restaurant trades, cannery workers, washing clothes, shopping with light load, golf, sailing, table tennis, volleyball	3	2.5–4.9	600 (2,520)	2.0–3.9	450 (1,890)
Moderate walking 3.5–4 mph, plastering, weeding and hoeing, loading and stacking bales, scrubbing floors, shopping with heavy load, cycling, skiing, tennis, dancing	1	5.0–7.4	300 (1,260)	4.0–5.9	240 (1,010)
Heavy walking with load uphill, tree felling, working with pick and shovel, basketball, swimming, climbing, football	0	7.5–12.0		6.0–10.0	
TOTAL	**24**		**2,740 (11,510)**		**2,030 (8,530)**

*Data from Durnin JVGA, Passmore R.[73]

Adherence

Despite the known health benefits of regular physical activity, the attrition rate among exercisers is high.[51] Therefore, an effective physical-activity prescription should include ways to keep clients motivated and to prevent relapse. *Table 9.4* provides motivational strategies for adherence to an exercise program; it can be used when prescribing a program. Having clients choose ways for making exercise more enjoyable helps ensure that long-term compliance is achieved. Asking them to identify reasons why they drop out may help them continue their participation in the program. It is important to emphasize permanent life-style changes, a strong need for follow-up, and positive reinforcement for effective life-style changes. To prescribe a program effectively it is also important for practitioners to maintain their own physical-activity programs and to serve as role models. The benefits of physical conditioning are not cumulative and may be quickly lost without regular activity.

Table 9.4
Motivational Strategies for Adherence to an Exercise Program

Maintenance

1. Get inspired by going to a health club or sports meet, or by subscribing to a sports magazine.
2. Consult reputable books, magazines, and health professionals or organizations for ideas on exercising without facilities or expensive equipment.
3. Enroll in a health club or make a commitment to a program.
4. Keep a daily log to record progress.
5. Set up nonfood rewards for attaining goals.
6. Make it a part of the daily routine.
7. Vary routines and locations to make exercise more interesting.
8. Incorporate fun activities like skating, skiing, dancing, and Frisbee tossing.

Progress

1. Define realistic goals.
2. Measure progress in terms of initial starting fitness.
3. Be willing to revise goals as progress is attained.
4. Monitor heart rates before, during, and after exercise.
5. Take weight measurements.
6. Have blood pressure checked.

EXERCISE TESTING AND CARDIAC REHABILITATION*

Exercise training is important in the rehabilitation of patients with CHD. This includes patients with ischemia (with and without angina) and those who have had a myocardial infarction, as well as those who have had coronary artery bypass graft surgery or angioplasty.[52] A vital component from diagnosis to rehabilitation of CHD is the multistage exercise-tolerance test.

Exercise-tolerance testing is the observation and recording of cardiovascular response during a measured exercise challenge in order to determine the subject's capacity to adapt to physical stress. Exercise tests are designed to use steps, treadmill, bicycle, or arm-crank ergometers[26] (see protocols in the appendix, Tables 14.31, 14.32, 14.33, and 14.35). Exercise testing is commonly used to identify patients in whom the possibility of coronary artery disease is high. While the diagnostic utility of exercise testing is well documented, recent attention has focused on its role in the evaluation and management of patients with existing CHD.[53,54]

Since evaluation of cardiac function during the resting state provides little information regarding cardiovascular reserve, complete assessment requires evaluation during conditions of enhanced metabolic demand. The standard exercise-tolerance test assesses the ability of both the coronary and systemic circulations to supply blood flow sufficient to meet the increased metabolic oxygen requirements generated by exercise. A variety of multistage protocols with progressive workloads can determine a client's capacity for circulatory oxygen transport (VO_2) for any given level of exercise.[53,54]

*By Randall Gretebeck

Maximum Systemic Oxygen Consumption

The best objective measure of exercise capacity and functional cardiovascular reserve is maximum oxygen consumption (VO_2max).[53,54] This parameter is defined as the maximum amount of oxygen (in mL/kg/min) consumed when no further increase in oxygen consumption occurs despite an increase in workload. Since the VO_2max provides an estimate of cardiovascular fitness, the higher this value, the more capable the subject is of high-intensity aerobic work. This value can be estimated from the endpoint workload of the test or may be measured directly through gas collection with a metabolic-measurement cart.

Metabolic Equivalents (METs)

The workload at various stages of a graded exercise test is often measured in metabolic equivalents (METs). One MET is defined as the VO_2 at rest and is equal to 3.5 mL/kg/min of oxygen consumed. Healthy sedentary people usually cannot exercise beyond 10 to 12 METs, whereas conditioned athletes often can exercise beyond 15 METs. Patients with congestive heart failure and left ventricular dysfunction are usually limited to 3 to 5 METs. The following formula may be used to determine the MET level for a particular exercise:

$$\text{METs} = \frac{\text{Oxygen Required for Exercise}}{\text{Oxygen Required at Rest (3.5 mL/kg/min)}}$$

Rate-Pressure Product

An exercise-tolerance test cannot directly measure myocardial oxygen consumption, however. The product of heart rate and systolic blood pressure, which is known as the rate-pressure product (double product), is closely correlated with myocardial oxygen consumption.[55] This parameter, derived through the use of an exercise test, can provide important diagnostic information. The following formula is used to determine rate-pressure product:

$$\text{Rate-Pressure Product} = \text{Heart Rate} \times \text{Systolic Blood Pressure}$$

Myocardial ischemia, with or without angina, usually occurs at a reproducible rate-pressure product. This helps to identify the ischemic threshold, which is necessary for prescribing an appropriate exercise program.

Rating of Perceived Exertion

A subjective measure of the level of effort expended during a symptom-limited exercise test is the rating of perceived exertion (RPE), developed by Borg (*Table 9.5*).[56] RPE and HR are linearly related to each other and to exercise intensity over a wide range of exercise modalities and conditions. A point categoric scale is used to rate the total amount of physical effort experienced during exercise. A rating of 6 indicates a minimal level of exertion, while a rating of 20 corresponds to a strenuous maximal effort. If the perceived effort at peak exercise is "very, very hard" (19 or 20) on the Borg scale, it can be reasonably assumed that a maximum effort has been expended by the subject.[53,54] RPE is useful in prescribing exercise for patients who have an irregular (and, therefore, difficult-to-count) pulse, as well as for patients who cannot find their pulse. (See Taking Your Pulse in the appendix, Table 14.34.) Many cardiac patients are in the training zone at an RPE of 12 to 16.[53,54]

Table 9.5
Rating of Perceived Exertion (RPE)

RPE		New Rating Scale	
6		0	Nothing at all
7	Very, very light	0.5	Very, very weak
8		1	Very weak
9	Very light	2	Weak
10		3	Moderate
11	Fairly light	4	Somewhat strong
12		5	Strong
13	Somewhat hard	6	
14		7	Very strong
15	Hard	8	
16		9	
17	Very hard	10	Very, very strong
18			Maximal
19	Very, very hard		
20			

Reprinted with permission from Borg GV. Guidelines for exercise testing and prescription. *Med Sci Sports Exer.* 1982;14:377. ©by American College of Sports Medicine.

PURPOSE OF STRESS TESTING*

The information received from an exercise tolerance test can be used for different purposes. In general, exercise testing is done for one of the following reasons[57]:

1. To aid in the diagnosis of CHD whether symptoms are present or not
2. To assess the safety of exercise prior to starting an exercise program
3. To assess the cardiopulmonary function capacity of apparently healthy or diseased persons
4. To follow the progress of known coronary or pulmonary disease
5. To assess the efficacy of various medical and surgical procedures including the effect of medications

Probably the most valuable use of the stress test is to estimate the severity and prognosis of coronary disease and to help provide guidelines for selecting patients who need more extensive diagnostic and therapeutic interventions such as cardiac catheterization and coronary artery bypass graft surgery.[58] The most important variables measured before, during, and immediately after a stress test are heart rate, blood pressure, and electrocardiogram (ECG). Maximal stress tests can only be performed in the presence of a physician, although submaximal stress tests and ECG monitoring of rehabilitation classes may be conducted by other health professionals.

Electrocardiogram Measurement

Many different ECG lead systems have been used for exercise testing. Single-lead systems may be adequate in young healthy populations where the primary purpose of testing is to measure fitness. In higher-risk populations, a 12-lead system that covers the inferior wall, anterior wall, and lateral precordial area of the heart is preferred.[57] A standard resting ECG performed both in the seated and supine positions should be obtained before the test is begun. The ECG should be continually displayed on an oscilloscope during testing, with

*By Randall Gretebeck

standard ECG strips recorded at periodic intervals. Monitoring should continue approximately 10 minutes into recovery after the stress test, since ECG changes may occur during the cool-down phase. If questionable abnormalities appear, readings should be taken at more-frequent intervals.[57]

Blood Pressure Measurement

Blood pressure should be taken in the sitting and standing positions prior to exercise. During the test, blood pressure should be measured every one to two minutes or at each stage of the test. During recovery, blood pressure is usually monitored at two- to three-minute intervals until it approaches resting levels; however, the heart rate and blood pressure do not come all the way back to resting values even at the end of the cool-down phase. If hypotensive or hypertensive readings are present, ie, if systolic blood pressure falls with continued exercise or rises too high, readings should be taken at more-frequent intervals.[57] Blood pressure should be taken with the subject's arm relaxed and not grasping a treadmill bar or cycle handlebar.

Submaximal Stress Testing

Submaximal stress testing may be useful for determining fitness when a diagnostic test is not required. In selecting patients who have had an uncomplicated myocardial infarction, a submaximal test may be used to[53,54]:

1. Promote patient confidence
2. Assess job-related work capacity
3. Determine appropriate out-of-hospital exercise prescription
4. Detect potentially serious cardiac arrhythmias
5. Determine posthospital prognosis
6. Monitor progress of a home exercise program

Most post–myocardial infarct exercise tests are performed 7 to 14 days following infarction and use a multistage treadmill protocol that begins at a low workload proceeding at small increments.[53,54] Heart-rate-limited tests usually use an HR max of 120 to 130 beats per minute (bpm) in patients not receiving beta-blockers. Workload-limited tests aim for a peak workload between 4 and 6 METs (the level of the usual activities of daily living). A submaximal test may be useful in monitoring changes in fitness resulting from an exercise program. As a subject becomes more fit, the HR at a given submaximal intensity decreases; therefore, a comparison of heart rates obtained during submaximal exercise will reflect changes in fitness level.[59]

Maximal Stress Testing

A maximal stress test is defined as one in which $\dot{V}O_2$ reaches a plateau before the test is terminated ($\dot{V}O_2$max is reached).[54,55,57,58] Serial measurements of oxygen consumption are required to be certain that maximum exertion has been achieved. Since these measurements are inconvenient to perform during routine exercise testing, maximum effort is usually approximated by having the patient exercise to a sympton-limited maximum exercise tolerance. The subject should be encouraged to continue as long as possible; the test ends when the subject signals that he or she can no longer continue. It can be assumed that a maximal effort has been achieved if the subject's HR reaches his or her age-adjusted maximum predicted heart rate (±10 bpm).[53,54,57] As a general rule, the value 220 minus age (in years) for men and women provides a reasonable approximation of the true HR max. In subjects with paced heart rhythms or in subjects receiving beta-adrenergic blocking agents, the maximum predicted heart rate is no longer useful. In these subjects the RPE scale by Borg can be used. If the perceived exertion at peak exercise is "very, very hard" (19 or 20) on the Borg scale, it can be reasonably assumed that a maximum effort has been achieved.[54,55,57,58] An outline of various protocols is included in the appendix (see Tables 14.31, 14.32, 14.33, and 14.35).

Observation and Integration

A diagnostic stress test should be an extension of an overall physical examination. The physician or other certified professional conducting the test gains the most information by observing the patient prior to, during, and following the test.[57] The patient's appearance, blood pressure, HR response, presence or absence of symptoms, functional capacity, as well as ECG, provide important information. It is important to use all available information in the interpretation of an exercise test in the diagnosis of coronary disease. In cardiac patients, the training response may not be as great as in nondiseased people. Since heart disease is a progressive disorder, stress-test results evaluated on a yearly basis may either show no improvement or a slight increase in exercise capacity. Nevertheless, simply halting or slowing down the progression of CHD through lifestyle modification enhances the quality of the patient's life.

Interpreting an exercise test requires knowledge of the risk factors and the clinical status of the person being tested, because false positivies and false negatives do occur with noninvasive stress testing. The ability of the stress test to predict coronary disease depends on the patient population on which it is used. Stone[58] showed that when the stress test is used on symptomatic patients, the predictive accuracy was 95%, while in asymptomatic patients, the ability of a stress test to predict significant coronary obstruction was only 36%. In other words, the stress test in asymptomatic patients showed 64% false-positive results.[58] These results illustrate that the diagnostic value of a stress test is limited to populations in which CHD may be most prevalent.

Nuclear Stress Testing*

Radioactive tracers can be used to assess myocardial function throughout the cardiac cycle. There are basically two types of stress tests that rely on radiation: thallium imaging and radionuclide ventriculography.

Although an extensive review of these tests is beyond the scope of this chapter, it is important to know some of the basics.

Thallium testing. In a thallium test the patient receives a symptom-limited maximum stress test. One minute before the test is stopped, a radioactive tracer (thallium 201) is injected intravenously into the bloodstream. As blood flows to the heart, it deposits the radioisotope within the cardiac muscle. Resting images of blood flow to the heart are compared with exercise images of the heart, and ischemic areas of the myocardium can be identified. In other words, if certain parts of the heart are not receiving enough blood, those areas will show little tracer deposited and are therefore known as "cold" areas. This may give the physician an idea as to which coronary artery may be occluded. During the stress test, the patient's ECG, blood pressure, and clinical findings must be carefully recorded. Thallium testing is particularly useful in special situations:

1. In the patient who has had a prior myocardial infarct, it can identify other areas of the heart that have not yet infarcted.

*By Patricia Volz-Clarke

2. When the ECG is difficult to interpret, such as left bundle branch block, left ventricular hypertrophy, or patients on digitalis.
3. To evaluate false-positive stress tests in populations that should not have heart disease, ie, young women with chest pain or young athletes or asymptomatic persons.

Radionuclide ventriculography (wall-motion studies). In a patient with coronary narrowing, marked changes can be seen in cardiac wall motion. A noninvasive test can be performed to assess these changes. It is usually performed with the patient in a supine position exercising on a cycle ergometer. An intravenous injection of a radiopharmaceutical allows the red blood cells to be "tagged" and counted as they exit the heart. Normal cardiac muscle increases its end diastolic volume and decreases its end systolic volume with exercise, causing an increase in ejection fraction and stroke volume. In a decreased coronary system, the ejection fraction falls and the overall efficiency of the system is reduced. Studies have shown that the presence of wall-motion abnormalities or a drop in the ejection fraction with exercise can predict coronary disease with a sensitivity of 93%. Radionuclide ventriculography is useful in predicting the magnitude and location of cardiac muscle loss in a patient who has had a myocardial infarct and it may also aid in diagnosing graft closure or the progression of an occlusion.

Stress testing with radioactive materials gives the physician the ability to study ventricular function under dynamic conditions and provides insight into the behavior of the heart with exercise. These tests are expensive, however, and are only used in patients with known cardiac disease or to provide additional information not received with regular stress tests.[55]

EXERCISE PRESCRIPTION FOR CARDIAC PATIENTS*

Regular exercise increases physical work capacity and may provide angina relief for many cardiac patients. The increase in aerobic capacity may be due to the increased central (heart rate or stroke volume) or peripheral (skeletal) oxygen transport and utilization, while relief of chest discomfort may be secondary to a decrease in myocardial oxygen demand[60] and/or an increase in oxygen delivery (*Table 9.6*). Peripheral adaptations come into play during the initial phases of rehabilitation, and central adaptations such as increased stroke volume and decreased heart rate occur after consistent moderate- to high-intensity training. Regular exercise may also increase the "ischemic threshold," allowing patients to exercise at higher levels before they feel angina.[60]

Exercise prescription for patients with coronary artery disease should be designed so that exercise is both safe and effective. Exercise, like medication, must be tailored to the individual patient's needs. A sound exercise prescription for the rehabilitation of patients with CHD including those with left ventricular dysfunction or acute ischemia and those who have undergone coronary artery bypass graft surgery (CABGS) or angioplasty requires that the medical history be reviewed. The physician or exercise physiologist who prescribes exercise for such patients, recommending optimal frequency, duration, intensity, and mode of exercise, must consider factors such as age, sex, clinical status, concomitant medical problems, previous physical activity, orthopedic and musculoskeletal integrity, and, most important, the data derived from a multistage exercise-tolerance test.[61] A comprehensive medical evaluation and graded exercise test to peak or symptom-limited effort will reveal the factors listed above as well as peak heart rate and oxygen uptake, ventilatory threshold,

*By Randall Gretebeck

rating of perceived exertion, limiting signs or symptoms, occurrences of ischemic ST-segment depression,* dysrhythmias, and an inappropriate blood pressure response.[52]

Table 9.6 Mechanisms Responsible for Increased VO_2max With Physical Conditioning

Central
1. Increased cardiac output and stroke volume at maximal exercise (predominantly normal individuals)
2. Increased size and number of skeletal muscle mitochondria

Peripheral
1. Increased size and number of skeletal muscle mitochondria
2. Increased myoglobin (increased O_2 storage)
3. Increased oxidative enzymes (for example, succinate dehydrogenase, cytochrome oxidase)
4. Increased capillary density in skeletal muscle
5. Decreased cardiac output (decreased muscle blood flow) at a given submaximal workload
6. Increased A-VO_2 difference at submaximal and maximal workloads

Reprinted with permission from Franklin B, Wisely D, et al. Chronic adaptations to physical conditioning in cardiac trainability. *Clin Sports Med.* 1984;3:471.

Intensity

The appropriate exercise intensity requires an individualized exercise prescription and adequate monitoring to ensure that the maximum prescribed intensity is not exceeded. The intensity of exercise may be expressed as a percentage of functional capacity, which may be obtained from a symptom-limited stress test. The average conditioning intensity for asymptomatic adults is usually between 60% and 70% of functional capacity. For most myocardial infarction patients, the threshold intensity for exercise training is approximately 40% to 60% of functional capacity.[57] The intensity of exercise may be prescribed by heart rate, relative perceived exertion, or by METs.

Training Session

Exercise training sessions should include a warm-up (10 minutes), a cooldown (5 minutes), and a conditioning phase (20 to 60 minutes) that involves aerobic-endurance exercise interspaced between the warm-up and cool-down phases. The exercise session can include a recreational game (10 to 15 minutes), a muscular conditioning strength-training period, and exercises for training specific body parts.

Warm-up

Warm-up exercises facilitate the transition from rest to aerobic-endurance training, the stretching of postural muscles, and an increase in blood flow.

*A depression of ST-segment of 2 mm or more below normal on an ECG signifies myocardial ischemia, which occurs when the heart muscle starves for oxygen, usually because of insufficient blood flow.

A warm-up period is particularly important for patients with CHD to allow sufficient time for autoregulation of myocardial blood flow. Subendocardial ischemia, secondary to a delay in autoregulation of myocardial blood flow, is an important mechanism in the response to sudden strenuous exertion and provides an important physiologic basis for warming up.[52] Stretching and flexibility movements should be followed by cardiorespiratory calesthenics that involve total body movements to increase the heart rate to within 20 beats per minute of the target heart rate recommended for endurance training. The best warm-up for any aerobic activity is the prescribed activity performed at a lower intensity. For example, a patient using fast walking as his or her mode of exercise should walk for ten minutes at a slower pace; a jogger should use brisk walking as a warm-up. For a swimmer, simply walking around in the pool before doing laps will gradually increase the heart rate, and using low tension on a stationary cycle is an ideal warm-up. Stretching and flexibility exercises can be incorporated into the program but are not sufficient by themselves to serve as the only warm-up activity. For patients on beta-blockers, heart rate will not serve as a guide to warm-up intensity; however, an RPE between 8 and 11 is usually a good guide.

Cool-down Phase

The cool-down involves slow walking or low-intensity exercise and provides a gradual recovery from the conditioning phase. This permits appropriate circulatory adjustments and the return of heart rate and blood pressure to near-resting values. The cool-down period enhances venous return, thereby reducing the potential for postexercise hypotension and dizziness; it also facilitates the dissipation of body heat, promotes more-rapid removal of lactic acid than stationary recovery,[61] and reduces the potentially deleterious effects of the postexercise rise in plasma catecholamines such as epinephrine.[62] This is particularly important in CHD patients in that postexercise hypotension and the resulting transient decrease in venous return may reduce coronary blood flow when myocardial oxygen demands may still be high.[52] Consequences may include angina pectoris, ischemic ST-segment depression, or malignant ventricular dysrhythmias. The importance of a gradual warm-up and cool-down period is emphasized in a study: of 61 cardiovascular complications reported during the exercise training of cardiac patients, 72% occurred during either the warm-up or cool-down phases.[63]

Conditioning Phase

The conditioning phase should follow the warm-up and must include aerobic-endurance exercise. Muscular-strength conditioning may also be included in the conditioning phase and is particularly important for CHD patients who want to return to occupations that require manual labor or frequent lifting.[64] Endurance exercise, which improves the patient's cardiorespiratory responses to submaximal and maximal exercise, should be prescribed in terms of intensity, duration, frequency, and type of activity. Another way to look at the prescription is by the FIT formula of frequency, intensity, and time.

TYPES OF TRAINING ACTIVITIES*

Weight training. Isometric or static exercises were once considered unsafe for cardiac patients. Recent studies, however, have shown that conventional weight-training programs using variable-resistance exercises are appropriate for some cardiac patients. Low to moderate weights with low repetitions do not seem to be associated with cardiac symptoms such as an inappropriate blood pressure reponse, ST depression, or ventricular ectopy. Selected forms of isometric exercises performed in a medically supervised setting will help cardiac patients perform both occupational and leisure-time activities.[52]

Arm exercises. Cardiac conditioning programs should include exercises for the upper extremities. Occupational and recreational activities rely more on arm work than on leg work, and walking or jogging programs, which rely primarily on lower-extremity conditioning, do not help with arm conditioning.[59] Recent studies have shown that the upper extremities respond to a conditioning program similar to the lower extremities.[52,60]

Using a treadmill workload to predict the heart rate required for upper-extremity conditioning may result in an inappropriately high recommendation for a target heart rate. An energy expenditure of approximately 50% of that used for leg exercises is suggested for arm training.[52] For example, a patient using a stationary cycle workload of 300 kilogram • meter per minute (kpm) for a leg workout would set the workload on the arm ergometer at 150 kpm. Although a stationary cycle (mounted on a table) or an arm-crank ergometer are the most easy to regulate, appropriate arm exercises may also be performed on a Schwinn Air-Dyne, Nautilus-type equipment, or with light dumbbells.

Aerobic conditioning. The most effective exercises for aerobic conditioning involve movement of the large muscles of the body, can be maintained continuously, and are rhythmic in nature. Walking, jogging, and cycling are particularly well suited for CHD patients because they can be closely regulated. Below are generalized guidelines for various modes of exercise. A combination of programs may increase compliance to the exercise program. Some of these exercises may be too strenuous; however, if a patient was accustomed to them prior to his or her heart problems, the patient may be able to modify the intensity and continue the activity.

Walking and jogging. These types of programs include very little equipment, have a low injury rate, are easily regulated, and have the lowest dropout rates of any exercise. Obviously, walking is considered the most appropriate for an unsupervised workout and in the early recovery stages of a heart attack.[52,60] Heart rate or perceived exertion ratings can be used to regulate exercise intensity closely. A combination walk/jog can be used as the next progression step to elicit a higher heart-rate response as the patient becomes more physically fit.

Swimming. Swimming incorporates both upper and lower body exercise and is an appropriate training modality for trained patients. However, swimming is difficult to prescribe because: (1) the energy output is based on skill and stroke and varies widely from patient to patient, and (2) training heart rates predicted from the maximal stress test may be 5 to 10 beats higher than appropriate.[52] As such, the target heart zone must be adjusted downward when establishing a swimming exercise prescription. Additionally, inappropriate heart-rate and blood pressure fluctuations may occur in water that is too cold or too hot.[52]

*By Patricia Volz-Clarke

Cycling. Stationary cycling has an obvious advantage over walking because it can be done during inclement weather. The workloads can also be accurately prescribed, especially if a cycle ergometer such as a Monark or Tunturi is used. Just as a walk/jog interval program can be used for patients as they become more physically fit, interval programs that alternate hard or easy tension levels can be used to increase the intensity of the cycle workout and to prevent boredom.

Cross-country skiing. Although this is an excellent activity for overall aerobic conditioning, the energy expended is considerably more than walking or jogging.[52] Myocardial oxygen demand is increased by the weight of the clothing, the arm motion, cold temperatures, and any inclines in terrain. Simulated cross-country machines may be too strenuous for untrained cardiac patients because the energy cost can be as great as 90% of the maximum achieved heart rate.[52]

Aerobic dancing. Dancing has been shown to induce favorable cardiovascular conditioning in men and women. Assuming that the appropriate intensity is maintained for 20 to 40 minutes and calisthenics do not involve breath holding or push-ups, some myocardial infarct patients should be able to incorporate aerobic dancing into their conditioning routines.

Rowing. Rowing is fast becoming a popular form of exercise. It may be hard for patients to do a full workout for 20 to 40 minutes because rowing involves quite a bit of arm work. However, the program could be designed so that a set period of rest (for example, 30 seconds every 3 minutes) would allow the program to be carried out in the target zone. Additionally, a rower could be incorporated into part of a circuit program* that includes walking or cycling.

Marathon running. Marathon running will not guarantee protection from CHD or sudden death, nor will it necessarily prevent progression of the disease. There are several factors to consider before marathon running is prescribed for cardiac patients:

- The training program requires a higher threshold for frequency, duration, and intensity than is usually recommended for most cardiac-conditioning programs.[52]
- The 26.2-mile run has limited application to patients, possibly due to restrictions of advanced age, disease progression, or the inability to achieve a high aerobic capacity.[52]
- The patient may require CPR, and personnel and equipment may not be available.[52,60]

Many cardiac patients can safely enter competitive running races if that is their goal, but marathon training needs to be carefully monitored. Additionally, adverse weather conditions may make the attempt at racing inadvisable.

Summary

Some patients, because of the underlying severity of their disease, may not be able to improve with a conditioning program. However, assuming no absolute medical contraindications exist, a low-level exercise program may benefit the patient psychologically. Additionally, serial exercise testing allows

*The overall objectives are total body fitness, muscular strength, and endurance of both the upper and lower body; the circuit program uses multiple exercise stations that vary between activities using upper- and lower-body exercise and between resistive and dynamic exercise.

the workout to be evaluated and is especially important if the patient is on a home program without direct supervision. A check approximately every three months by a health professional not only helps the patient with compliance, but also allows for an adjustment in workload as the patient becomes more physically fit.

ENVIRONMENTAL CONDITIONS*

Cold weather. Patients who have had a myocardial infarction can participate safely in cold-weather activity if appropriate precautions are observed. Inhalation of cold air may aggravate angina pectoris in susceptible cardiac patients. A mask or scarf will help warm inhaled air and may prevent discomfort. The wind-chill factor as well as the air temperature must be considered as indices for inappropriate cold stress. Wet clothing (especially hat and gloves) must be changed immediately and the head and feet must be covered.[52]

Warm weather. Myocardial oxygen demand is increased during hot weather due to an increase in body temperature and a drop in circulating blood volume due to increased sweating.[52] The training heart rate is a useful guide in setting the appropriate pace of the workout. Heart rate increases in hot weather and, if the patient is monitoring it correctly, it should automatically slow down to within the training zone. Additionally, excessive sweating may cause electrolyte imbalance in sodium and potassium and may cause ventricular ectopy. Warm-weather recommendations[52] for outside exercise include:

- Drinking plenty of fluids before, during, and after the workout
- Decrease or discontinue the exercise at temperatures greater than 80 °F and 75% relative humidity
- Exercise in the cooler part of the day
- Allow for gradual acclimation, which may take 4 to 14 days

EXERCISE PRESCRIPTION CRITERIA†

Exercise Prescription by Heart Rate

In general, unless disturbed by environmental conditions, psychological stimuli, or disease, a linear relationship exists between heart rate and exercise intensity.[57] This relationship has led to various methods for determining a "target" or training heart rate. The first method for calculating exercise heart rate is to plot the line that shows the relationship between exercise heart rate and exercise intensity in either METs or V_{O_2}. The maximum heart rate is usually the heart rate measured at the highest exercise intensity. From this relationship, the heart rate associated with a given percentage of functional capacity (usually 60% to 70%) can be determined. This heart-rate value may be used for regulating intensity during conditioning. Another method is to determine the target heart rate for a subject by multiplying the difference between the maximum and resting heart rate by a percentage based on a 60% intensity adjusted upward in proportion to functional capacity measured in METs. For example[57]:

Functional Capacity (METs)	Percentage of Heart-Rate Range
3	60 + 3 = 63
5	60 + 5 = 65
10	60 + 10 = 70
15	60 + 15 = 75
20	60 + 20 = 80

*By Patricia Volz-Clarke
†By Randall Gretebeck

Target heart rate can then be computed as follows for a person whose exercise capacity is 10 METs:

Maximum heart rate	180	
Resting heart rate	– 60	
Conditioning intensity	120	
percentage heart rate range	×0.7	(60 + 10 MET capacity)
	84	
Resting heart rate	+ 60	
Training heart rate	144	

A third method, the one used most frequently for determining target heart rate, is to calculate a specified percentage of maximum heart rate. If the maximum heart rate is 180 beats per minute, the target heart rate might be 70% of 180 (180 × 0.70), or 126 bpm. An upper limit would be 85% (0.85 × 180), or 153. In an exercise setting, subjects can monitor their pulse by palpation either at the carotid or radial pulse. The radial pulse is the preferred method since carotid pressure may cause the patient to become lightheaded and may, in fact, slow the pulse rate down. Counting the pulse for ten seconds immediately after a bout of exercise and multiplying by 6 gives a good estimate of exercise heart rate. (See Table 14.34 in the appendix.)

Exercise Prescription by Rating of Perceived Exertion

As shown previously, the original rating of perceived exertion (RPE) scale is a 15-point numerical scale ranging from 6 to 20 with a verbal description provided at every odd number. The RPE response to a graded exercise test correlates highly with cardiorespiratory and metabolic measures such as VO_2, HR, ventilation, and blood lactate concentration. RPE is a valid and reliable indicator of the level of physical exertion during constant-intensity exercise and therefore can be used to establish an exercise intensity for endurance training. Using the Borg scale, a perceived exertion rating of 12 to 13 corresponds to approximately 60% of the heart-rate range. A rating of 16 corresponds to approximately 90% of heart-rate range. Consequently, most participants should exercise at an intensity rated between 12 and 16 ("somewhat hard" to "hard") depending on their functional capacity. RPE can also be used in conjunction with heart-rate prescription methods. At the onset of a training program the participant can be instructed to exercise at a specified heart rate and to self-monitor the RPE at that intensity. Once the participant has developed a knowledge of the heart rate–RPE relationship, heart rate can be monitored less frequently and RPE can be employed as the primary method for regulating exercise intensity.

Exercise Prescription by METs

The intensity of exercise may be prescribed by determining a specified percentage (50% to 85%) of the client's functional capacity and then selecting activities that are known to require energy expenditures at the desired level.[30] The same procedure as described with the heart-rate method can be employed when designating exercise intensity in terms of METs. The baseline intensity is

6. Over prolonged periods, electrodes tend to become relatively fixed. Nonetheless, caution is advised regarding excessive stretching and body manipulation.

Beta-Blockers

The relationship between the percentage relative $\dot{V}O_2max$ and percentage of maximum heart rate (HR max) is remarkably consistent (that is, 57% to 78% $\dot{V}O_2max$ is proportional to 70% to 85% HR max) regardless of subject age, sex, aerobic capacity, presence or absence of cardiovascular disease, and the use of upper or lower extremity exercise.[66] Although beta-blockers lower resting heart rate, blood pressure, and exercising heart rate at any given exercise intensity, cross-sectional and longitudinal studies have shown that propranolol does not alter the regression of percentage $\dot{V}O_2max$ on percentage HR max,[40] ie, $\dot{V}O_2max$ can be increased without an increase in heart rate[67] (*Figure 9.4*). To set an appropriate exercise intensity for subjects taking beta-blockers, a stress test should be conducted with the subject on the prescribed dosage. The resulting regression line can then be used to prescribe an appropriate target heart rate. Perceived exertion and exercise intensity derived from a stress test may also be used to prescribe exercise intensity. Paying close attention to MET equivalents is particularly useful in adjusting a training program if the drug dose is altered.

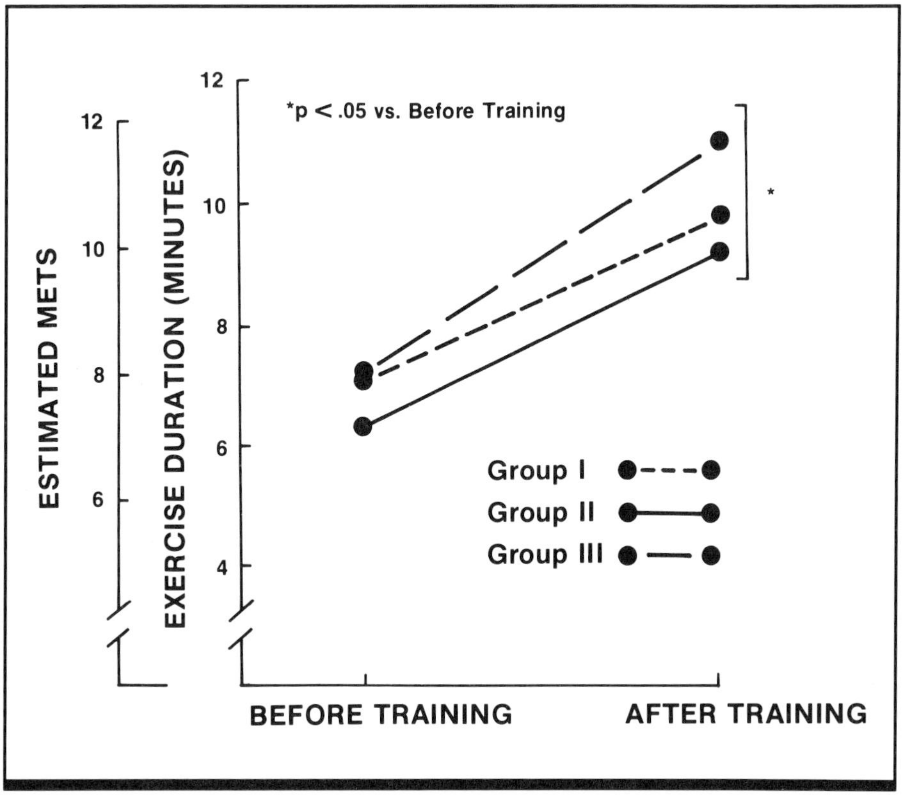

Fig 9.4
Duration of exercise according to the Bruce protocol and estimated aerobic capacity (METs) before and after a 12-week training program. Results were measured in patients receiving no propranolol (group I), patients receiving low-dose propranolol (group II), and patients receiving high-dose propranolol (group III). Adapted with permission from Pratt CM, Welton DE, et al. Demonstration of training effect during chronic beta and adrenergic blockade in patients with coronary artery disease.* Circulation. *1981;64:1125.

Calcium Channel Blockers (Calcium Antagonists)

Calcium antagonists such as nifedipine, verapamil, and diltiazem block calcium-dependent contraction in vascular smooth muscle and myocardial cells.[57] These drugs are used as antianginal agents. In patients limited by angina, calcium antagonists may increase exercise capacity. In patients without angina, little effect on peak exercise intensity would be expected. Because of peripheral vasodilation, nifedipine, in particular, sometimes causes resting tachycardia.[57] On the other hand, verapamil may lower resting heart rate.[57] As with beta-blockers, the agent and dose used must be noted at the time of exercise testing, and changes in rest and exercise heart rate should be anticipated if medication changes occur.

Nitrates

Nitrate preparations include short-acting sublingual nitroglycerin, nitroglycerin ointment or discs, and long-acting nitrates. These agents act as coronary artery vasodilators, but their principal antianginal effect is probably a result of venous dilatation, which reduces cardiac preload and thus myocardial oxygen consumption.[57] Nitrates may alter exercise capacity in patients limited by angina by increasing the anginal threshold, ie, they can exercise longer before they feel discomfort. In patients who develop exertional angina, sublingual nitroglycerin will potentiate exercise-induced venous dilatation and may result in hypotension, so blood pressure needs to be monitored while they exercise.[57] Such patients should cool down slowly following exercise testing or training session.

Monitoring for three months is suggested for patients who are exercising in a community-based center or at home. This will help with patient adherence to the program as well as allow the counselor to upgrade the workout as the patient becomes more physically fit.

Summary

Prescribing exercise guidelines for the patient with CHD relies on the results of a progressive exercise test. The exercise recommendations derived from this test should be validated and verified according to the patient's ability to implement the activity program through observation of warm-up and cool-down procedures, pulse monitoring, RPE responses, and work-intensity selection.[52] A realistic exercise intensity should be one that can be attained without inducing extreme dyspnea, lightheadedness, chest pain, dysrhythmias, nausea, or musculoskeletal trauma. The patient's own sensing of discomfor or distress is a key component. The prescription for physical activity should be adapted to the patient, rather than the patient to the prescription. Increased functional capacity, relief of angina, risk-factor reduction, enhanced psychological status, and improved quality of life are justifiable ends to recommend a physical-training program for CHD patients. Registered dietitians with an expertise in fitness appraisal and exercise prescription may play a major role in making exercise recommendations and implementing exercise programs.

EXERCISE EQUIPMENT*

Equipment for Cardiac Rehabilitation

The type of equipment that is used in a cardiac rehabilitation unit often depends on personal preferences and budgetary restraints. Equipment in a center or unit that is used professionally is different from that purchased for home use. Both, however, serve similar functions. Ongoing equipment maintenance is essential. The equipment mentioned below and in the appendix (see Table 14.36) is not an exhaustive listing. Additional manufacturers may be available and preferred in specific instances.

*By Ann R. Semenske

Essential equipment for a cardiac rehabilitation unit can be grouped into exercise equipment and monitoring equipment. Patients can be encouraged to purchase some equipment for home use to facilitate long-term compliance to the exercise program year-round. However, it is important for patients to understand that only exercise equipment that makes the body work is of benefit physiologically. For example, there is a common misconception that vibrating belts cause fat-tissue break-down. All of the equipment listed serves a vital but distinct role in the unit.

Treadmills. Essential aerobic-exercise equipment for a cardiac rehabilitation unit, treadmills are often used for stress testing after myocardial infarcts and surgery. Exercise prescriptions are often based on treadmill performance. Oxygen consumption, cardiac output, and a VO_2 difference are all higher when patients are tested on a treadmill than when they are tested on a bicycle. A list of treadmill suppliers appears in the appendix.

Exercise bicycles. Bicycles offer some advantages over treadmills. Oxygen uptake can be predicted with greater accuracy than with any other type of exercise equipment, and mechanical efficiency is independent of body weight.[68] Exercise bicycles are a good form of exercise for patients unable to use a treadmill[69] or for patients whose exercise prescription is based on METs because of heart-rate-lowering medications. A list of exercise-bicycle manufacturers and suppliers appears in the appendix.

Arm ergometers. This type of equipment produces a peak workload that is significantly less than that produced by leg exercise equipment. In addition, heart rate, systolic blood pressure, and rate-pressure product are higher for a given workload due to small muscle groups used in arm work. Arm ergometers are less sensitive than other exercise equipment in detecting CHD.[70] However, some patients such as hemiplegics and paraplegics are unable to perform leg work. For these patients, arm ergometery is a reasonable alternative.*

Rowing machines. During maximal exercise, rowing slightly lowers heart rate. Oxygen uptake is significantly lower; however, a training effect is possible by exercising between 70% and 90% of the maximal predicted heart rate. A high Vo_2max can be achieved with a rowing machine.[71] A list of rowing-machine manufacturers appears in the appendix.

Stair machines. Stair machines are the newest form of exercise equipment. Using the equipment backward also may help patients with chronic lower-back problems. Exercise on a stair machine has shown comparable increases in Vo_2max compared with walking, running, and cycling. Heart rate and oxygen consumption rise rapidly with this form of exercise, so any stair-climbing program should be started slowly.[72]

The Stair Master stair machine is one of the hottest items in health clubs today. The address for Stair Master is in the Appendix (see Table 14.36).

Fitness Monitors

Cardiac rehabilitation requires that patients be monitored constantly to determine responses such as heart rate, blood pressure, and changes in body weight. The following monitoring equipment covers the basic needs of a cardiac rehabilitation unit and is not inclusive.

*One popular arm ergometer is from Engineering Dynamics Corp, 120 Stedman St, Lowell, MA 01851-2797

Basic monitoring equipment. Items such as blood pressure cuffs, stethoscopes, electrodes, and electrocardiogram supplies are among the basic materials needed in a cardiac rehabilitation unit. The best place to purchase these items in your area is through hospital-supply companies, which will provide the names of different products on the market.*

Medical Electronic Products† provides the latest product news of medical research and diagnostic instrumentation. It offers product descriptions of cardiovascular equipment including cardiac stimulators, ECG, EEG, halters, monitors, stress-test equipment, and treadmills.

Heart-rate monitors. Heart-rate monitors are used during exercise so that safe levels of exertion prescribed by an attending physician may be maintained. A study in Canada evaluated several heart-rate monitors and found that those devices that measure the cardiac electrical potential or that incorporate a light transmission device attached to the earlobe were accurate and provided a suitable monitor of heart rate during exercise. The most accurate monitors were those that were strapped to the chest and monitored by a watch placed on the wrist.[70] One US supplier is listed in the appendix (see Table 14.36).

References

1. Haskell WL. Exercise-induced changes in plasma lipids and lipoproteins. *Prev Med.* 1984;13:23.
2. Kopitsky RG, Switzer ME, Williams RS, et al. The basis for the increase in factor VIII procoagulant activity during exercise. *Thromb Haemost.* 1983;49:53.
3. Williams RS, Logue, EE, Lewis JL, et al. Physical conditioning augments the fibrinolytic response to venous occlusion in healthy adults. *N Engl J Med.* 1980;302:987.
4. Rauramaa R, Salonen JT, Seppanen K, et al. Inhibition of platelet aggregability by moderate-intensity physical exercise. *Circulation.* 1986;74:939.
5. Rauramaa R, Salonen JT, Kukkonen-Harjula K, et al. Effects of mild physical exercise on serum lipoproteins and metabolites of arachidonic acid. *Br Med J.* 1984;288:603.
6. Eklund LG, Haskell WL, Johnson JL, et al. Physical fitness as a predictor of cardiovascular mortality in asymptomatic North American men. *N Engl J Med.* 1988;319:1379.
7. Lehtonen A, Viikari J. Serum triglycerides and cholesterol and serum high-density lipoprotein cholesterol in highly physically active men. *Acta Med Scand.* 1978;204:111.
8. Adner MM, Castelli WP. Elevated high-density lipoprotein levels in marathon runners. *JAMA.* 1980;243:534.
9. Krauss RM, Williams PT, Lindgren FT, Wood PD. Coordinate changes in levels of human serum low and high density lipoprotein subclasses in healthy men. *Arteriosclerosis.* 1988;8:155.
10. Goldberg L, Elliot DL, Schutz RW, et al. Changes in lipid and lipoprotein levels after weight training. *JAMA.* 1984;252:504.
11. Kiens B, Jorgensen I, Lewis S, et al. Increased plasma HDL-cholesterol and apo A-1 in sedentary middle-aged men after physical conditioning. *Europ J Clin Invest.* 1980;10:203.
12. Wood PD, Haskell WL, Blair SN, et al. Increased exercise level and plasma lipoprotein concentrations: one-year, randomized, controlled study in sedentary, middle-aged men. *Metabolism.* 1983;32:31.
13. Hurley BF, Seals DR, Hagberg JM, et al. High-density-lipoprotein cholesterol in bodybuilders v powerlifters: negative effects of androgen use. *JAMA.* 1984;254:507.

*One company that provides rehabilitation equipment and supplies through catalog services is Vital Signs, Country Technology, Inc, PO Box 87, Gay Mills, WI 54631.
†Medical Electronics, 2994 W Liberty Ave, Pittsburgh, PA 15216.

14. Huttunen JK, Lansimies E, Voutilainen E, et al. Effect of moderate physical exercise on serum lipids: controlled clinical trial with special reference to serum high-density lipoproteins. *Circulation.* 1979;60:1220.
15. Gaesser GA, Rich RG. Effects of high- and low-intensity exercise training on aerobic capacity and blood lipids. *Med Sci Sports Exer.* 1984;16:269.
16. Deshaies Y, Allard C. Serum high-density lipoprotein cholesterol in male and female Olympic athletes. *Med Sci Sports Exer.* 1982;14:207.
17. Vodak PA, Wood PD, Haskell WL, et al. HDL-cholesterol and other plasma lipid and lipoprotein concentrations in middle-aged male and female tennis players. *Metabolism.* 1980;29:745-752.
18. Herbert PN, Bernier DN, Cullinane EM, et al. High-density lipoprotein metabolism in runners and sedentary men. *JAMA.* 1984;252:1034.
19. Farrell PA, Maksud MG, Pollock ML, et al. A comparison of plasma cholesterol, triglycerides, and high density lipoprotein-cholesterol in speed skaters, weightlifters and non-athletes. *Europ J Appl Physiol.* 1982;48:77
20. Goldberg L, Elliot DL. The effect of physical activity on lipid and lipoprotein levels. *Med Clin North Am.* 1985;69:41.
21. Cook TC, Laporte RE, Washburn RA, et al. Chronic low level physical activity as a determinant of high density lipoprotein cholesterol and subfractions. *Med Sci Sports Exer.* 1986;18:653.
22. Williams PT, Wood PD, Haskell WL, et al. The effects of running mileage and duration on plasma lipoprotein levels. *JAMA.* 1982;247:2674.
23. Frey MAB, Doerr BM, Laubach LL, et al. Exercise does not change high-density lipoprotein cholesterol in women after ten weeks of training. *Metabolism.* 1982;31:1142.
24. Thompson PD, Cullinane EM, Sady SP, et al. Modest changes in high-density lipoprotein concentration and metabolism with prolonged exercise training. *Circulation.* 1988;78:25.
25. Wood PD, Haskell WL. The effect of exercise on plasma high density lipoproteins. *Lipids.* 1979;14:417.
26. Frey MAB, Doerr BM, Srivastava LS, et al. Exercise training, sex hormones, and lipoprotein relationships in men. *J Appl Physiol.* 1983;54:757.
27. Brownell, KD, Bachorik PS, Ayerle RS. Changes in plasma lipid and lipoprotein levels in men and women after a program of moderate exercise. *Circulation.* 1982;65:477.
28. Moore CE, Hartung H, Mitchell RE, et al. The relationship of exercise and diet on high-density lipoprotein cholesterol levels in women. *Metabolism.* 1983;32:189.
29. Levy RI, Rifkind BM. The structure, function and metabolism of high-density lipoproteins: a status report. *Circulation.* 1980;62 (suppl IV):IV-4.
30. Curfman GD, Thomas GS, Paffenbarger RS. Physical activity and primary prevention of cardiovascular disease. *Cardiol Clin.* 1985;3:203.
31. Sady SP, Cullinane EM, Saritelli A, et al. Elevated high density lipoprotein cholesterol in endurance athletes is related to enhanced plasma triglyceride clearance. *Metabolism.* 1988;37:568.
32. Kris-Etherton PM. The effect of exercise on lipid and lipoprotein metabolism. *Am Chem Soc Symp Series.* 1986;294:59.
33. McCunney RJ. Fitness, heart disease, and high-density lipoproteins: a look at the relationships. *Phys Sports Med.* 1987;15:67.
34. McArdle WD, Katch FI, Katch VL. *Exercise Physiology: Energy, Nutrition, and Human Performance.* Philadelphia, Pa: Lea & Febiger; 1986.
35. Rauramaa R. Relationship of physical activity, glucose tolerance, and weight management. *Prev Med.* 1984;13:37.
36. Leon AS. The diabetic patient and athletic performance. In: Haskell W, Scala J, Whitman J, eds. *Nutrition and Athletic Performance.* Palo Alto, Calif: Bull Publishing Co; 1982.
37. Seals DR, Hagberg JM, Hurley et al. Effects of endurance training on glucose tolerance and plasma lipid levels in older men and women. *JAMA.* 1984;252:645.
38. Vranic M, Berger M. Exercise and diabetes mellitus. *Diabetes.* 1979;28:147.
39. Zinman B, Vranic M. Diabetes and exercise. *Med Clin North Am.* 1985;69:145.
40. Duncan JJ, Farr JE, Upton SJ, et al. The effects of aerobic exercise on plasma catecholamines and blood pressure in patients with mild essential hypertension. *JAMA.* 1985;254:2609.
41. Fox EL, Mathews DK. *The Physiological Basis of Physical Education and Athletics.* 3rd ed. Philadelphia, Pa: Saunders College Publishing; 1981.

42. Froelicher VF. Exercise and the heart. *Cardiol Clin.* 1978;9:13.
43. Wilson PK, Fardy PS, Froelicher VF. *Cardiac Rehabilitation, Adult Fitness, and Exercise Testing.* Philadelphia, Pa: Lea & Febiger; 1981.
44. American College of Sports Medicine. *Guidelines for Exercise Testing and Prescription.* 3rd ed. Philadelphia, Pa: Lea & Febiger; 1986.
45. McMahan M, Palmer RM. Exercise and hypertension. *Med Clin North Am.* 1985;69:57.
46. Roman O, Camuzz AL, Villalon E, et al. Physical training program in arterial hypertension: a long term prospective follow-up. *Cardiology.* 1981;67:230.
47. Seals DR, Hagberg JM. The effect of exercise training on human hypertension: a review. *Med Sci Sports Exer.* 1984;16:207.
48. American Heart Association Committee on Exercise. *Exercise Testing and Training of Apparently Healthy Individuals: A Handbook for Physicians.* New York, NY: American Heart Association; 1972.
49. *The Y's Way to Physical Fitness.* Revised. Rosemont, Ill: YMCA of the USA; 1982.
50. Paffenbarger RS, Hyde RT, Wing AL, et al. Physical activity, all-cause mortality, and longevity of college alumni. *N Engl J Med.* 1968;314:605.
51. Pollock ML, Gettman LR, Milesis CA. Effects of frequency and duration of training on attrition and incidence of injury. *Med Sci Sports Exer.* 1979;9:31.
52. Franklin BA, Hellerstein HK, Gordon S, et al. Exercise prescription for the myocardial infarction patient. *J Cardiopulmonary Rehab.* 1986;6:62.
53. American Heart Association. *Exercise Testing and Training of Individuals with Heart Disease or at High Risk for its Development: A Handbook for Physicians.* American Heart Association; 1975.
54. Dec GW, Curfman GD. Exercise testing in cardiac rehabilitation. *Cardiol Clin.* 1985;3:223.
55. Ellestad MH. *Stress Testing: Principals and Practice.* 2nd ed. Philadelphia, Pa: Davis Co; 1980.
56. Borg GV. Subjective effort in relation to physical performance and working capacity. In: Pick HL, ed. *Psychology: From Research to Practice.* New York, NY: Plenum Publishing Co; 1978.
57. American College of Sports Medicine. *Guidelines for Graded Exercise Testing and Exercise Prescription.* 3rd ed. Philadelphia, Pa: Lea & Febiger; 1986.
58. Stone PH. Exercise testing in perspective. *Cardiac Rehab.* 1980;11:1.
59. Astrand P, Rodahl K. *Textbook of Work Physiology.* New York, NY: McGraw-Hill Book Co; 1977.
60. Franklin B, Wisley D, et al. Chronic adaptations to physical conditioning in cardiac trainability. *Clin Sports Med.* 1984;3:471.
61. Hellerstein HK, Franklin BA. Exercise testing and prescription. In: Wenger NK, Hellerstein HK, eds. *Rehabilitation of the Coronary Patient.* 2nd ed. New York, NY: John Wiley & Sons; 1984.
62. Dimsdale JE, Hartley H, Guiney T, et al. Post exercise peril: plasma catecholamines and exercise. *JAMA.* 1984;251:630.
63. Franklin BA. Motivating and educating adults to exercise. *J Phys Educ Recreation.* 1978;49:13.
64. Pollock ML, Peis AE. Exercise prescription for the cardiac patient. In: Franklin BA, Rubenfire M, eds. *Cardiac Rehabilitation.* Philadelphia, Pa: WB Saunders Co; 1984.
65. Pollock ML, Gettman LR, Milesis CA, et al. Effects of frequency and duration of training on attrition and incidence of injury. *Med Sci Sports Exer.* 1977;9:31.
66. Franklin B, Hodgson J, Buskirk ER. Relationship between percent maximal oxygen uptake and percent maximum heart rate in females. *Res Quar Exer Sports.* 1980;51:616.
67. Pratt CM, Welton DE, et al. Demonstration of training effect during chronic beta and adrenergic blockade in patients with coronary artery disease. *Circulation.* 1981;64:1125.
68. Smodlaka V. Treadmills vs bicycle ergometers. *Phys Sports Med.* 1982;10:75.
69. Stuller J. Considering the stationary cycle. *Phys Sports Med.* 1985;13:161.
70. Humen D, Boughner D. Evaluation of commercially available heart rate monitors. *Can Med Assoc J.* 1984;131:585.
71. Petratis M, Williams F, Ryschon K, et al. Comparison of maximal and submaximal cardiovascular responses to rowing vs treadmill exercise in cardiac patients. *Med Sci Sports Exer.* 1986;18:S27.

72. Koszuta L. Can fitness be found at the top of the stairs? *Phys Sports Med.* 1987;15,165.
73. Durnin JVGA, Passmore R. *Energy, Work and Leisure.* London, England: Heinemann Educational Books; 1967.
74. Borg GV. Guidelines for exercise testing and prescription. *Med Sci Sports Exer.* 1982;14:377.

10. STRATEGIES FOR MODIFYING BEHAVIOR TO REDUCE CARDIAC RISK

THE IMPORTANCE AND CHALLENGE OF DIETARY BEHAVIOR CHANGE*

Dietary change is a treatment goal for a broad spectrum of chronic diseases. Changes in eating patterns are central to the reduction of cardiovascular risk in both treatment and preventive care situations. Furthermore, the provision of guidance, assistance, and counseling for dietary behavior change is the largest area of cardiovascular disease (CVD) prevention and treatment in which dietitians must assume leadership.

Dietary behavior changes are only truly effective in preventing cardiovascular disease and its complications when they are sustained over the long term. This presents challenges to patients and dietitians as well. In order to be effective in promoting patients' health, nutrition counselors need to understand both the principles of nutrition management and a variety of behavioral issues.

Several earlier chapters in this manual described the nutrient composition of cholesterol-lowering diets and offered suggestions for foods and ways of fitting them into patients' life styles, such as when shopping, cooking, and eating out. This chapter focuses not on the content of behavior-change advice, but on the context, concepts, and methods that can be used to help patients adopt the recommended eating patterns.

The technical expertise that dietitians possess can only make a difference in patients' health if it is communicated in a way that enhances patient motivation, skills, and problem-solving ability. For example, the dietitian may see a patient who is referred for counseling about a Step Two Diet because the Step One Diet did not achieve a desired cholesterol reduction. But if the ineffectiveness of previous diet therapy was due to the patient's inability to follow the diet, and not to a lack of physiological response, the more-restrictive Step Two Diet will probably not be successful, either. Thus, the dietitian must be able to evaluate factors related to the patient's behavior and to devise a practical method for overcoming barriers to behavior change.

Eating patterns are habitual life-style behaviors requiring long-term behavior change for successful reduction of cardiac risk. Dietary recommendations are often restrictive, they may be only one aspect of a complex medical regimen, and they may be incompatible with individual or family eating habits. Barriers such as food costs, access, time, effort, or skill necessary for preparation may further increase the likelihood of noncompliance with special diets.[1] For many, consistent and long-term adherence to a low-fat diet requires dramatic changes in shopping, meal-planning, cooking, and eating habits.[2]

In recent years, awareness and concern about problems associated with elevated blood cholesterol have rapidly gained momentum.[3,4] There is an increasing recognition that elevated plasma cholesterol is widespread and that hypercholesterolemia can be reduced through dietary change. Thus, it is necessary to develop individualized strategies for specific patients as well as general procedures intended to reach broader audiences. These strategies should include more affordable and usable counseling methods than those traditionally employed.

*By Karen Glanz

Adults with elevated plasma cholesterol levels are likely to be motivated to attempt eating-pattern changes primarily because of health concerns, rather than cosmetic or psychosocial factors.[5] Thus, for those who understand the health risks associated with elevated plasma lipid levels, the goals of patient nutrition education are primarily to build a useful knowledge base and enhance skills for adherence.[1]

This chapter has the following objectives:

1. To acquaint nutritionists with the practical constraints of nutrition counseling for CVD risk reduction and the various counseling models that are available
2. To present key concepts behind strategies for changing dietary behavior and maintaining behavior change to reduce CVD risk
3. To describe a practical model for brief dietary counseling
4. To delineate the counseling principles and techniques for comprehensive dietary counseling
5. To address the supporting role of written patient-education materials in encouraging dietary behavior change

Although the focus of this chapter is on promoting adoption of a low-fat, cholesterol-lowering diet, weight loss also promotes cholesterol-lowering for many overweight patients,[6] and adherence to low-fat eating patterns is compatible with safe weight-loss regimens. Since much of the research on facilitating patient eating-behavior change has been based on work with weight management, the body of knowledge about nutrition counseling has been heavily influenced by weight-management models. Chapter 8 on nutrition intervention for weight management provides additional detail on this topic.

NUTRITION COUNSELING: PRACTICAL CONSTRAINTS AND ALTERNATIVES*

A "traditional" model of nutrition counseling includes referral by a physician, a one-to-one counseling relationship between patient and dietitian, and repeated sessions over a period of time. This model, however, is not feasible for many patients. Application of guidelines for management of hyperlipidemia is likely to be based on the judgment of the physician, the preferences of the patient, and the context of the health care situation.[7] Many physicians do not follow aggressive treatment approaches for CVD risk reduction through diet,[4,8] although more say that they are doing so now than in the past.

Most outpatient medical practices do not employ dietitians on a regular basis. Inpatient nutrition consultations are limited by other medical needs, the length of the hospital stay, and, often, the inability to follow up after discharge.

Financial barriers to clinical management of dietary risks for CVD are also of great concern. The lack of reimbursement for outpatient nutrition education and the difficulty of obtaining insurance coverage for nonphysician health counselors' time present further challenges.[8] Furthermore, patients and physicians may not appreciate the need for return counseling visits when no medication prescription is involved.

Thus, it is essential to consider alternative models for patient nutrition counseling to reduce cardiac risk. Three basic models are: (1) brief individual counseling, (2) comprehensive individual counseling, and (3) group education, either brief or long-term. Combinations of group and individual counseling are also possible. Various models have been discussed previously.[9] This chapter emphasizes the availability of various options and encourages nutritionists to

*By Karen Glanz

consider development of systematic and structured methods that they can implement themselves or train other health professionals to use as part of a health care team.

In addition to considering various models of nutrition counseling in clinical settings, complementary educational efforts in community settings are becoming increasingly common. Dietitians can and should establish links with educational programs in food outlets (eg, supermarkets and restaurants) and other community and work settings. This can extend the reach of nutrition behavior-change efforts and improve the success of cardiac risk reduction.

THE PATIENT'S SITUATION: DIETARY CHANGE EXPERIENCE AND COEXISTING RISK FACTORS*

At the beginning of every patient encounter that focuses on dietary behavior change to reduce cardiac risk, two important factors in the patient's situation should be considered, regardless of the model for or length of counseling. These are prior dietary change experience and coexisting risk factors. These two factors can have a major impact on the patient's efforts to make dietary changes, and the dietitian will likely be much more effective if these are considered at the outset.

Many adults, particularly those with a history of overweight, have made one or more attempts to modify their eating patterns. In addition, many more have had some involvement in dietary change or therapeutic diets through a family member or close friend. Their personal efforts, involvement with others' dietary changes, and experience of success or failure set the stage for their motivation and confidence in the present situation.

At a minimum, the patient should be asked about past experiences, the nature of the change effort, and the level of success or experience with that effort (or efforts). A more detailed inquiry might include these questions:

- Have you ever thought about changing your diet to . . . ?
- Have you ever tried to change the way you eat . . . ?
- How did you do it? Did you seek outside help? What kind?
- How successful were you in making those changes . . . ?
- What problems did you encounter?
- What did you do to deal with those problems?
- What do you think you can do now to be successful at changing your eating patterns?

These questions, adapted from a brief clinical approach for smoking-cessation counseling,[10] allow both patient and dietitian to learn from and build on prior experiences. They focus on overcoming the stumbling blocks or barriers to change in a personal and relevant manner.

The existence of other risk factors may affect patient motivation and ability to change eating patterns in paradoxical ways. The other risk factors may make the need for change very compelling for the patient (for example, after coronary artery bypass surgery or a myocardial infarction). Alternatively, the patient may be overwhelmed by the many aspects of his or her life style that need modification. In the Multiple Risk Factor Intervention Trial (MRFIT), men with concurrent CVD risk factors (smoking and/or hypertension) were less successful at adhering to low-fat diets and reducing their lipids.[11]

*By Karen Glanz

The clinical judgment of both the dietitian and the physician and a patient's interest in attempting dietary change should be based on an understanding of the total risk-factor profile. One option is to postpone dietary change efforts until other changes have been accomplished (for example, smoking cessation). Another option is to emphasize only the changes that the patient feels will be easy to make (for example, eating more fish and poultry). A third approach is to focus on changing the patient's diet, but to deemphasize the reduction of other risks for the time being.

MODELS FOR CHANGING DIETARY BEHAVIOR*

Comprehensive models for nutrition education and counseling have been proposed by Mason et al[12] and Snetselaar,[5] who describe a cyclical sequence of assessment, treatment, and evaluation and monitoring. Also, the NHLBI has published a manual for nutrition counseling for CVD risk reduction.[9] Efforts to assist in modifying eating behavior have historically been eclectic, drawing on a variety of theories from psychology, education, sociology, communications, and anthropology.[1,5] This section highlights a few of the currently prominent models for changing dietary behavior.

Dietary behavior-change strategies have often been based on principles of behavior modification, using strategies that include goal setting, behavioral contracting, monitoring, and reinforcement.[8,13] More recently, social learning theory (SLT; also known as social cognitive theory) has provided a framework for organizing eating-behavior-change strategies. SLT includes behavior-change strategies and also addresses cognitive (knowledge and attitude), interpersonal, and environmental influences on the learning process.[14,15]

The basic components of *behavioral approaches* are (1) self-monitoring and analysis of behavior; (2) stimulus control, or external cues that set the occasion for eating high-fat foods; and (3) reinforcement of desired behaviors. These strategies have been widely used in weight-management programs and are a central component of comprehensive counseling for low-fat eating.

SLT provides a model in which interpersonal and environmental factors also receive attention. There may be real supports or barriers in family and work situations; using SLT, opportunities or constraints on dietary change can be addressed and modified.

The variable of *self-efficacy* from SLT appears to be useful as a basis for fostering behavior change.[15,16] Self-efficacy is defined as a person's estimate of his or her chances of success at mastering a given behavior; it is synonymous with "self-confidence" about performing a specific type of behavior. Behavioral and cognitive strategies such as setting small goals, monitoring, and self-reward can be used to increase self-efficacy and ultimately improve motivation to initiate or maintain behavior changes.

Researchers in the areas of substance abuse and smoking cessation have developed a model of *stages of change* that may be fruitful to apply in nutrition-behavior change and especially in brief counseling situations. This model suggests that people are in various locations along a continuum of change-proneness: precontemplation (unaware, not interested in change); contemplation (thinking about changing); decision (becoming determined to change); action (actively modifying habits and/or environment); and maintenance (maintaining the new, healthier habits).[17,18] People are not considered always to move through the stages in a straight line, but rather to recycle often and repeat. The

*By Karen Glanz

stages-of-change model has a unique implication for the definition of success in health counseling: It suggests that movement through the stages is a mark of success, and not merely the endpoints of behavior change and maintenance. If we consider the possibility that people might attempt to change several times before thay make "permanent" changes, this model permits a wider range of outcomes to be seen as successes.

A final model for dietary behavior change strategies is called *relapse prevention*. It comes from the field of cognitive behavior modification and is consistent with Bandura's cognitive social learning theory.[15] Relapse prevention is a generic term that refers to a wide range of strategies designed to prevent a return to former habits, and it was developed mainly in the area of addictive behaviors.[19] Its primary focus is the maintenance of the habit-change process through self-management or self-control procedures. Relapse prevention encourages client or patient decision making and provides a framework for skills to help strengthen a person's commitment and ability to continue new habits. Three major techniques for improving self-management using relapse prevention training are: (1) acquiring adaptive coping skills, or ways to deal with stressful and challenging situations; (2) fostering new cognitions (attitudes, attributions) concerning the nature of habit change and one's ability to control the habits; and (3) developing a daily life style that includes positive and constructive self-care habits that help continue desirable behaviors.[19]

There is great potential for applying these behavior-change models to dietary behavior change to reduce cardiac risk. Behavior-change research in areas such as smoking cessation and weight management offers precedents that can be adapted to nutrition counseling. For example, self-management guides based on the stages-of-change model have been developed for smoking cessation.[20] A series of studies of self-help smoking cessation provides promising evidence that behavior change can be facilitated with a minimum of face-to-face professional contact.[21] There are major public health benefits from training programs on counseling techniques for physicians[10]—making it possible to reach smokers who would be unlikely to participate in more intensive interventions.

An important caveat in applying these models is in order. Dietary change for cardiovascular risk reduction involves qualitative dietary change for reducing an identifiable health risk, which, by itself, does not share the cosmetic or addictive properties of changes in body weight or smoking. There may be less reason to pay attention to intrapsychic factors in low-fat diet counseling (eg, emotional eating, self-esteem, stress as a trigger) than for behaviors involved in weight control or smoking cessation. There may be a larger knowledge or informational component to be concerned about; this issue will be addressed later in relation to written educational materials. However, coexisting risk factors may bring the psychodynamic issues back to the forefront. So the dietitian must recognize the possible range of individual factors involved in individual patients' attempts to modify their eating practices to reduce cardiac risk.

The following sections will focus on how the models described here can be applied in various nutrition counseling and education strategies for reducing cardiac risk.

BRIEF DIETARY COUNSELING*

Brief dietary counseling is the best technique when either patient or staff time is limited, when it is possible that the patient will not return for more in-depth counseling, or as a first step toward comprehensive counseling. It can be implemented by trained health professionals other than dietitians, but ideally a dietitian will train and collaborate with the other professionals (eg, physician, nurse, health educator).

Brief dietary counseling includes four major components: assessment of risks, assessment of readiness to change behavior, motivation or action planning, and follow-up. One unique feature of this approach is that it does not imply an assumption that all patients are equally motivated, ready, or interested in attempting dietary changes. Thus, through a decision-tree approach, the counselor makes a triage assignment to help move the patient to begin to change immediately.

Assessment of risks. Before meeting with the patient/client, the dietitian reviews his or her risk indicators, including concurrent risk factors, family history, lipid profile, and eating-pattern assessment, and positive dietary habits (to the extent that information about these is available). This provides a starting point for the counselor, who can emphasize the need for change or anticipate the multiple problems facing the patient (eg, the need to stop smoking as well as the need to reduce dietary fat). A brief discussion of the risks with the patient or verification that he or she understands the health problems establishes an initial contact.

Assessment of readiness to change behavior. After explaining to the patient that a lower-fat or cholesterol-lowering diet will reduce his or her cardiac risk, the counselor asks if the patient is interested in attempting change at this time. (In other words, is he or she at the contemplation or decision stage?) This can be asked simply: "Are you interested in developing a cholesterol-lowering, or low-fat, eating pattern at this time?" If the patient says yes or maybe, the counselor proceeds to an assessment of past dietary change experience, barriers counseling, and action planning. If the patient says no, the counselor moves quickly to the motivation phase and follows up at a later date.

Motivating the precontemplator. Motivation includes two basic elements: personalizing the benefits of change and increasing awareness and opportunities for thinking about change efforts. A key approach is to emphasize the benefits of dietary change, rather than to stress the risks of not changing. To increase awareness, available sources of information can be suggested, and everyday opportunities for trying small changes can be pointed out (for example, trying frozen yogurt next time the urge for ice cream strikes). Patients should be encouraged to think about when (not whether) they will be willing to try some dietary changes. Follow-up can be a phone call or raising the possibility of change at the next medical visit.

Assessment of past dietary change experience. If the patient is definitely or possibly interested in changing his or her eating pattern, motivation involves assessment of past dietary change experience and barriers counseling. First the counselor should ask about previous efforts to make dietary changes. The nature of the changes, whether outside help was sought, and the success or problems with change provide important information for the next step, barriers counseling.

*By Karen Glanz

Barriers counseling. A discussion of the most important obstacles or barriers that the patient thinks will stand in the way of adopting a low-fat eating pattern is useful in anticipating and dealing with problem situations. The counselor can be prepared with suggestions and ways to overcome the most common barriers (*Table 10.1*). Unique individual barriers can also be discussed and the counselor can help the patient problem-solve and develop his or her own solutions.

Table 10.1
Barriers Counseling

1. *I like the foods I eat now; I would have to give up my favorite foods.*
2. *I don't know how to fit low-fat foods into the way I eat.*
   - Even though adopting a low-fat eating pattern means making changes in how you eat, you don't have to *give up* the foods you like. You might have to cut down on the foods you like or plan for those choices, though.
   - Small, gradual changes are the key.
   - Often you can eat the same *type* of foods by only having to change the way the food is prepared or the portion size.
3. *I don't know which foods I can eat on a low-fat diet; there are too many things to remember.*
   - It seems complicated at first, but once you learn some basic ideas and begin to pay attention to what you eat, choosing foods will get easier.
   - Some of the guides, books, manuals you can read or classes you can attend will include convenient wallet-size reminder cards; the tipsheet from our office should be helpful also.
   - Learning to read labels can go a long way in helping you choose low-fat foods.
4. *I'm too rushed; it's too much work to buy or fix low-fat foods.*
5. *I eat out a lot.*
   - It's easy to learn ways to cook low-fat foods without too much work; once you pick out some low-fat foods that are your favorites, you will find it even easier.
   - Often you can partially prepare foods in advance and save time in the long run.
   - Some of the foods need *less* preparation; for example, fresh fruit and those that do not need heavy sauces or frying.
   - Once you learn some basic ideas and tips you will find it easy to choose low-fat foods when eating out.
6. *Someone else buys and prepares my food.*
   - In that case, you will want to have that person work with you as you try to develop a low-fat eating plan.
7. *I enjoy having a drink with my friends.*
8. *I drink when I feel anxious.*
   - If you usually have more than two drinks (or the equivalent) at one occasion, try drinking nonalcoholic beverages (juice, mineral water, soda) instead of alcohol some of the time.
   - If "binge" drinking, even periodic, is present, consider referral for counseling.

Action planning. During this phase of brief counseling, a few suggestions for beginning to make dietary change are given. The counselor should recommend suitable intervention modalities for the patient, such as written educational materials, comprehensive individual counseling, group education, or a combination. Set at least one specific patient goal and specify a referral, if appropriate at this time. The goal and referral should be written down—not only on the patient's chart, but also on a card or sheet of paper that the patient will take home.

Follow-up. It is helpful to advise the patient that you will follow up on this discussion with either a phone call or a later medical visit. This follow-up should be routine and should involve reinforcement and encouragement, as well as counseling if unanticipated difficulties arise as the patient tries to make changes.

Figure 10.1 summarizes the sequence, flow, and decision points for brief dietary counseling. This example can be adapted to fit specific nutrition-education settings and patient populations.

Fig. 10.1
Brief dietary counseling for low-fat eating.

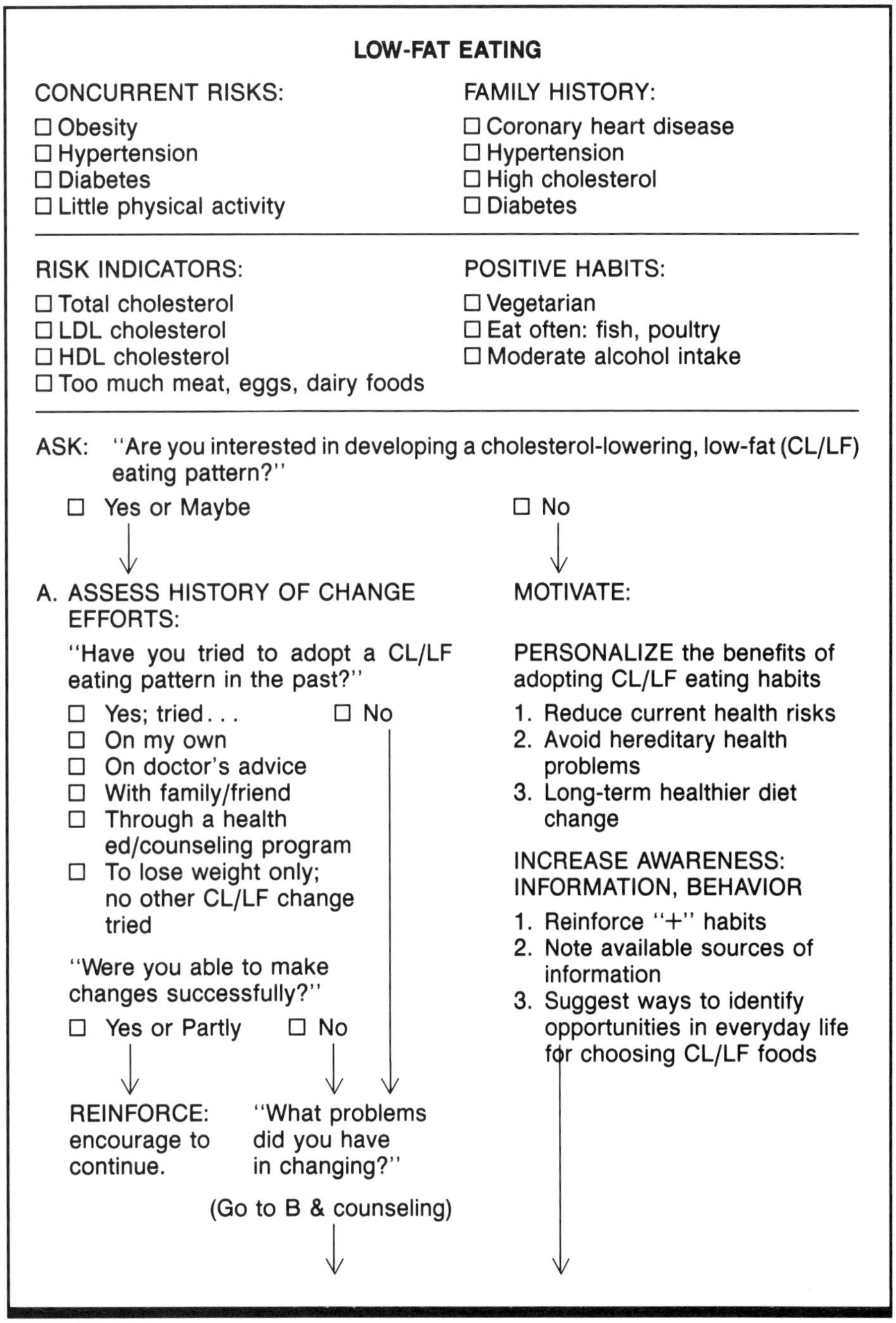

Fig. 10.1
Brief dietary counseling for low-fat eating—(Cont.)

B. ASSESS OBSTACLES TO ADOPTING A CL/LF EATING PATTERN:

- ☐ 1. I like the foods I eat now; I would have to give up favorites.
- ☐ 2. I don't know how to fit CL/LF foods into the way I eat.
- ☐ 3. I don't know which foods I can eat on a CL/LF diet. There are too many things to remember.
- ☐ 4. I'm too rushed; it's too much work to buy or fix CL/LF foods.
- ☐ 5. I eat out a lot.
- ☐ 6. Someone else buys and prepares my food.
- ☐ 7. I enjoy drinking with my friends.
- ☐ 8. I drink when I feel anxious.

FOLLOW-UP

If not motivated to change, check on motivation at next visit or call.

↓

COUNSEL PATIENT ON BARRIERS

CONSIDER SUITABLE INTERVENTION MODALITY/MODALITIES

↓

C. SUGGEST A SPECIFIC APPROACH TO CHANGE

Advise the person to attempt changes gradually; each change will help.
Suggest signing up for a class, reading, or meeting with a nutritionist for individualized counseling.

Suggest keeping track of eating patterns most closely related to CL/LF eating pattern: meat, dairy, eggs, poultry, fish, alcohol, etc.

Reinforce positive habits.
Encourage the person to discuss with family and friends the changes he or she is trying to make.
Remind the person that he or she can learn *easy* ways to adopt CL/LF eating patterns.

GIVE OUT WRITTEN EDUCATIONAL MATERIAL

↓

D. FOLLOW-UP

Check on change at next visit or call.
Reinforce/encourage and counsel if problems arise.

PRINCIPLES AND METHODS OF COMPREHENSIVE NUTRITION COUNSELING*

Comprehensive nutrition counseling involves a cyclical process of assessment, treatment, and evaluation.[1,5] It reflects a continuum of approaches ranging from a single, "full-length" encounter of 30 to 45 minutes to regular and repeated individual sessions over a period of six months or more. The goals of comprehensive nutrition counseling are to work with the client/patient to set goals, solve problems, and take action to make dietary changes that reduce cardiovascular risk. The process is ideally one in which responsibility is shared and the patient is an active participant; eventually the patient adopts and maintains new behavior patterns so that treatment is no longer needed.[22,23]

Counseling relationships. The core of comprehensive counseling is in the "therapeutic alliance," a relationship between the patient/client and counselor that is based on liking, respect, and trust and is conducive to positive client change.[22] Several qualities of the counselor, or helper, are important: expertness, credibility, empathy, warmth, self-disclosure, and a compatible match with the client.[22] The progression from relationship enhancement to client change is summarized in *Table 10.2.*

Table 10.2
Counseling Relationships to Enhance Client Change

Relationship Enhancers	→	**Relationship Components**	→	**Relationship Consequences**	→	**Outcome**
Client structuring						
Client imitation						
Client conformity		Liking		Communication		
Helper expertness						
Helper credibility						
Helper empathy		Respect		Openness		Client Change
Helper warmth						
Helper self-disclosure						
Helper-client matching		Trust		Persuasibility		
Helper-client physical closeness and posture						

Adapted with permission from Kanfer FH, Goldstein AP. *Helping People Change: A Textbook of Methods.* 3rd ed. ©1986, Pergamon Press PLC.

Counseling methods. A wide variety of methods is available to help people change—the past two decades have brought rapid development in the research and conceptual base of behavior-change methods.[22] The most prominent conceptual models were described earlier in the chapter; here, they are described in terms of action techniques for comprehensive nutrition counseling.

Figure 10.2 presents the cyclical counseling process and its context for the nutrition counselor. Kanfer and Schefft[23] have described the seven phases of counseling: relationship development, developing commitment for change, behavioral analysis, treatment decisions, treatment implementation, monitoring, and maintenance and termination (*Table 10.3*).

*By Karen Glanz

Fig. 10.2
Model for nutrition counseling. Reprinted from* Nutrition Counseling Skills: Assessment, Treatment, and Evaluation, *2nd ed, by L.G. Snetselaar, p 19, with permission of Aspen Publishers, Inc, © 1989.

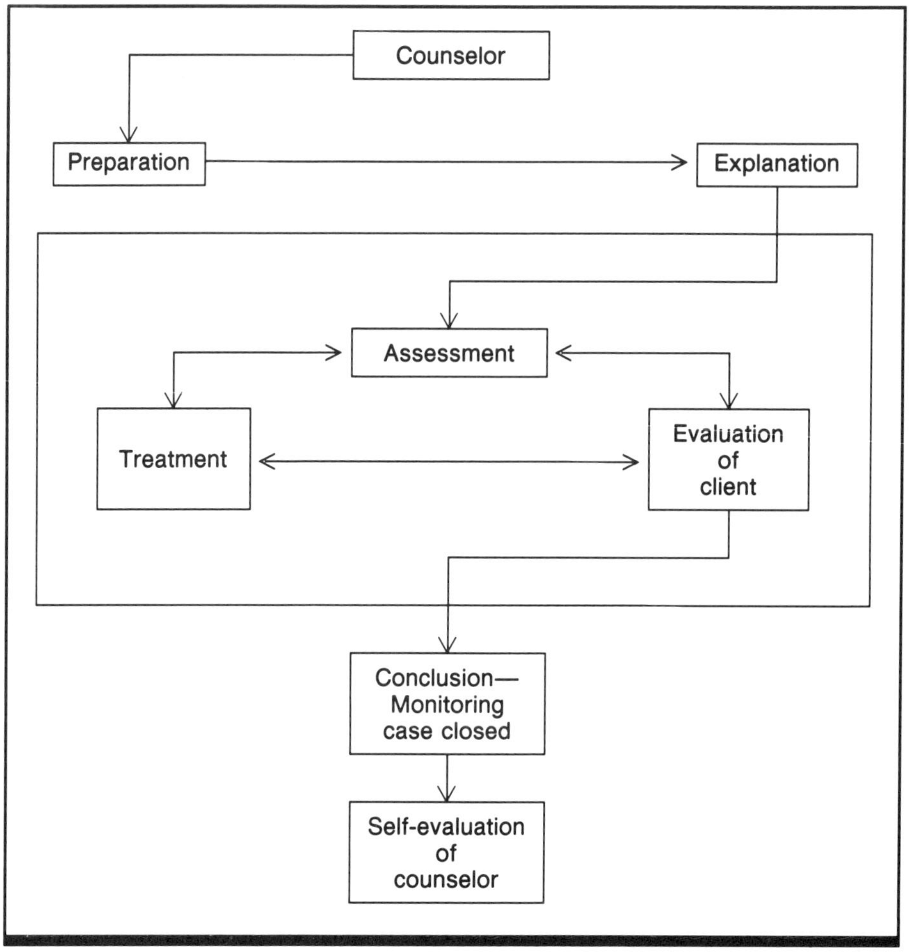

Table 10.3
Seven Phases of Counseling

1. Role structuring and creating a therapeutic alliance
2. Developing a commitment for change
3. Behavioral analysis
4. Negotiating treatment objectives and methods
5. Implementing treatment and maintaining motivation
6. Monitoring and evaluating progress
7. Maintenance, generalization, and termination of treatment

Adapted from Kanfer FH, Schefft BK. *Guiding the Process of Therapeutic Change.* Champaign, Ill: Research Press; 1988.

These phases of counseling encompass the intervention strategies of behavior modification and social learning theory in that they include attention not only to behavior per se but to interpersonal processes as well. *Analysis of behavior* usually involves eating-pattern assessment, often in the form of a food diary. This aids the understanding of eating patterns and relevant situational triggers. *Goal setting* occurs next, often with small, achievable goals at first. *Behavioral contracting* is a frequently used formal method of setting goals and making a commitment for change. Rewards can be planned as *reinforcements* for reaching goals. Most patients find that long-term change is best achieved through gradual, stepwise goal attainment rather than by attempting major changes all at once.

Throughout, the mutuality of the counseling relationship plays an important role. Social learning theory suggests considering the *totality of the client's food environment* as an adjunct to the client-counselor relationship. This means that interpersonal relationships, family, work, and community are viewed as important to adherence to a low-fat dietary regimen and are viewed as potential foci of goals and participants in rewarding behavior change.

A number of counselor actions can increase the chances of the client's commitment to change and his or her acceptance of ultimate responsibility for maintaining long-term behavior modification. These actions include focusing on the client, fostering commitment, and developing an effective working relationship.[23] *Table 10.4* summarizes the actions and the "think rules" that increase counseling effectiveness.

Table 10.4
Counselor's Action Checklist and Think Rules

1. Remember the principle of *least intervention* when planning treatment.
2. Give the *client's goals* priority in treatment, if possible.
3. Assist the client from the first session onward in gradually assuming responsibility for treatment.
4. Focus on developing a working relationship so that the client returns for later sessions.
5. From the first session onward, get the client's commitment to some small between-session tasks to increase involvement in treatment and help establish a participative relationship.
6. Use the *think rules* for yourself and for the client to promote problem solving and motivation:

   Think behavior—Assist the client to redefine problems in terms of behaviors.

   Think solution—Get the client to ask continuously, "What is the least I can do to improve the situation?"

   Think positive—Have the client identify personal strengths and positive aspects of any event or effort to change.

   Think small steps—Set limited goals to enhance the possibility of success and permit continuing reappraisal.

   Think flexible—Help the client to develop alternatives and back-up plans and to be prepared for the unexpected.

   Think future—Focus on the future and encourage rehearsal and planning.

From *Guiding the Process of Therapeutic Change* (p 122) by F.H. Kanfer and B.K. Schefft, 1988, Champaign, Ill: Research Press. Copyright 1988 by the authors. Adapted by permission.

Group and family counseling methods. Many of the counseling methods described here can be adapted for use with groups and families. Group education can also include one or more individual sessions to set and monitor personal goals. Family-education and group programs may enhance the social support, both emotional and practical, for putting dietary changes into action. One example of a multimethod group education/counseling program is the Family Heart Study, which includes group sessions, cooking demonstrations, family involvement, and group decision methods to overcome barriers to adherence. It also mobilizes group support by encouraging changes in group norms for dietary changes.[24]

MAINTAINING BEHAVIOR CHANGE*

Initial behavior change is only the first step in achieving cardiovascular risk reduction through diet. Maintaining behavior change is crucial to improved health. A major challenge in promoting long-term adherence to low-fat, low-cholesterol eating patterns involves methods to prevent relapse to former eating habits.[2]

We cannot realistically expect long-term behavior changes with short-term programs of finite length. It has been found repeatedly that when an intervention is not sustained, improved eating habits and reduced lipid levels do not persist.[1] Use of self-management techniques such as those included in relapse-prevention training and periodic reinforcement from counselors (by telephone or in person) are the most promising methods for enhancing behavior-change maintenance. The use of support groups and related strategies like buddy systems are additional ways to extend the supportive aspect of counseling beyond the formal treatment period.

Self-management techniques to prevent relapse can be built in to the end of counseling programs or used in postcounseling "booster sessions." These might include teaching behavioral rehearsal, "self-talk" for coping with minor slips, and practicing skills for coping with difficult or challenging eating situations.[19]

Just as there are organizational and situational barriers to comprehensive counseling, there are often administrative and financial obstacles to implementing maintenance strategies. It is worth the effort to devise methods to overcome these barriers, because nutrition counseling and dietary behavior change will only yield long-term health benefits when they are sustained. Individual nutritionists may need to enlist the aid of other health professionals to propose and establish creative strategies for maintenance that work in their health care settings.

WRITTEN PATIENT-EDUCATION MATERIALS*

An important part of cholesterol-reduction education involves designing methods of presenting information that can be understood and used in day-to-day food choices. Even the best oral communication to a patient can result in misunderstandings and memory failures over time.[25] Thus, written cholesterol-education materials are important for education and counseling for changing dietary behavior. Since these are the aids to self-management that patients take with them when counseling ends, the nutrition educator must pay attention to their development and selection.

It is essential that educational materials be accessible and understandable to the clients for whom they are intended. In nutrition education, however, concern about the technical accuracy of the content often takes priority over readability and understandability.[26] Educational materials may be written at a level that is too sophisticated in terms of wording and concepts. A recent analysis of readability levels of 38 publicly available, print materials for cholesterol education revealed that the average reading level was close to grade 11, which is too difficult for many adults.[27]

Nutrition counselors should become familiar with their patients' average reading levels and should evaluate written education materials with them in

*By Karen Glanz

mind. If new materials are developed, they should be pretested with a population that is similar to the patients who will receive them. The counselor can even go through, mark, and "translate" some difficult words so the patient will not find them confusing once he or she brings the material home.

IMPLEMENTING THE NUTRITION CARE PLAN*

Important considerations in the development of a successful nutrition care plan are listed below. The dietitian should:

1. Prioritize problems.
2. Set realistic and measurable short- and long-term goals that are negotiated with the client. Consider the client's personal goals, perhaps implementing a staged approach consisting of small steps. Work with one goal at a time. When appropriate, allow clients to change behavior at a self-guided pace.
3. Write action plans for each goal. The client should learn skills to manage appropriate nutrition behavior.
4. Identify appropriate resource materials for each action plan if appropriate.
5. Identify an evaluation strategy for each goal to assess whether it has been achieved. Provide frequent feedback.
6. Consider alternative strategies when a goal has not been met.
7. Set time lines.
8. Be flexible.
9. Plan a long-term follow-up and maintenance program.
10. At all stages have the client actively involved in the development, implementation, evaluation, and revision of the nutrition care plan. Change is more likely to be permanent when clients are actively involved.
11. Facilitate social support.

Implicit to the development of a successful nutrition care plan is one that is individualized to each client. It is also important that the clients assume responsibility for the nutrition care plan so they can take credit for the success they achieve. Clients then accept responsibility for the outcome of the nutrition care plan.

During the implementation of the nutrition care plan, dietitians are encouraged to use the following techniques selectively to keep the client both motivated and actively involved in the intervention program.

1. Have the client write a contract.
2. List the long-term risks of maintaining the present behavior.
3. List the outcomes from changing the behavior.
4. Discuss the importance of the expected outcomes.
5. Use a reward system, eg, money or prizes.
6. Discuss previous strategies that have been successful.
7. Encourage the client to discuss change with significant others or with others who have made the changes.

Other strategies can be employed to elicit behavior change and maintain a high level of patient motivation and involvement:

Have clients periodically keep food records. This makes them aware of their eating habits and helps monitor progress. Instruct clients to include information on when food was eaten, the associated activity, their mood while eating, where and with whom the food was eaten, and so on. Self-monitoring will not only provide feedback on progress but will also help identify problems and strategies for dealing with them.

*By Anastasia Snelling

Encourage positive thinking. The nutrition educator should encourage clients to speak in positive terms about their nutrition care–related accomplishments. This approach nurtures the idea that clients believe they can achieve their objectives.

Have clients work toward environmental control. Controlling the environment may mean adopting one or more of the following strategies:
1. Place allowable foods in view while making other foods inaccessible.
2. Repackage foods in different containers.
3. Serve food from the stove or store leftovers before starting the meal.
4. Allow others to prepare their own meals, desserts, and snacks.
5. Eat in a designated space.
6. Shop from a list.
7. Choose restaurants that serve appropriate food choices.
8. List alternate activities that can be done during unstructured time.

Recommend support groups to your clients. Support groups are one of the most influential techniques used in changing behavior. Such groups encourage individuals to work together, intensifying efforts that lead to behavior change. Participants share concerns, problems, solutions, and the knowledge that they are not alone.

Create new scenarios. The dietitian and client should work together in developing options when changing behavior. The client then chooses the option that is best suited to him or her. This reinforces the concept of "ownership" of the nutrition care plan.

MODIFICATION OF SMOKING BEHAVIOR*

Since many people who start smoking continue the habit for a lifetime, the emphasis should be on prevention. Only about one fourth of those who become habituated to smoking quit, even though most want to quit. At the present time, it is not possible to predict who will become habituated.

Most of the techniques employed at the prevention stage (*Table 10.5*) have a social or political emphasis because these are, indeed, the influential factors.

Cessation

Smoking cessation is a top priority for coronary heart disease (CHD) risk reduction.[28] People who participate in a smoking-cessation program often have been unsuccessful in their attempts to quit. Approximately 95% of the ex-smokers in the United States quit smoking without the aid of a formal cessation program.[29] Thus, people who enter a smoking-cessation program represent a special challenge for achieving success. Techniques and strategies that have been successful are discussed below.

Smoking cessation requires behavior modification. The focus of this section is on those techniques in conjunction with cognitive methods. Using the cognitive approach, the smokers identify why they started to smoke, why they continued, what is pleasurable and distasteful about the habit, and why they want and do not want to stop. This is accomplished through group discussions and making lists.[30]

*By Donna Payne

Table 10.5
Techniques for Prevention of Smoking Onset and/or Habituation

Short videotapes:	Emphasizing short- and long-term benefits of not smoking
	Explaining peer pressure and its influence on smoking behavior
	Using relevant peer role models
Health professionals setting examples by not smoking	
Restriction of smoking in all enclosed public places to ensure the rights of nonsmokers	
Increased social pressure against smoking	
Restriction of tobacco advertising and prohibiting those that glamorize smoking	
Use of mass media to convey antismoking messages	
Increase taxes on cigarettes to raise cost of smoking	
Discontinue government support of tobacco industry	
Make cigarette purchase difficult for children	

Adapted with permission from Aronow WS, Kaplan NM. Smoking. In: Kaplan NM, Stamler JS, eds. *Prevention of Coronary Heart Disease—Practical Management of the Risk Factors.* Philadelphia, Pa: WB Saunders Co; 1983.

The behavior-modification approach requires that the participant keep a daily record of smoking with regard to all or some of the following: time, place, mode, what was being done and with whom, and the level of need or craving for smoking (usually rated on a number scale). A discussion follows that focuses on the behavioral patterns illustrated in the record and how the participant can begin to change by substituting a response that does not include smoking. The new response may be oriented more toward problem solving or toward disruption of the habit sequence.

The participant must learn to recognize and control three factors through practice and repetition: the stimuli or cues that trigger the behavior; the response, which is smoking; and the reinforcement or consequences of this behavioral response. Some specific behavioral techniques used to aid smoking cessation appear in *Table 10.6.*

The focus is on changing the stimulus-response-reinforcement pattern. Generally, the objective is a gradual reduction in the number of cigarettes smoked and a targeted quit date during the program.[31]

The leader should praise and reinforce positive achievements; negative behavior or failure should not be emphasized. Instead, strategies for dealing with negative behavior should be discussed.

During the new ex-smoker phase, it is important that participants have one or more accessible persons for support. Follow-up should be conducted at 3, 6, 12, 18, and 24 months. On questionnaires used to assess success at smoking cessation, the response ratio should not be less than 80%.

Table 10.6
Behavioral Techniques for Aiding Smoking Cessation

1. Change brands.
2. Keep a daily smoking record attached to cigarette package.
3. Use a large jar to collect cigarette butts.
4. Buy one pack of cigarettes at a time.
5. Scatter antismoking literature around the house.
6. Do not carry matches or a lighter.
7. Change the hand used for smoking.
8. Put the cigarette down between puffs.
9. Keep a daily progress chart or graph.
10. Keep a piggy bank for money saved by not buying cigarettes.
11. Have ashtrays, house, clothes, and teeth cleaned.
12. Throw out extra cigarettes.
13. Write a contract with a friend, professional, or group about decreasing or quitting smoking.
14. Do not smoke in certain places such as the car, office, and kitchen.
15. Gradually eliminate cigarettes by starting with those that have the lowest rating for craving.
16. Try relaxation and mental imagery, either positive or negative.

Adapted with permission from Eliot RS, Bond MB, Brandenbert RO, et al. Bethesda Conference, task force 3: the physician in the work setting. *Am J Cardiol.* 1981;47:751.

Caution is necessary for the person with CHD who has become habituated to smoking, because some of the techniques commonly employed are not acceptable even though they may aid in the actual cessation of smoking. For example, the rapid-smoking technique, which produces nausea, is effective for some smokers, but it should not be used with people with CHD because it can cause tachycardia and electrocardiographic changes. Snuff and nicotine chewing gum have been shown to be effective for smoking cessation, but they still provide nicotine. In addition, snuff increases risk of cancer of the oropharynx. Lobeline does not appear to be effective. Of the methods listed in *Table 10.7*, "cold turkey" (quitting smoking on a specified date) is considered the most effective.[32]

Table 10.7
Techniques for Aiding People Habituated to Smoking

1. May be useful for persons with CHD

Counseling sessions:	Individual
	Group, with spouses or significant others
Self-help programs and hypnosis	
Cold turkey	

2. Should not be used for persons with CHD

Other sources of nicotine:	Lobeline
	Nicotine chewing gum
	Snuff
Adverse conditioning:	Rapid smoking

Adapted with permission from Aronow WS, Kaplan NM. Smoking. In: Kaplan NM, Stamler JS, eds. *Prevention of Coronary Heart Disease—Practical Management of the Risk Factors.* Philadelphia, Pa: WB Saunders Co; 1983.

Smokers who cannot quit. People who cannot quit should still be given advice to offset, at least partially, some of the effects of smoking. Techniques they may use include inhaling less, smoking less of each cigarette, taking fewer puffs from each cigarette, and taking the cigarette out of the mouth between puffs.[32] These people should know that filter cigarettes do not decrease risk of CHD, and they may actually increase CHD risk while decreasing the risk of lung cancer.

Maintenance. The majority of smokers resume smoking within a few months of termination. Thus, maintenance requires attention. Three maintenance strategies are described in *Table 10.8.*

General Considerations

A smoking-cessation program requires a minimum of six weeks, and reinforcement requires 6 to 12 months with emphasis on the first three months.

Table 10.8
Smoking Cessation Maintenance Strategies

Social support:	Group, individual
Coping skills:	Dealing with discomfort of depriving oneself, developing substitute responses, recognizing and modifying cues
Cognitive restructuring:	Dealing with attitude, self-perception, covert verbalization

Adapted by permission from Lichtenstein E. The smoking problem: a behavioral perspective. *J Con Clin Psy.* 1982;50:804. ©1982 by the American Psychological Association.

Smoking intervention programs should: provide specific information for the health consequences of smoking and skills helpful in coping (specifically what can be done); reinforce early changes in behavior; identify models in the community and long-term social reinforcements of the behavior; involve the family, not just the person participating in the health education program; formulate messages in ways that link the behavior change with self-respect; use schools and work sites; use specific media for certain audiences such as the television or radio for adolescents; and use the leadership of health professionals in the spirit of collaboration.[31] Smoking-intervention leaders can be self-trained* or have received outside training. Training requires reading, discussion, and practice.

The work site can be an especially useful setting for smoking intervention for several reasons[29,31]:

1. Most adult smokers can be reached in the workplace.
2. Among men who smoke, the problem is most significant among blue-collar workers who tend not to seek outside help even though their desire to stop smoking is similar to that of other smokers.

*Some self-training references are:

I Quit Kit. American Cancer Society; 1977.

Danaher BG, Lichtenstein E. *Become an Ex-Smoker.* Englewood Cliffs, NJ: Prentice-Hall; 1977.

Pomerleau DE, Pomerleau CS. *Break the Smoking Habit.* Champaign, Ill: Research Press, Inc; 1977.

Other training resources are available from agencies such as the American Cancer Society and the American Heart Association.

3. The incidence of smoking among women who work outside of the home is higher than among women who work in the home.
4. Smokers in certain occupations have an increased risk of CHD because of exposure to other hazardous substances.
5. The workplace provides an environment for long-term social reinforcement.
6. The workplace facilitates the development of social support systems through organizations such as labor unions, ethnic societies, and social organizations.

Some considerations for smoking-cessation programs include, among others: confidentiality of records and threats to job security; suspicion about the motivation of the employer or others; potential costs; and perceived threats to private practices.

MODIFICATION OF EXERCISE HABITS*

Strategies to promote adherence to an exercise prescription or program are also discussed in Chapter 9. Despite the positive effects of exercise, it has been reported that 40% to 60% of the patients in exercise rehabilitation programs drop out within 6 to 12 months.[30] Most of the dropout occurs early; 70% of the total dropout occurs within 2 to 5 months of a 12-month program.[33] Factors associated with a high level of adherence to an exercise program include high self-motivation, active spouse support for the exerciser's program, proximity to the exercise facility, and group-based exercise.[34]

Successful adherence to an exercise regimen has been demonstrated in group-based programs. One technique employs contracting for aerobic points.[35] Participants receive points for varying amounts of aerobic exercise. Monetary rewards, winning back personal items, and social reinforcement are exchanged for points.[34] Other successful strategies include using the buddy system, booster sessions and phone calls, flexible goal setting, and participation in games.[34] Any technique designed to increase compliance should also increase self-motivation, provide additional support systems, or reduce problems that interfere with the exercise program.[36]

Although motivating the patient to comply with the exercise program is often challenging, it is essential for long-term adherence. Factors that affect patient motivation are defined in the Porter-Lawler model (*Table 10.9*).

The Porter-Lawler model can be used throughout the cardiac rehabilitation process to increase motivation. When the patient first begins the program, the value and potential outcomes of the program should be discussed. The patient should be given exercise options. Role-perception acquisition can lead to goal setting and establishing contracts that are written commitments of the performance the client is expected to attain. It is the responsibility of the exercise specialist to reinforce that patient's behavior and to offer rewards as an incentive to compliance. Permanent changes in behavior occur gradually. Goals, both short- and long-term, must be attainable and realistic.

Patient motivation is perhaps the most important factor in successful behavior change. Together exercise leaders and patients must identify needs, negotiate goals, identify exercise opportunities and choices, evaluate the program or plan, and provide an adequate reward system to increase patient compliance.

*By Ann R. Semenske

Table 10.9
Porter-Lawler Model: Factors That Affect Patient Motivation

1. Value of reward: attractiveness of the outcome options of an exercise program available to the patient
2. Perceived effort reward probability: subjective determination by the patient that exercise effort will lead to some valued reward
3. Effort: how hard a patient works toward a goal or performance level
4. Abilities and traits: characteristics of the patient such as personality, physical and motor skills, and so forth
5. Role perceptions: a patient's interpretation of what constitutes successful performance, such as skill acquisition, distance jogged, and so forth
6. Performance: level of achievement that the patient attains
7. Rewards: intrinsic rewards meet higher-order needs such as self-esteem; that is, those that are internal in nature. Extrinsic rewards are those administered by an external source
8. Perceived equitable rewards: the level of award that the patient feels is appropriate based on his or her perception of effort and performance
9. Satisfaction: how the patient perceives what he or she considers to be an equitable reward, compared with the amount of actual reward

Reprinted with permission from Oldridge N, Stoedefalke K. Compliance and motivation in cardiac exercise programs. *Clin Sports Med.* 1984;3:443.

STRESS*

Stress is difficult to define. According to Glass,[37] stress includes certain events that are perceived as a threat, and it includes the coping processes that follow the perceived threat. A threat is the anticipation of future harm, whether physical or psychological.[37] Stress is the combination of a stressor and stress reactivity.

Three classes of psychological stressors have been studied as they relate to CHD: general dissatisfaction with various aspects of life; chronic or relatively long-term stressful life events; and acute stressful life events.[37]

A number of questionnaires and rating scales have been developed to measure a variety of stressful life events,[38] but the assignment of values weighted in terms of importance may be inappropriate when applied to an individual client.

Stress Intervention

The purposes of a stress-management program are: (1) to reduce the incidence of stress-related illnesses, perhaps in a particular setting (eg, the work site) through scientifically based stress-management techniques; and (2) to reduce self-destructive behavioral patterns that may lead to illness and interpersonal and other incompatibilities.

Types of Stress-Intervention Programs

Several types of common intervention programs are listed in *Table 10.10.* Cognitive reorganization is a restructuring of beliefs and attitudes. It involves

*By Donna Payne

the unlearning of unrewarding and self-defeating attitudes. This type of program is strongly associated with the learning curve for memory retention. Accomplishments must be reinforced through feedback and practiced until they significantly influence behavior.

Table 10.10
Types of Programs for Stress Management

1. Cognitive reorganization
2. Assertiveness training
3. Relaxation techniques
4. Time-management strategies
5. Modification of undesirable features of type A life style
6. Environmental restructuring

Adapted with permission from Jaffe DT, Scott CD, Orioli EM, et al. Stress management: programs and prospects. *Am J Health Promotion.* 1986;1:29.

Assertiveness training facilitates decision making and the expression of thoughts and feelings. Programs examine supervisor-supervisee relationships, coworker interactions, and group-participative activities and provide training in conflict-resolution skills and problem-solving strategies.

Relaxation techniques may use progressive muscle relaxation, meditative techniques, and biofeedback-assisted relaxation. Participants are encouraged to become aware of their levels of muscle tone in various situations and to develop countermeasures.

Time management can assist in analyzing and reorganizing current time expenditures. Environmental modification can be very difficult because there are many environmental stressors.[31]

Specific how-to information on stress-intervention techniques is not often addressed in terms of the defined structure of behavior-modification methodology. Even when behavior-modification techniques are presented, they are for modifying behaviors other than those related to stress.

Greenberg[39] suggests a number of practical how-to techniques and offers theoretical information (such as the psychophysiology of stress and stress-illness relationships) that is useful in modifying stress-related behaviors. Techniques that evoke a relaxation response may be helpful, at least for a short time.[32] To deal with stress, the daily practice of yoga and meditation techniques, particularly those that evoke the relaxation response, are recommended.[32] Relaxation techniques described by Greenberg include meditation, autogenic training, progressive relaxation, and biofeedback.

Meditation can significantly slow heart rate and breathing rate. Brief instructions are included in *Table 10.11.* Environmental requirements become less restrictive once one has learned the meditation process. When seated there should be only a minimum of muscle contraction. Preferably, the chair supports the back and spine, but it should not allow meditators to fall asleep. The head position is up to the meditator. A clock is required to time the session (with experience, however, there is little need for a clock). The phone and other distractions should be removed. A passive attitude with a focus on breathing is recommended. (Avoid focusing on meditating.) Meditation is recommended daily, but not after a meal, after consuming coffee or other stimulants, or after cigarette smoking. Before breakfast and dinner are often good times.

Table 10.11
A Meditation Technique

Environment	Quiet, comfortable
	Comfortable, straight-backed chair; preferably, one that supports back and head
Position	Buttocks pushed against chair back
	Feet slightly forward of knees
	Hands rested on arms of chair or lap
	Muscles relaxed to greatest extent possible
Procedure	1. Close eyes
	2. Repeat in mind the word *one* each time you inhale, and *two* each time you exhale
	3. Breathe regularly; do not alter breathing
	4. Continue for 20 minutes
	5. When you realize you are thinking, gently go back repeating the words *one* and *two* without feeling as though you are doing something wrong
	6. When finished meditating, "come back" gradually: a. Open eyes gradually b. Focus on one object in the room c. Focus on several objects in the room d. Take several deep breaths e. Stretch while seated f. When ready, stand and stretch

Adapted from Greenberg JS. *Comprehensive Stress Management.* Dubuque, Ia: Wm. C. Brown Publishers; 1983.

TYPE A BEHAVIOR PATTERN*

Some do not consider type A behavior to be synonymous with "stress" because "the behavior is neither an unpleasant stimulus nor a reaction of discomfort."[28] Several instruments are used in assessing the type A behavior pattern.[28]

Several methods for changing type A behavior have been developed. Friedman and Ulman[40] have written a book on this topic. Recent evidence, however, questions the value of modifying type A behavior in people who have suffered myocardial infarct. In a recent study,[41] postcoronary patients who participated in an intervention program to modify type A behavior had a higher incidence of subsequent coronary incidents than control subjects. This study, together with others, demonstrates a need to assess the relative effects of stress and type A personality on CHD risk. It is also essential to determine the benefit of modifying stress and behavior on the incidence of primary and secondary CHD events.

When type A behavior is present, current recommendations call for rigorous intervention directed at established CHD risk factors such as smoking, elevated plasma total-cholesterol level, and hypertension.[32]

CONCLUSION†

Behavior change is central to the reduction of cardiovascular risk. Dietitians should take leadership responsibility in implementing behavior-change programs and training and working with other health professionals to assist in guiding patients toward improved health habits.

*By Donna Payne
†By Karen Glanz

No single approach will work for all patients or in all health care settings. Thus, it is necessary to recognize and provide for a range of choices for intervention. The suitability of different educational formats (eg, brief counseling, comprehensive counseling, group programs) varies among individual patients and clinical situations.[8]

For patient education to be successful in reducing cardiac risk it is important to identify the barriers to compliance and also the opportunities for encouraging behavior changes; to tailor behavior-change strategies to the patient's situation and needs; and to communicate effectively within the constraints of the interaction. Attention to follow-up, monitoring, and reinforcement is basic to effective behavior-change interventions.

The strongest health-enhancing initiatives embody an approach with interventions directed not only at individual patients, but also toward the groups to which they belong, including their families, workplaces, and communities.[43] In the ideal scenario, behavior change is supported in the family, at work, and in the community.[44,45] The dietitian is the catalyst and facilitator, initiating and guiding the process of behavior change to improve cardiovascular health.

References

1. Glanz K. Nutrition education for risk factor reduction and patient education: a review. *Prev Med.* 1985;14:721.
2. Carmody TP, Matarazzo JD, Istvan JA. Promoting adherence to heart-healthy diets: a review of the literature. *J Compl Health Care.* 1987;2:105.
3. Schucker B, Bailey K, Heimbach JT, et al. Change in public perspective on cholesterol and heart disease: results from two national surveys. *JAMA.* 1987;258:3527.
4. Schucker B, Wittes JT, Cutler JA, et al. Change in physician perspective on cholesterol and heart disease: results from two national surveys. *JAMA.* 1987;258:3521.
5. Snetselaar LG. *Nutrition Counseling Skills: Assessment, Treatment, and Evaluation.* 2nd ed. Rockville, Md: Aspen Systems Corp; 1989.
6. National Cholesterol Education Program Expert Panel. Report on detection, evaluation, and treatment of high blood cholesterol in adults. *Arch Intern Med.* 1988;148:36.
7. Palumbo PJ. Cholesterol lowering for all: a closer look. *JAMA.* 1989;262:91.
8. Glanz K. Patient and public education for cholesterol reduction: a review of strategies and issues. *Pat Educ Couns.* 1988;12:235.
9. Raab C, Tillotson JL, eds. *Heart to Heart: A Manual on Nutrition Counseling for the Reduction of Cardiovascular Disease Risk Factors.* Bethesda, Md; 1983. US Dept of Health and Human Services publication, NIH 83-1528.
10. Ockene JK. Physician-delivered interventions for smoking cessation: strategies for increasing effectiveness. *Prev Med.* 1987;16:723.
11. Dolecek TA, Milas NC, Van Horn LV, et al. A long-term nutrition intervention experience: lipid responses and dietary adherence patterns in the Multiple Risk Factor Intervention Trial (MRFIT). *J Am Diet Assoc.* 1986;86:752.
12. Mason M, Wenberg B, Welch PK. *The Dynamics of Clinical Dietetics.* New York, NY: John Wiley & Sons; 1977.
13. Glanz K. Compliance with dietary regimens: its magnitude, measurement, and determinants. *Prev Med.* 1980;9:787.
14. Bandura A. *Social Learning Theory.* Englewood Cliffs, NJ: Prentice-Hall Inc; 1977.
15. Bandura A. *Social Foundations of Thought and Action: A Social Cognitive Theory.* Englewood Cliffs, NJ: Prentice-Hall Inc; 1986.
16. Strecher VJ, DeVellis BM, Becker MH, Rosenstock IM. The role of self-efficacy in achieving health behavior change. *Health Educ Quar.* 1986;13:73.
17. DiClemente C, Prochaska JO. Self-change and therapy change of smoking behavior: a comparison of processes of change in cessation and maintenance. *Addict Behav.* 1982;7:133.

18. Prochaska JO, DiClemente CC. Transtheoretical therapy: toward a more integrative model of change. *Psychotherapy: Theory, Res, Prac.* 1982;19:276.
19. Marlatt GA, Gordon JR. *Relapse Prevention.* New York, NY: Guilford Press; 1985.
20. Rimer BK, Glanz K, Lerman C. Contributions of public health to patient compliance with preventive medical regimens. 1990. In review.
21. Cohen S, Lichtenstein E, Prochaska JO, et al. Debunking myths about self-quitting: evidence from ten prospective studies of persons quitting smoking by themselves. *Am Psychol.* 1989;44:1355.
22. Kanfer FH, Goldstein AP, eds. *Helping People Change: A Textbook of Methods.* 3rd ed. New York, NY: Pergamon Press; 1986.
23. Kanfer FH, Schefft BK. *Guiding the Process of Therapeutic Change.* Champaign, Ill: Research Press; 1988.
24. Carmody TP, Istvan J, Matarazzo JD, et al. Applications of social learning theory in the promotion of heart-healthy diets: the Family Heart Study dietary intervention model. *Health Educ Res.* 1986;1:13.
25. Ley P. Cognitive variables and noncompliance. *J Compl Health Care.* 1987;1:171.
26. McCabe BJ, Tysinger JW, Kreger M, Currwin AC. A strategy for designing effective patient education materials. *J Am Diet Assoc.* 1989;89:1290, 1295.
27. Glanz K, Rudd J. Readability and content analysis of written cholesterol education materials. *Pat Educ Couns.* 1990. In press.
28. Jenkins CD. Psychological and behavioral factors. In: Kaplan NM, Stamler JS, eds. *Prevention of Coronary Heart Disease: Practical Management of the Risk Factors.* Philadelphia, Pa: WB Saunders Co; 1983.
29. Lichtenstein E. The smoking problem: a behavioral perspective. *J Con Clin Psy.* 1982;50:804.
30. Oldridge N. Compliance and exercise in primary and secondary prevention of coronary heart disease: a review. *Prev Med.* 1982;11:56.
31. Eliot RS, Bond MB, Brandenbert RO, et al. Bethesda Conference, task force 3: the physician in the work setting. *Am J Cardiol.* 1981;47:751.
32. Aronow WS, Kaplan NM. Smoking. In: Kaplan NM, Stamler JS, eds. *Prevention of Coronary Heart Disease—Practical Management of the Risk Factors.* Philadelphia, Pa: WB Saunders Co; 1983.
33. Oldridge N, Wisks J, Hanley C. Non-compliance in an exercise rehabilitation program for men who have suffered a myocardial infarction. *Can Med Assoc J.* 1978;118:361.
34. Martin J, Dubbert P. Exercise and health: the adherence problem. *Behav Med Update.* 1981;4:16.
35. Wysocki I, Hall G, Iwata B, et al. Behavioral management of exercise: contracting for aerobic points. *J Appl Behav Anal.* 1979;12:55.
36. Oldridge N, Stoedefalke K. Compliance and motivation in cardiac exercise programs. *Clin Sports Med.* 1984;3:443.
37. Glass DC. *Behavior Patterns, Stress and Coronary Heart Disease.* Hillsdale, NJ: Lawrence Erlbawm Associates; 1977.
38. Hamburg DA. Bethesda Conference, keynote address: changing behavior for health. *Am J Cardiol.* 1981;47:736.
39. Greenberg JS. *Comprehensive Stress Management.* Dubuque, Ia: Wm. C. Brown Co; 1983.
40. Friedman M, Ulmer D. *Treating Type A Behavior and Your Heart.* New York, NY: Ballantine Books; 1985.
41. Kolman P. The value of group psychotherapy after myocardial infarction: a critical review. *J Cardiol Rehab.* 1983;3:360.
42. Jaffe DT, Scott CD, Orioli EM. Stress management: programs and prospects. *Am J Health Promotion.* 1986;1:29.
43. Glanz K, Mullis RM. Environmental interventions to promote healthy eating: a review of models, programs, and evidence. *Health Educ Quar.* 1988;15:395.
44. McLeroy KR, Bibeau D, Steckler A, Glanz K. An ecological perspective on health promotion programs. *Health Educ Quar.* 1988;15:351.
45. Glanz K, Marcus F, eds. *Health Behavior and Health Education: Theory, Research and Practice.* San Francisco, Calif: Jossey-Bass Inc; 1990.

11. DRUG TREATMENT

DRUG THERAPY FOR LOWERING PLASMA LIPIDS*

LDL Cholesterol

Three classical clinical trials[1–3] established that pharmacological therapy is beneficial in decreasing CHD mortality. Patients who have elevated plasma LDL-cholesterol levels after intensive dietary therapy are candidates for drug treatment. Prior to commencing drug therapy, patients should follow a blood cholesterol–lowering diet for at least six months.[4] In patients with marked elevations in plasma LDL cholesterol (> 225 mg/dL) or CHD, it may be appropriate to initiate drug therapy sooner than six months. It is important to have an accurate assessment of the plasma LDL-cholesterol level to assess the efficacy of subsequent drug treatment.

The National Cholesterol Education Program (NCEP)[4] has identified LDL-cholesterol levels at which drug therapy should be considered (after an appropriate dietary intervention). The levels are:

- 190 mg/dL or more (very-high-risk LDL cholesterol) — All patients with LDL-cholesterol levels above 190 mg/dL are candidates for drug therapy even though they may not have CHD. The minimal goal for this group is to lower LDL cholesterol to less than 160 mg/dL.
- 160 mg/dL or more (high-risk LDL cholesterol) — Patients who have CHD or two other risk factors are candidates for drug therapy. The minimal goal for this group is to lower LDL cholesterol to less than 130 mg/dL.

Selection and use of drugs. These drugs are currently recommended for the treatment of elevated LDL cholesterol:

1. Bile-acid sequestrants (cholestyramine, colestipol)
2. Nicotinic acid
3. Hydroxymethylglutaryl coenzyme-A (HMG-CoA) reductase inhibitors (lovastatin)
4. Gemfibrozil
5. Probucol

The therapeutic results of these drugs, side effects, and other characteristics are listed in *Table 11.1.* The drugs of first choice for treating patients who do not have hypertriglyceridemia are the bile-acid sequestrants and nicotinic acid. This is because these drugs have been shown to be effective and are generally safe for long-term use. Lovastatin effectively lowers plasma LDL-cholesterol levels. It is not currently classified as a drug of first choice because it has only been used for a few years, and its long-term safety is not known. Gemfibrozil and probucol are not considered to be drugs of first choice because they are less effective in lowering plasma LDL-cholesterol levels. The effects of selected drugs on serum lipids are outlined in *Table 11.2.*

Familial Hypercholesterolemia

Patients with familial hypercholesterolemia rarely respond adequately to diet therapy alone. In these patients it is not necessary to wait six months before initiating drug therapy. Frequently, these patients are treated with two drugs. Presently, the use of a bile-acid sequestrant and nicotinic acid is the most effective treatment available.

*By Sally Ortiz

Cholesterol levels in patients with homozygous familial hypercholesterolemia are markedly elevated (600 to 1,000 mg/dL), and severe and fatal CHD frequently develops in the teen years. These patients respond poorly to drug therapy. Other intensive treatments are used (such as portacaval shunt, liver transplantation, plasmapheresis).

Table 11.1
Drug Treatment of Hyperlipidemia

Category	Drug Name (Brand Names)	Mechanism of Action	Therapeutic Result	Nutritional Side Effects
I. Resin	cholestyramine (Questran)	Binds bile acids in the intestine and prevents reabsorption	Low-density lipoproteins (LDL) decreased 25%–35% in type IIb heterozygotes and type IIa and b homozygotes	Never take dry, or with carbonated beverages. Decreased absorption of fat; vitamins A, D, K, B_{12}; folic acid; medium-chain triglycerides; and glucose. Decreased iron reserves. In long-term use, possible osteomalacia and hyperchoremic acidosis. Nausea, indigestion, anorexia, flatulence, edema, constipation.
	colestipol (Colestid)	Same as cholestyramine	Alternative to cholestyramine in type II patients	Similar to cholestyramine.
II. Nicotinic acid	(Nico-400, Nicobid)	Decreases synthesis of LDL and apoprotein B (apo B) by decreasing very-low-density lipoprotein (VLDL) synthesis	Effective in all types of hyperlipoproteinemia except type I (for which no drug treatment is effective). LDL decreased 15%–35%, VLDL decreased 35%–50%	Take with food. Decreased glucose tolerance, hyperuricemia and hyperglycemia. Nausea, vomiting, cramps, diarrhea, flatulence.
III. Fibrate	clofibrate (Atromid-S)	Not well understood. May inhibit release of liproproteins from the liver and possibly increases hydrolysis of VLDL by lipoprotein lipase.	In type IIb, LDL decreased 5% and VLDL decreased 35%–50%	Take with meals. Decreased absorption of carotene, glucose, iron, medium-chain triglycerides, vitamin B_{12}, and electrolytes. Possible decreased taste acuity. Increased appetite. Nausea, diarrhea, flatulence.
	gemfibrozil (Lopid)	Also increases lipolysis of VLDL	In type IV, decreased VLDL $> 30\%$. May increase HDL levels. In type V, decreased VLDL $> 70\%$ and increased HDL.	Take 1/2 hour before meals. May cause anemia, cramps, nausea, vomiting, diarrhea.

Table 11.1
Drug Treatment of Hyperlipidemia—(Cont.)

Category	Drug Name (Brand Names)	Mechanism of Action	Therapeutic Result	Nutritional Side Effects
IV. Other agents	probucol (Lorelco)	Decreases serum cholesterol by reducing LDL concentrations. Also lowers HDL concentrations.	LDL decreased 10%–20% and HDL also decreased 10%–20% in type IIa. A drug of second choice because of decreased HDL.	Take with food. Decreased sense of smell and taste. Nausea, vomiting, anorexia.
	Neomycin sulfate (Mycifradin Sulfate; Neobiotic)	Prevents bile acids from being reabsorbed in the intestine	LDL decreased as much as 22% in type IIa. A drug of second choice because of less information on safety and efficacy.	Decrease consumption of sweets. Decreased absorption of carotene; glucose; lactose; sodium; calcium; iron; vitamins A, D, K, B_{12}; folic acid. Nausea, vomiting, diarrhea.
	dextrothyroxine sodium (Choloxin)	Lowers LDL by increasing peripheral LDL receptor activity in both euthyroid and hypothyroid patients	LDL decreased 15%–30% in type II (no effect on VLDL)	Avoid large amounts of goitrogenic foods. Altered taste. Constipation, diarrhea, dyspepsia, anorexia, weight loss.
	norethindrone acetate (Aygestin, Norlutate)	Decreases VLDL and chylomicrons. Also HDL and apolipoprotein A.	In type V, decreased VLDL 10%–50%. Used only in women because of estrogenic activity.	Possible altered glucose tolerance and decreased or increased appetite
	lovastatin (Mevacor)	Decreases serum cholesterol by inhibiting cholesterol synthesis	LDL decreased 25%–45%	Take with meals. Constipation, flatulence, abdominal pain, nausea, diarrhea.

Adapted with permission from the *Annual Review of Medicine*, vol 37, ©1986 by Annual Reviews Inc; from Powers D, Moore AD. *Food-Medication Interactions.* 6th ed. Tempe, Ariz: FMI Publishers; 1988; and from *Physicians' Desk Reference.* 41st ed. Oradell, NJ: Medical Economics Co; 1987.

Familial Combined Hyperlipidemia (FCHL)

Diet therapy is important in the treatment of FCHL. In many patients drug therapy is necessary to control plasma lipid levels adequately. The drug of choice for FCHL is nicotinic acid. Patients with FCHL who have elevated LDL-cholesterol levels and normal triglyceride levels have been treated effectively with nicotinic acid, bile-acid-binding resins, and lovastatin. These drugs alone, however, may not be effective in patients with elevated plasma triglyceride levels, as noted in a later section.

Table 11.2
Effects of Selected Drugs on Serum Lipids

Drug	Effect
Alcohol	Increases triglycerides (TG), may increase HDL cholesterol
Androgens, anabolic steroids	Decreases HDL cholesterol
Corticosteroids (cortisol, prednisone)	Decreases HDL cholesterol
Diuretics*	Increases TG, increases total and LDL cholesterol, decreases HDL cholesterol
Estrogens†	Increases TG at higher doses, decreases LDL cholesterol
Isotretinoin (Accutane)	Increases TG, increases total and LDL cholesterol
Progestins†	Increases TG, decreases total and LDL cholesterol

*Effects from diuretics are dose-related and may only be transitory. Less problem with doses of 25 mg or less of hydrochlorothiazide.
†Oral contraceptives contain varying ratios of estrogens to progestins. Unpredictable effects on lipids.
Adapted with permission from Kradjan WA. Drug and food interactions, effects of drugs on serum lipids. *RD.* 1983; 3:2.

Severe Primary Hypercholesterolemia

Many patients with severe primary hypercholesterolemia do not respond well to dietary intervention and must be treated with drugs. The drug-therapy strategy employed is identical to that described above for treating elevated plasma LDL-cholesterol levels.

Familial Dysbetalipoproteinemia (Type III Hyperlipoproteinemia)

If patients are overweight, caloric restriction frequently reduces the plasma total-cholesterol to normal levels. If the condition persists despite dietary intervention, drug therapy is used. Nicotinic acid is the preferred drug. The fibric acids (gemfibrozil and clofibrate) are also effective.

Hypertriglyceridemia

The NIH Consensus Development Conference on Treatment of Hypertriglyceridemia defined definite hypertriglyceridemia as a fasting triglyceride level exceeding 500 mg/dL. For patients with severe hypertriglyceridemia and chylomicronemia, a very-low-fat diet (10% to 20% of calories) should be prescribed to prevent pancreatitis. For patients with definite hypertriglyceridemia, drug therapy can be used to reduce the risk of acute pancreatitis. Nicotinic acid is the drug of choice. If this is not tolerated by the patient, gemfibrozil or clofibrate are used. In borderline hypertriglyceridemia (250 to 500 mg/dL) the use of drugs has been a controversial subject. If a hypertriglyceridemic patient also has FCHL, then drug therapy is warranted. Nicotinic acid is the drug of choice for FCHL since it inhibits the production of lipoproteins that are characteristic of this disorder.

Fig. 11.1
Recommended protocols for drug treatment of hypercholesterolemia. From National Cholesterol Education Program Expert Panel. Report on detection, evaluation and treatment of high blood cholesterol in adults. **Arch Intern Med.** ***1988;148:36.***

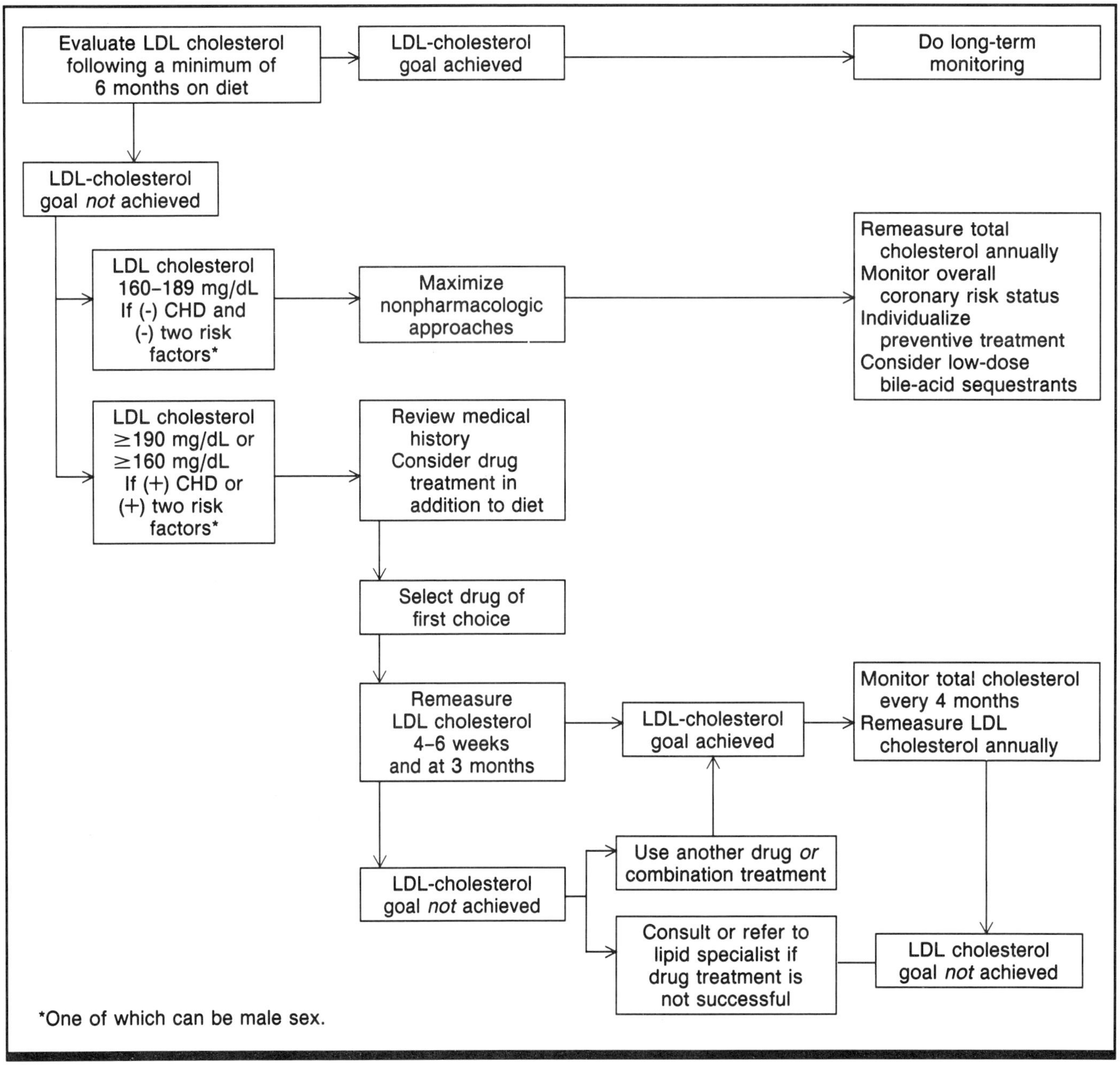

Patient Monitoring and Follow-up

The recommended protocol for monitoring patients is presented in *Figure 11.1*. It is important to have at least two measurements of the lipoprotein profile prior to initiating drug therapy. If patients follow the recommended protocol for taking the drug, the maximum lowering of LDL cholesterol is achieved within four weeks after initiation of therapy. If the patient achieves a decrease in LDL cholesterol that is less than the minimum target goal, consideration should be given to switching drugs or adding an additional drug for combination therapy.

It is important for patients to realize that drug therapy will likely continue for a lifetime. The patient must be well informed of the clinical goals of the therapy and the side effects of the medication. It is important for health professionals to be actively involved in patient education and to provide information in a timely and understandable manner. This is important for patients who may have problems with side effects. In many instances the patients' initial experience with the drug regimen is predictive of long-term adherence. It should also be underscored that sound, aggressive diet therapy must be continued with the drug therapy.

HYPERTENSION*

Hypertension may not only be a primary disease but also may be a sign of many disorders. Primary or essential hypertension has no identifiable cause and affects well over 90% of all hypertensive patients. When hypertension occurs as a result of an underlying primary disease it is called secondary hypertension. Causes of secondary hypertension include coarctation, Cushing's syndrome, certain drugs, increased intercranial pressure, pheochromocytoma, primary aldosteronism, renal parenchymal disease, and renovascular hypertension.

Elevated blood pressure is a major cause of heart failure, renal failure, and stroke. Persons with untreated high blood pressure are likely to have substantially elevated levels of plasma lipid or lipoprotein cholesterol levels.[9]

As of 1984, one half of the hypertensive population was properly diagnosed and one third was receiving some form of antihypertensive therapy.[10] These statistics have improved since 1970 due to a worldwide effort in educating physicians and patients on the detection and treatment of hypertension. The availabilty of a wide variety of antihypertensive agents has also contributed to patient and physician compliance.

The benefits of antihypertensive drug therapy for moderate to severe hypertension have been demonstrated.[11,12] Recent studies have indicated that antihypertensive drug treatment reduces mortality and morbidity even in people with mild hypertension.[13-15] Therefore, it is now advisable that the millions of Americans with relatively milder degrees of hypertension also be treated. The Hypertension Detection and Follow-up Program (HDFP) and the Australian Trials have prompted the 1984 Third Joint National Committee (JNC) to establish recommendations on drug therapy for mildly hypertensive patients.[16] The following is an excerpt from that report:

> The benefits of drug therapy appear to outweigh any known risks from such therapy for those with a diastolic pressure persistently elevated above 95 mm Hg and for those with lesser elevations who are at high risk (eg, patients with target organ damage, diabetes mellitus, or other major risk factors for CHD). For those with diastolic pressure in the 90 to 94

*By Janice Daly

mm Hg range who are otherwise at low risk, nonpharmacologic therapy should be pursued aggressively. If blood pressure remains above 90 mm Hg with nonpharmacologic therapy, however, antihypertensive drugs are indicated. However, some experts would delay drug therapy in this group if blood pressure is not constantly above 94 mm Hg and there is no evidence of target organ disease or other risk factors for CVD (male sex, cigarette smoking, hypercholesterolemia, or diabetes mellitus). Physicians who elect not to use drug therapy for patients with diastolic pressures of 90 to 94 mm Hg should follow these patients as closely as if they were on drugs, because many will progress to higher levels of diastolic pressure that all agree should be treated with antihypertensive agents.

Patients with a diastolic blood pressure greater than 105 mm Hg should be treated aggressively.[10] The goal of therapy is to reduce diastolic blood pressure to 90 mm Hg with minimal adverse effects. In these patients, therapy reduces morbidity and mortality from congestive heart failure, renal failure, stroke, and ischemic cardiac events.[11,12] Even partial reduction of blood pressure can reduce any hypertensive complications significantly.[17]

For mild hypertension (whether a diastolic blood pressure of 90, 95, or 100 mm Hg is used as an indication of drug therapy) it is paramount for the patient to be monitored while following the general guidelines listed in *Table 11.3.*[16] Nonpharmacologic therapies are advocated during the initial three- to six-month period of monitoring. These therapies should be offered and encouraged irrespective of whether drugs are needed. The nondrug therapies for reducing blood pressure have been discussed previously.

Table 11.3
Guidelines for Therapy for Mild Hypertension

1. Recheck blood pressure over 3–6 months while using nondrug therapy:
   - Weight reduction, if overweight
   - Moderate sodium restriction (2 g sodium = 88 mmol/day)
   - Relaxation
   - Isotonic exercise
   - Moderate alcohol intake (1–2 oz ethanol per day)
2. If diastolic blood pressure remains above 95 mm Hg, start drug therapy:
   - Consider adrenergic inhibitors instead of diuretics
   - Use small doses initially
   - Avoid metabolic side effects
3. If diastolic blood pressure is 90–95:
   - Low-risk patients: continue on nondrug therapy
   - High-risk patients: start drug therapy

Adapted with permission from Management Committee of the Australian Therapeutic Trial in Mild Hypertension. Untreated mild hypertension. *Lancet.* 1982;1:185.

Pharmacological Intervention

Drug therapy is usually initiated after a trial period of nonpharmacological intervention has failed. The benefits of therapy outweigh the risks for people with persistently elevated diastolic blood pressure (> 94 mm Hg) or isolated elevated systolic blood pressure readings (> 160 mm Hg). A stepped-care approach, in which a combination of antihypertensive drugs with different modes of action is used, may allow for smaller doses and fewer side effects. Once control is established for a consistent period, attempts should be made to reduce the dose and possibly eliminate some of the drugs. Drug therapy, however, is most beneficial when dietary or life-style modifications are also incorporated into the treatment plan.

Once the decision is made to treat with drugs, the choice will depend on the presence and absence of specific contraindications and the occurrence of adverse effects in the individual patient. Drugs used to treat hypertension include diuretics, sympatholytics, vasodilators, angiotension-converting enzyme inhibitors, and calcium channel blockers. A comprehensive listing of the antihypertensive drugs is provided in *Table 11.4.*[10] For a more detailed explanation of side effects, the drug packet inserts or a reputable reference text should be consulted.

Table 11.4
Effect of Antihypertensives on Serum Lipids

Drug	Effect
Postsynaptic alpha-blocker	
prazosin	Decreases total cholesterol
trimazosin	Decreases total cholesterol
Combined postsynaptic alpha-blocker and central sympatholytic	
urapidil	Decreases total cholesterol, LDL cholesterol, increases HDL cholesterol
Combined alpha-beta-blocker	
labetalol	Increases total cholesterol, increases triglycerides
Beta-blockers	
propranolol	Increases total cholesterol, triglycerides
Agents that lower sympatholytic activity	
reserpine	No effect on lipids
methyldopa	Decreases HDL cholesterol
clonidine	Decreases total cholesterol
debrisoquin	Decreases total, LDL, and HDL cholesterol, decreases triglycerides
Calcium channel blockers	
nifedipine	No change

Data from Weidmann P, Vehlinger DE, Gerber A[39]; Weidmann P, Gerber A[40]; Ames RP, Hill P[41]; Kirkendall WM, Hammond JJ, Thomas JC, et al[42]; Sommers DEK, Villiers LS, Van Wyk M[43]; Singleton W, Taylor CR[44]; Gerber A, Weidmann P, Marone C.[45]

Experimental studies have shown that various antihypertensive drugs have adverse effects on plasma lipid and lipoprotein levels. Methyldopa has been shown to decrease HDL-cholesterol levels.[18,19] Thiazide and loop diuretics may increase the levels of plasma total cholesterol, LDL cholesterol, and triglycerides.[20–22] Beta-blockers have been shown to decrease HDL cholesterol and increase triglyceride levels.[23–25] When beta-blockers and diuretics are given concurrently, HDL cholesterol decreases and total cholesterol increases; however, diuretic-induced changes in LDL cholesterol and total cholesterol are prevented. It is apparent that there is a need to monitor lipid and lipoprotein levels before and during hypertensive therapy. An evaluation of the benefit of using antihypertensive drug(s) to lower cardiovascular risk versus the risk of adverse effects on lipid and lipoprotein levels is warranted.

A growing realization of the adverse effects of the most commonly employed first-line agents and the new knowledge of the role that calcium plays in hypertension have prompted the consideration of calcium channel blockers as first-line therapy. Calcium channel–blocking drugs appear to decrease peripheral resistance in hypertension by specifically reversing a functional abnormality that maintains the hypertensive state, ie, excessive intracellular calcium concentrations in vascular smooth muscle.[26] These drugs may also reduce blood pressure through antisympathetic actions at adrenergic receptors[27] and through a natriuretic effect.[28] Serious adverse reactions to the drugs were not seen.[13,16,29,30] One of the most advantageous effects of diltiazem is that it may increase HDL-cholesterol levels.[29] Diltiazem shows no adverse effects on other blood chemistries, and it does not impair exercise performance; it does not cause orthostatic effects, fluid retention, or tachycardia. The major disadvantages are cost and the two-times-a-day dosage regimen. It has been concluded that diltiazem is an acceptable monotherapy in patients with moderate essential hypertension.[29]

One facet of patient care that is often given little consideration is the drug-induced nutrition-related effects. Medications can be affected by food, and nourishment may be affected by medication. The increasing emphasis on nutrition and multidisciplinary patient care has prompted the development of references on food and medication interaction. To facilitate the care of hypertensive patients, a list has been compiled (*Table 11.5*) of the common antihypertensive drugs and their nutrition-related effects as documented in the manual.[31] Many of the recommendations advise against the use of natural licorice when using antihypertensive drugs. Natural licorice flavoring is an extract from the sweet root of the glycrrhiza plant, a plant in the pea family. Glycyrrhizin, a chemical in the saponin group, has corticosteroid-like effects. Imported licorice (as little as two to four twists per day) can complicate antihypertensive therapy and cause hypokalemia and sodium retention. Glycyrrhizin can also raise blood pressure and could conceivably induce heart failure if doses are high enough.[32] Ninety percent of licorice imported into the United States is used in tobacco products. People who chew tobacco and swallow the saliva are at risk for licorice toxicity.[32] Thus, people with hypertension should avoid chewing tobacco as well as licorice. It is important to note that anise oil, a licorice-like flavoring agent, does not have the harmful effects of natural licorice and is used in most products made in the United States. Ingredients on labels should be checked.

Hypertension is a significant risk factor for CHD. Antihypertensive drug therapy has been shown to be beneficial in reducing and preventing the CVD complications of hypertension. Calcium channel blockers as a monotherapy in essential hypertension will likely increase in popularity as more supportive research on their minimal side effects is reported.

Table 11.5
Nutrition-Related Effects of Antihypertensive Drugs (Generic and Brand Names)

Drug Name	Nutrition and Related Effects
Aldactazide (HCTZ-spironolactone)	Take with food 6 or more hours before bedtime. Avoid natural licorice. Monitor diabetes, electrolytes. Diet important: sodium- and calorie-restricted diet may be recommended. Anorexia, dry mouth, gastrointestinal distress.
Aldactone (spironolactone)	Take with food 6 or more hours before bedtime. Avoid natural licorice. Possible fluid and electrolyte imbalance. Diet important: monitor potassium, potassium retention possible. Dry mouth, thirst, gastrointestinal distress.
Apresoline (hydralazine)	Take with food same time each day. Limit alcohol: 1–2 oz with physician's permission. Avoid natural licorice. Sodium- and calorie-restricted diet may be recommended. Anorexia, gastrointestinal distress, constipation.
Blocadren (timolol)	Take with food same time each day. Avoid natural licorice. Monitor diabetes. Diet important: sodium-and calorie-restricted diet may be recommended. Weight loss, nausea, edema.
Calan, Isoptin (verapamil)	Take on empty stomach. Limit alcohol: 1–2 oz with physician's permission. Constipation, edema.
Capoten, (captopril)	Take on empty stomach, 1 hour before meals. Hyperkalemia. Diet important: sodium- and calorie-restricted diet may be recommended. Decreased taste acuity, weight loss or gain.
Cardizem (diltiazem)	Take drug 1 or 2 hours after meals. Limit alcohol: 1–2 oz. with physician's permission. Nausea, edema, dry mouth, constipation.
Catapres (clonidine)	Limit alcohol: 1–2 oz with physician's permission. Diet important: sodium and/or calorie restriction may be recommended. Dry mouth, nausea, constipation, vomiting, weight gain, edema.
Corgard (nadolol)	Take with food same time each day. Avoid natural licorice. Monitor diabetes; decreased carbohydrate tolerance. Diet important: possible sodium- and calorie-restricted diet. Constipation, gastrointestinal distress, dry mouth, nausea.
Diuril (chlorothiazide)	Take with food 6 or more hours before bedtime. Limit alcohol: 1–2 oz with physician's permission. Avoid natural licorice. Monitor electrolytes, diabetes. Long-term use: increases serum calcium. Diet important: sodium restriction/high potassium may be recommended. Increased need for foods high in zinc. Anorexia, nausea, vomiting, diarrhea, constipation, dry mouth.
Dyazide, Maxzide (triamterene)	Take with food 6 hours before bedtime. Limit alcohol: 1–2 oz with physician's permission. Avoid natural licorice. Monitor electrolytes, diabetes. Long-term use: increases serum calcium and decreases absorption of magnesium. May decrease serum folate, conserves potassium. May need low-sodium diet with foods high in magnesium. Decreased utilization of dietary folate. Nausea, vomiting, dry mouth, diarrhea, gastrointestinal distress, constipation.
Dyrenium (triamterene)	Take with food. Monitor diabetes, electrolytes. May decrease serum folate, may increase calcium excretion. Conserves iodine, possibly serum potassium. Avoid diet high in potassium. Nausea, vomiting, dry mouth, diarrhea, gastrointestinal distress.
Edecrin (ethacrynic acid)	Take with meals or milk 6 or more hours before bedtime. Limit alcohol: 1–2 oz with physician's permission. Monitor diabetes: decreased carbohydrate tolerance. Hypokalemia. Need foods high in potassium and magnesium. Gastrointestinal distress, nausea, vomiting, diarrhea, anorexia.
Enduron (methylclothiazide)	Take with food 6 or more hours before bedtime. Limit alcohol: 1–2 oz with physician's permission. Avoid natural licorice. Monitor diabetes, electrolytes. Long-term use: increases bone calcium, decreases absorption of magnesium, possible hypokalemia. Concurrent use with calcium supplements may result in hypercalcemia; with magnesium supplements may result in the formation of an insoluble complex. Diet important: may need a sodium-restricted, high-potassium diet. Need of foods high in magnesium. Anorexia, nausea, vomiting, diarrhea, constipation, dizziness, dry mouth.

Table 11.5
Nutrition-Related Effects of Antihypertensive Drugs (Generic and Brand Names)—(Cont.)

Drug Name	Nutrition and Related Effects
Esidrix (HCTZ hydrochlorothiazide)	See Enduron
HydroDIURIL (HCTZ)	See Enduron
Hygroton (chlorthalidone)	Take with food 6 hours or more before bedtime. Limit alcohol: 1–2 oz with physician's permission. Avoid natural licorice. Monitor electrolytes, diabetes. Long-term use: decreases carbohydrate tolerance. Diet important: sodium-restricted, high-potassium diet may be recommended. Anorexia, gastrointestinal irritation, nausea, vomiting, diarrhea, constipation, dizziness, dry mouth.
Inderal (propranolol)	Take with food same time each day. Avoid natural licorice. Monitor diabetes: decreased carbohydrate tolerance. Diet important: sodium- and calorie-restricted diet. Constipation, gastrointestinal distress, dry mouth, nausea.
Ismelin (guanethidine)	Avoid natural licorice. Limit alcohol: 1–2 oz with physician's permission. Monitor diabetes. Diet important: sodium and calorie restriction may be recommended. Edema, diarrhea, nausea, dry mouth, weight gain.
Lasix (furosemide)	Take with food before 6 PM. Limit alcohol: 1–2 oz with physician's permission. Sorbitol content may increase possibility of diarrhea in children. Oral solution: 11.5% alcohol. Monitor diabetes: decreased carbohydrate tolerance. Monitor electrolytes. Decreased zinc in liver. Need foods high in potassium and magnesium. Anorexia, vomiting, nausea, dry mouth, increased thirst. Magnesium: depletion may occur in selected patients on long-term diuretic therapy.
Lopressor (metoprolol)	Take with food same time each day. Monitor diabetes. Diet important: sodium and calorie restriction may be recommended. Metallic taste, epigastric distress, dry mouth, constipation.
Lozol (indapamide)	Take with food same time of day and before 6 PM. Limit alcohol: 1–2 oz with physician's permission. Monitor diabetes, electrolytes. Diet important: consider sodium-restricted, high-potassium, calorie-controlled diet. Dry mouth, constipation, gastrointestinal distress, weight loss.
Minipress (prazosin)	Limit alcohol: 1–2 oz with physician's permission. Dizziness, drowsiness, nausea, edema, weight gain, decrease in appetite, dry mouth, diarrhea, constipation, gastrointestinal distress.
Moduretic (amiloride)	Take with food. Limit alcohol: 1–2 oz with physician's permission. Monitor diabetes. Electrolyte imbalance: monitor potassium. Diet important: sodium- and calorie-restricted diet may be recommended. Nausea, anorexia, diarrhea, gastrointestinal pain, dry mouth, constipation.
Normodyne (labetalol)	Take with food. Monitor diabetes. Diet important: sodium- and calorie-restricted diet may be prescribed. Nausea, vomiting, dyspepsia, altered taste.
Oretic (HCTZ)	See Enduron
Procardia (nifedipine)	Take with meals. Monitor diabetes: decreased glucose tolerance. Nausea, diarrhea, constipation, cramps, flatulence, edema.
Renese (polythiazide)	See Enduron
Sandril, Serpasil (reserpine)	Take with meals. Limit alcohol: 1–2 oz with physician's permission. Sodium and water retention, decreased carbohydrate tolerance, increased gastrointestinal motility and gastric acid secretion. Diet important: sodium- and calorie-restricted diet may be recommended. Diarrhea, nausea, vomiting, anorexia, weight gain, dry mouth.
Tenormin (atenolol)	Take with food same time each day. Monitor diabetes. Diarrhea, nausea, dry mouth.
Thiuretic (HCTZ)	See Enduron
Trandate (labetalol)	See Normodyne
Visken (pindolol)	Monitor diabetes. Edema, weight gain, nausea, vomiting.
Zaroxolyn (metolazone)	Take in the morning after breakfast or last dose before 6 PM. Limit alcohol: 1–2 oz with physician's permission. Monitor diabetes. Monitor electrolytes: possible hypokalemia, hyponatremia. High-potassium diet may be recommended. Hypochloremic alkalosis, dry mouth, constipation, anorexia, nausea, bloating, dizziness.

Adapted with permission from *Physicians' Desk Reference*. 41st ed. Oradell, NJ: Medical Economics Co; 1987.

DIABETES*

When diet and regular exercise are ineffective in achieving glycemic control, pharmacological therapy is indicated. Numerous investigations have shown the benefits of tight glycemic control as a preventive measure against the complications of diabetes. There is less controversy now over the safety and rigors of tight glycemic control as the benefits continue to be identified.

In considering the best pharmacologic alternative, the following factors should be considered: the severity of the disease (ie, hyperglycemia, presence or absence of symptoms); the overall condition of the patient; the patient's age, weight, motivation, and preference; the expected treatments; and the side effects of oral agents and insulin.

Insulin Types

Insulin is available from different sources (eg, beef, pork, human, or a mixture).[33] Differences also exist in purity, concentration, solubility, and time of onset and duration of biologic action. Many different insulin formulations are available in the United States (*Table 11.6*). As the use of recombinant human insulin (eg, humulin) increases, the use of other types of insulin from animal sources is expected to decrease.

While the majority of patients continue to take insulin via injection, other delivery systems are being tested (ie, air-jet injection and via nasal spray). Continuous subcutaneous infusion devices (insulin pumps) are also an option. These instruments have become smaller and more reliable.[34]

Complications of insulin therapy may include hypoglycemia and the accompanying sequelae, insulin allergy or resistance, and lipodystrophy (ie, atrophy of the subcutaneous fatty tissue) at the injection site.

Table 11.6
Currently Available Insulin Preparations

Product Name	Manufacturer	Form
Rapid-Acting (onset, ½–4 hr; duration 5–12 hr)		
Humulin BR (for external insulin pumps only)	Lilly	human
Humulin regular	Lilly	human
Iletin I regular	Lilly	beef/pork
Iletin I semilente	Lilly	beef/pork
Iletin II regular	Lilly	beef
Iletin II regular	Lilly	pork
Novolin R penfill (regular) (only for Squibb-Novo Novo Pen)	Squibb-Novo	human
Novolin R (regular) (formerly Acrapid human)	Squibb-Novo	pork
Purified Pork R (regular) (formerly Semitard)	Squibb-Novo	pork
Regular	Squibb-Novo	beef/pork
Semilente	Squibb-Novo	beef
Velosulin (regular)	Nordisk-USA	human
Velosulin (regular)	Nordisk-USA	pork

*By Ann M. Sherry

Table 11.6
Currently Available Insulin Preparations—(Cont.)

Product Name	Manufacturer	Form
Intermediate-Acting (onset, 1–4 hr; duration, 16–24 hr)		
Humulin lente	Lilly	human
Humulin NPH	Lilly	human
Iletin II lente	Lilly	pork
Iletin II NPH	Lilly	pork
Iletin I lente	Lilly	beef/pork
Iletin I NPH	Lilly	beef/pork
Iletin II lente	Lilly	beef
Iletin II NPH	Lilly	beef
Insulatard (NPH)	Nordisk-USA	pork
Insulatard + (NPH)	Nordisk-USA	human
Novolin L (lente) (formerly Monotard human)	Squibb-Novo	human
Novolin N (NPH)	Squibb-Novo	human
NPH	Squibb-Novo	beef
Purified Pork Lente (formerly Monotard)	Squibb-Novo	pork
Purified Pork N (NPH) (formerly Protaphane)	Squibb-Novo	pork
Long-Acting (Onset, 4–6 hr; duration, 36+ hr)		
Humulin U (Ultralente)—duration only 24–36 hr	Lilly	human
Iletin I PZI	Lilly	beef/pork
Iletin I ultralente	Lilly	beef/pork
Iletin II PZI	Lilly	beef
Iletin II PZI	Lilly	pork
Purified beef U (Ultralente) (formerly Ultratard)	Squibb-Novo	beef
Ultralente	Squibb-Novo	beef
Mixtures		
Humulin 70/30	Lilly	human
Mixtard 70/30	Nordisk-USA	pork or human
Novolin 70/30	Squibb-Novo	human

Adapted with permission from Campbell RK. Clinical uses of insulin: its types and characteristics. *J Pract Nurs.* 1989;9:17.

Circumstances requiring insulin use in type II diabetes mellitus include: periods of acute injury, stress, or infection; surgery; pregnancy; and allergic or serious reactions to sulfonylurea agents. Patients may need exogenous insulin to manage hyperglycemia; it may be the only effective treatment. In others, insulin may be an alternative to oral hypoglycemic agent therapy.[35]

Oral Hypoglycemic Agents

A large number of substances are capable of affecting insulin release (*Table 11.7*), including drugs useful in the treatment of diabetes mellitus. Sulfonylureas increase the release of endogenous insulin and increase its peripheral effectiveness. Biguanides were removed from the market in 1977 because phenformin was associated with an increased incidence of lactic acidosis.[33] The pharmacokinetics of the oral hypoglycemic agents differ (*Table 11.8*).

Table 11.7
Stimulants, Amplifiers, and Inhibitors of Insulin Release in Humans

Stimulants of insulin release
- Glucose, mannose
- Leucine
- Vagal stimulation
- Sulfonylureas

Amplifiers of glucose-induced insulin release
- Enteric hormones:
  - Gastrin inhibitory polypeptide
  - Cholecystokinin secretion, gastrin
- Neutral amplifiers:
  - β-Adrenoceptor stimulation
- Amino acids:
  - Arginine

Inhibitors of insulin release
- Neutral: α-Sympathomimetic effect of catecholamines
- Humoral: Somatostatin
- Drugs: Diazoxide, phenytoin, vinblastine, colchicine

Reprinted with permission from Greenspan FS, Forsham PH, eds. *Basic and Clinical Endocrinology.* 2nd ed. San Mateo, Calif: Lange Medical Books; 1986.

Table 11.8
Pharmacokinetics of the Oral Hypoglycemic Drugs

Category	Drug	Activity: Onset, hr	Activity: Duration, hr	Nutritional Side Effects
First-generation sulfonylureas	acetohexamide (Dymelor)	1	10–14	*Note:* All drugs have similar side effects, including:
	chlorpropamide (Diabinese)	1	72	Hypoglycemia; increased by alcohol and low-caloric diets GI distress
	tolazamide (Tolinase)	4–6	10–14	Aplastic and hematologic anemia hepatic porphyria
	tolbutamide (Orinase)	1	6–12	Hyperglycemia; caused by thiazide diuretics, nicotinic acid, calcium channel blockers, oral contraceptives
Second-generation sulfonylureas	glyburide (Micronase) (DiaBeta)	1.5	24	May increase risk of heart disease
	glipizide (Glucotrol)	1	12–16	

Adapted with permission from Campbell RK. How oral agents are used in type II diabetes mellitus. *Pharm Times.* 1987;53:32; and from *Physicians' Desk Reference.* 41st ed. Oradell, NJ: Medical Economics Co; 1987.

An oral hypoglycemic agent may be prescribed as an adjunct to, and not a substitute for, dietary modification and exercise for people with non–insulin-dependent diabetes.[34] Patients most likely to respond to sulfonylureas are over 40 years of age, have had diabetes mellitus less than five years, or have had mild to moderate diabetes mellitus (ie, fasting glucose of less than 200 to 250 mg/dL). They may be of normal body weight or obese.[35,36]

Sulfonylurea agents are not indicated for people with type I diabetes mellitus, children, pregnant women, lactating women, or in patients with severe hepatic or renal failure. Patients with stressful concurrent diseases or conditions (eg, infection, trauma, an acute myocardial infarction, or an allergy to sulfonylurea compounds) should not be given sulfonylurea agents.[36]

Hypoglycemia, hyponatremia, and edema (only seen with chlorpropamide), skin and hematological reactions, gastrointestinal disturbances, and the unique disulfiram-like reaction (tachycardia, flushing, headache, and so on) after the ingestion of ethanol[36,37] are the most common side effects of the sulfonylurea agents and other drugs. There are extensive interactions between sulfonylureas and other drugs. Those that potentiate hypoglycemia include alcohol, phenylbutazone, beta-adrenergic blockers, salicylates, sulfonamides, coumarin, chloramphenicol, and sympathetic nervous system depressants. Medications that decrease their hypoglycemic effect include thiazides, corticosteroids, phenothiazines, thyroid medications, estrogens, oral contraceptive agents, phenytoin, nicotinic acid, calcium channel blockers, isoniazid, and sympathomimetics.[37] Patients with hepatic or renal insufficiency should be monitored for signs of toxicity of possible drug accumulation. The effects of certain drugs on plasma glucose levels are outlined in *Table 11.9*.

Table 11.9
Effect of Drugs on Plasma Glucose Levels

Drug	Effect
Alcohol	Decreases glucose
Anabolic steroids	Decreases glucose
Beta-blockers	Decreases glucose
Caffeine (large quantities)	Increases glucose
Diuretics	Increases glucose
Diazoxide	Increases glucose
Estrogens	Increases glucose
Epinephrine-like drugs	Increases glucose
Lithium	Increases glucose
Phenytoin	Increases glucose
Salicylates (large quantities)	Decreases glucose
Thyroid preparations	Increases glucose

Adapted with permission from Campbell RK. Clinical uses of insulin: side effects and dosing factors. *J Pract Nurs.* 1989;12:22.

References

1. Blankenhorn DH, Nessim SA, Johnson RL, et al. Beneficial effects of combined colestipol-niacin therapy on coronary atherosclerosis and coronary venous bypass grafts. *JAMA.* 1987;257:3233.
2. Lipid Research Clinics. *Population Studies Data Book, I: The Prevalence Study.* 1980. Dept of Health and Human Services publication NIC 80-157.
3. Grundy SM. Lessons from the Helsinki Heart Study. *Postgrad Med.* 1988;84:217.
4. National Cholesterol Education Program Expert Panel. Report on detection, evaluation, and treatment of high blood cholesterol in adults. *Arch Intern Med.* 1988;148:36.
5. Kane JP, Havel RJ. Treatment of hypercholesterolemia. *Ann Rev Med.* 1986;37:427.
6. American Medical Association. *Drug Evaluations.* 5th ed. Philadelphia, Pa: WB Saunders Co; 1983.

7. Powers D, Moore AD. *Food-Medication Interactions.* 6th ed. Tempe, Ariz: FMI Publishers; 1988.
8. *Physicians' Desk Reference.* 41st ed. Oradell, NJ: Medical Economics Co; 1987.
9. MacMahon SW, MacDonald GJ. Antihypertensive treatment and plasma lipoprotein levels. *Am J Med.* 1986;80:40.
10. *Cardiology, VII: High Blood Pressure.* New York, NY: Scientific American Inc; 1986.
11. Freis ED, Calabresi M, Castle CH, et al. Veterans Administration Cooperative Study Group on Antihypertensive Agents. Effects of treatment on morbidity in hypertension: results in patients with diastolic blood pressures averaging 115 through 129 mm Hg. *JAMA.* 1967;202:1028.
12. Freis ED, Calabresi M, Castle CH, et al. Veterans Administration Cooperative Study Group on Antihypertensive Agents. Effects of treatment on morbidity in hypertension, II: results in patients with diastolic blood pressures averaging 90 through 114 mm Hg. *JAMA.* 1970;213:1143.
13. Lewis GRJ. Long-term results with verapamil in essential hypertension and its influence on serum lipids. *Am J Cardiol.* 1986;57:35D.
14. Hypertension Detection and Follow-Up Program Co-operative Group. Five-year findings of the hypertensive detection and follow-up program. *JAMA.* 1979;242:2562.
15. Management Committee, Australian Therapeutic Trial in Mild Hypertension. Untreated mild hypertension. *Lancet.* 1982;1:185.
16. Kaplan N. Hypertension. In: Frackel RE, ed. *Conn's Current Therapy.* Philadelphia, Pa: WB Saunders Co; 1985:202.
17. Taguchi J, Freis ED. Partial reduction of blood pressure and prevention of complications in hypertension. *N Engl J Med.* 1974;291:329.
18. Ames RP, Hill P. Antihypertensive therapy and the risk of coronary heart disease. *J Cardiovasc Pharmacol.* 1982;4:S206.
19. Leon AS, Agre J, Grimm R, et al. Plasma lipid changes with Aldomet and propranolol during treatment of hypertension. *Circulation.* 1982;66:37. Abstract.
20. Ames RP, Hill P. Increase in serum lipids during treatment of hypertension with chlorthalidone. *Lancet.* 1976;1:721.
21. Goldman AL, Steele BW, Schnaper HW, et al. Serum lipoprotein levels during chlorthalidone therapy. *JAMA.* 1980;224:1691.
22. Ames RP. Metabolic disturbances increasing the risk of coronary heart disease during diuretic-based antihypertensive therapy: lipid alterations and glucose intolerance. *Am Heart J.* 1983;106:1207.
23. Kjeldsen SE, Eidel I, Leren P, et al. The effect on HDL cholesterol of oxprenolol and atenolol. *Scan J Clin Lab Invest.* 1982;42:449.
24. Day JL, Matcalfe J, Simpson CN. Adrenergic mechanisms in control of plasma lipid concentrations. *Br Med J.* 1982;284:1145.
25. Rouffy J, Jaillard J. Comparative effects of prazosin and atenolol on plasma lipids in hypertensive patients. *Am J Med.* 1984;76:105.
26. Frishman WH, Shlomo C, Michelson EL. Calcium channel blockers in systemic hypertension. *Am J Cardiol.* 1986;58:157.
27. Motulsky HJ, Snavely MD, Hughes RJ, et al. Interactions of verapamil and other calcium-channel blockers with alpha and alpha adrenergic receptors. *Circ Res.* 1983;82:226.
28. Laragh J, Buhler F, De Leeuw PW, et al. Calcium metabolism and calcium-channel blockers for understanding and treating hypertension. *Am J Med.* 1984;77:1.
29. Pool PE, Seagren SC, Salel AF. Effects of diltiazem on serum lipids, exercise performance and blood pressure: randomized, double-blind placebo-controlled evaluation for systemic hypertension. *Am J Cardiol.* 1985;56:86H.
30. Doyle AE. Comparison of calcium antagonists with other antihypertensive agents. *Am J Cardiol.* 1986;57:90D.
31. *Food-Medication Interactions.* Phoenix, Ariz: FMI Publishing; 1986.
32. Gershoff SN. Licorice and high blood pressure. *Tufts Univ Diet Nutr Ltr.* 1986;4:7.
33. Karam J. Pancreatic hormones and antidiabetic drugs. In: Katzung B, ed. *Basic and Clinical Pharmacology.* 3rd ed. Norwalk, Conn: Appleton & Lange; 1987:484.
34. American Diabetes Association. *Physician's Guide to Non–Insulin-Dependent (Type II) Diabetes: Diagnosis and Treatment.* 2nd ed. Alexandria, Va: American Diabetes Association Inc; 1988.
35. Vinicor F. An update on diabetes. *Pharm Times.* 1986;52:140.

36. Orland MJ. Diabetes mellitus. In: Orland M, Saltman R, eds. *Manual of Medical Therapeutics.* 24th ed. Boston, Mass: Little, Brown & Co; 1986:314.
37. Greenspan FS, Forsham PH, eds. *Basic and Clinical Endocrinology.* 2nd ed. San Mateo, Calif: Lange Medical Books; 1986.
38. Kradjan WA. Drug and food interactions, effects of drugs on serum lipids. *RD.* 1983;3:2.
39. Weidmann P, Vehlinger DE, Gerber A. Antihypertensive treatment and serum lipids. *J Hypertension.* 1985;3:297.
40. Weidmann P, Gerber A. Effects of antihypertensive therapy on serum lipoproteins. *Hypertension.* 1983;5(suppl III):120.
41. Ames RP, Hill P. Antihypertensive therapy and the risk of coronary heart disease. *J Cardiovasc. Pharmacol.* 1982;4(suppl 2):S206.
42. Kirkendall WM, Hammond JJ, Thomas JC, et al. Prazosin and chloridine for moderately severe hypertension. *JAMA.* 1978;240:2553.
43. Sommers DEK, Villiers LS, Van Wyk M, et al. The effect of labetalol and prenolol on blood lipids. *S Afr Med J.* 1980;60:379.
44. Singleton W, Taylor CR. Effect of trimazosin on serum lipid profiles in hypertensive patients. *Am Heart J.* 1983;106:1265.
45. Gerber A, Weidmann P, Marone C, et al. Cardiovascular and metabolic profile during intervention with urapidil in man. *Hypertension.* 1985;7:963.
46. Campbell RK. How oral agents are used in type II diabetes mellitus. *Pharm Times.* 1987;53:32.
47. Campbell RK. Clinical use of insulin: its types and characteristics. *J Pract Nurs.* 1989;9:17.
48. Campbell RK. Clinical uses of insulin: side effects and dosing factors. *J Pract Nurs.* 1989;12:22.

12. OVERVIEW OF CARDIAC REHABILITATION

REHABILITATION GOALS*

"In individuals with a prior history of CHD, including myocardial infarction or revascularization surgery, cardiac rehabilitation can be considered the process of restoring psychological, physical, and social function to optimal levels."[1]

Until 25 years ago, the early mobilization of the acute coronary patient was not recommended; after a myocardial infarction, six weeks of bed rest was common practice. Fortunately, many cardiologists questioned this approach. As early as the 1940s, a reduction in complications and mortality was demonstrated in patients who were mobilized during the acute care phase. Since then, the safety of activity for the patient with angina, the early use of bedside chairs for stabilized patients who have had a myocardial infarct, and progressive endurance-exercise regimens for those recovering from a myocardial infarction or coronary artery bypass grafts have been demonstrated.[2] Physical conditioning can improve heart rate, arterial blood pressure, myocardial oxygen uptake, and maximum cardiac output. Improvement in peripheral circulation, pulmonary ventilation, and autonomic nervous system balance further benefit physical work tolerance. Parallel with physical improvement are greater emotional stability and a return to productivity.[3] The goals of cardiac rehabilitation are summarized in *Table 12.1.*[4]

Table 12.1
Objectives of the Exercise Component of the University of Wisconsin-LaCrosse Cardiac Rehabilitation Program

A. To provide an opportunity for cardiac patients (nonoperative and postoperative) and those at high risk for CHD to become involved in a scientifically sound and medically supervised exercise program.
B. To provide guidance and supervision in the use of exercise as a form of therapy in the rehabilitation of patients with cardiac disease.
C. To periodically determine, through laboratory evaluation, the most advantageous exercise level for the program participants.
D. To educate the program participants with regard to cardiovascular and related benefits available through controlled, progressive, physical exercise.
E. To provide physicians of the LaCrosse area with an opportunity to refer cardiac patients and those at high risk for CHD to a quality exercise program, from which they would receive data pertinent to the patients' laboratory evaluations and monthly exercise progress.

Reprinted with permission from Wilson WK, Winga ER, Edgett JW, et al. *Policies and Procedures of a Cardiac Rehabilitation Program: Intermediate to Long-Term Care.* Philadelphia, Pa: Lea & Febiger; 1978.

FLOWCHART*

The rehabilitation of the cardiac patient should begin at the onset of illness and remain as a continuing feature in the long-term care of the patient.[2] A typical cardiac rehabilitation program is charted in *Figure 12.1.* At the onset of illness or surgery, the patient's primary care physician writes an order in the chart for cardiac rehabilitation. Inpatient rehabilitation progresses through several steps until discharge. A home exercise program is prescribed during the interim or until the patient returns for outpatient cardiac rehabilitation, as

*By Patricia Peterson

early as two weeks later. The initial visit involves a submaximal exercise treadmill test. If the patient is accepted into the program, he or she is given an exercise prescription for intensity (target heart rate), duration, and frequency. The program, with supervised progressive exercise, education, and counseling, will last approximately six to eight weeks. At the completion of the outpatient program, a maximal exercise test and biochemical assessment are done, and the patient is discharged with an exercise prescription and returned to the care of the referring physician.

Fig. 12.1
Cardiac rehabilitation program flowchart. GXT, graded exercise testing.

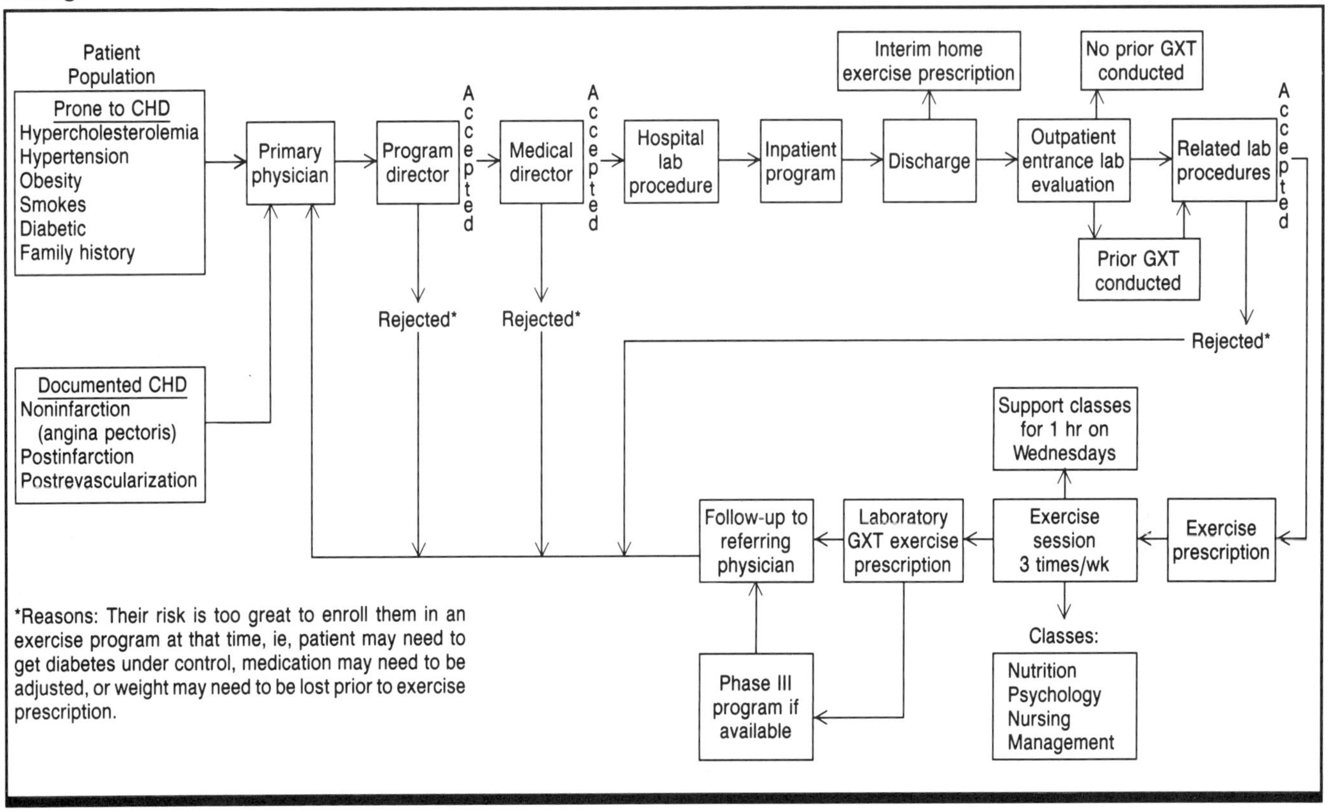

Phases of Cardiac Rehabilitation

The rehabilitation procedure can be described in phases, beginning during the acute stage as an inpatient in the hospital (phase I), the intermediate stage, usually the first two to 12 weeks after discharge (phase II), and the long-term program, usually conducted in a community-based facility (phase III). The phases of the Mount Sinai Medical Center Program[5] and the exercise prescription for each phase are shown in *Table 12.2.*

Table 12.2
Guidelines for Exercise Prescription for Cardiac Patients

Prescription	Phase I (Inpatient Program)	Phase II (Discharge to 3 mo)	Phase III (3 mo After Discharge)	Healthy Adults
Frequency	2–3 times/day	1–2 times/day	3–5 times/wk	3–5 times/wk
Intensity	MI: RHR + 20	MI: RHR + 20* RPE 13	70%–85% max	60%–90% max
	CABG: RHR + 20	CABG: RHR + 20* RPE 13	HR reserve	HR reserve
Duration	MI: 5–20 min CABG: 10–30 min	MI: 20–60 min CABG: 30–60 min	30–60 min	15–60 min
Mode-activity, sports	ROM, TDM, bike, 1 flight of stairs, wgt trg	ROM, TDM (walk, walk-jog), bike, arm erg, endurance sports	Walk, bike, jog, swim, cal, wgt trg cal	Walk, jog, run, bike, swim, endurance sports

MI indicates myocardial infarction patient; CABG, coronary artery bypass graft surgery patient; HR, heart rate, beats per minute; RHR, standing resting HR; ROM, range of motion exercise; TDM, treadmill; arm erg, arm ergometer; cal, calisthenics; wgt trg, weight training; RPE, rate of perceived exertion.
*Six to eight weeks after surgery or event, a symptom-limited exercise test is performed. Heart-rate intensity is then based on70% of maximum heart rate reserve.
Adapted with permission from Pollock M, Foster C, Ward A. Exercise prescription for rehabilitation of the cardiac patient. In: Pollock ML, Schmidt DH, eds. *Heart Disease and Rehabilitation.* New York, NY: Churchill-Livingstone; 1986:480.

Wenger[2] discusses cardiac rehabilitation in four phases and describes at each phase both the patient's changing need for care by various members of the rehabilitation team and the facilities needed for delivery of these services:

Phase I. The patient is admitted into an intensive care unit or coronary care unit to receive continuous electrocardiographic monitoring. Primary care is provided by the physician and nurses with specialized training in acute cardiac care. Initial emphasis is on prevention and control of dysrhythmias and management of chest pain, heart failure, and shock. The coronary artery bypass graft patient also receives intensive care and monitoring following surgery. During this time of intensive care, emotional reactions must be dealt with by the rehabilitation team.

Phase II. The convalescent period is characterized by a lessening in the roles of the physician and hospital-based nurse as the patient returns home. During this phase, the goal of the rehabilitation efforts is to restore the physical, emotional, and social well-being of the patient in preparation for the resumption of pre-illness activities, including a return to work. The patient assumes more responsibility for his or her health care with support from family and friends. The primary care physician continues to access and direct the patient's physical performance by exercise testing and pharmacological intervention. In large centers, outpatient cardiac rehabilitation programs provide six- to 12-week programs. Patients attend three sessions per week and receive counseling in addition to specific physical activity and education. During this time, the patient gains strength and emotional stability under the guidance of the rehabilitation team and physician.

Phase III. Beginning at the time of transfer from intensive care and for the duration of the hospital stay, other team members' responsibilities increase. Progressive levels of physical activity are begun. Phase III can be described in steps as outlined in *Table 12.3*.[6] Simple calisthenics and walking can be performed in the hospital room or corridor. Education and activities are provided by nurses, physical therapists, social workers, psychologists, and dietitians, but are directed by the physician (see team roles, below).

Table 12.3
Post-Myocardial Infarction Exercise Program

	Physical Activity	Activities of Daily Living (ADLs)
Step I* BID†	Passive ROM† Active plantar and dorsiflexion Diaphragmatic breathing	Bed rest Self-feed (bed at 45 degrees) Commode Sponge bath
Step II BID	Passive/active ROM Shoulder shrugs Deep breathing	Bedside chair for bed changes Dangle legs for meals Commode Sponge bath, self-grooming
Step III BID	Active ROM Deep breathing Supine flex knees to 75 degrees	TID† sitting 10 minutes Bedside chair for meals Walk to bathroom with assistance Sponge bath, self-grooming
Step IV BID 1 min	Supine flex knees to 75 degrees Sitting knee extender Sitting push-and-pull 3-minute walk TID	Bedside chair QID† 15 minutes Chair for meals Bathroom with assistance Sponge bath, self-grooming
Step V BID 1.25 min	Supine flex knees to 75 degrees Sitting lateral trunk bender Standing push-and-pull 4-minute walk TID	Bedside chair QID 20 minutes Sitting self-grooming Bathroom with assistance Tub or shower as indicated
Step VI BID 1.5 min	Sitting hip flexion Standing arm extender Standing lateral trunk bender 5-minute walk TID	Bedside chair ad lib Standing self-care Tub bath or shower
Step VII 1.5 min	Standing knee flexion Standing arms overhead Standing lateral bend 6-minute walk TID One flight stairs Home exercise program	Up ad lib

*Step levels are progressed by attending physician. Exercises and ADLs can be adjusted within different step levels as needed (ie, pain, nausea, etc) by the patient under the discretion of the professional staff.
†ROM = range of motion; BID = two times daily; TID = three times daily; QID = four times daily.
Adapted with permission from McKay-Dee Hospital Cardiac Fitness Institute. *Cardiac Rehabilitation Program*. Ogden, Utah; 1987.

Phase IV. The recovery-maintenance phase is characterized by an adaptation to a normal or near-normal life style. The vocational counselor, employee, and industrial physician assume dominant roles. The patient's cardiovascular status has improved enough to allow a return to prior levels of work and daily activities. Nearly half of the survivors of a myocardial infarct have mild, uncomplicated illness without significant residual disability. Eighty-five percent return to work within two to four months and work for an average of five years. During this phase it is important that an individualized physical-activity prescription be given to enhance cardiopulmonary function and promote a sense of well-being.

COMMUNITY-BASED CARDIAC REHABILITATION*

A supervised community-based program† is generally conducted in a YMCA, a community or private rehabilitation or prevention center, a university campus facility, or a health club. These programs are typically based on physician referral. Most patients attending these programs have returned to work and, as a result, seek convenient locations and times (ie, lunch or evening hours). These programs are patterned after hospital-based programs.[1,7]

PATIENT SELECTION*

Two categories of patients are accepted into a cardiac rehabilitation program after appropriate physician referral and approval of the referral by the program's medical director[4]:

1. Cardiac-prone patient—This includes people with hyperlipidemia, hypertension, diabetes mellitus, and/or a strong family history of premature CHD.
2. Cardiac patients—This includes patients with known CHD, past myocardial infarction, or coronary revascularization. These patients will ideally have passed through phase I of cardiac rehabilitation while inpatients.

Table 12.4
Contraindications for Entry Into Inpatient and Outpatient Exercise Programs

1. Unstable angina
2. Resting systolic blood pressure over 200 mm Hg or resting diastolic blood pressure over 100 mm Hg
3. Significant drop (20 mm Hg or more) in resting systolic blood pressure from the patient's average level that cannot be explained by medications
4. Moderate to severe aortic stenosis
5. Acute systemic illness or fever
6. Uncontrolled atrial or ventricular arrhythmias
7. Uncontrolled tachycardia (greater than 100 beats/minute)
8. Symptomatic congestive heart failure
9. Third-degree heart block
10. Active pericarditis or myocarditis
11. Recent embolism
12. Thrombophlebitis
13. Resting ST displacement (greater than 3 mm)
14. Uncontrolled diabetes
15. Orthopedic problems that would prohibit exercise

Reprinted with permission from Wilson WK, Winga ER, Edgett JW, et al. *Policies and Procedures of a Cardiac Rehabilitation Program: Intermediate to Long-Term Care.* Philadelphia, Pa: Lea & Febiger; 1978.

People at higher risk are those with at least one major coronary risk factor and/or symptoms suggestive of cardiopulmonary or metabolic disease. An exercise test prior to beginning a vigorous exercise program is necessary for high-risk participants of any age. For people who are younger than 35 years and are without symptoms, an exercise test prior to beginning an exercise program may not be necessary if appropriate guidance is available and if exercise is undertaken gradually and competitive participation is avoided. If maximal

*By Patricia Peterson
†For specific guidelines for developing a community-based cardiac rehabilitation program, see Fardy PS, Yanowitz F, Wilson PK. *Cardiac Rehabilitation, Adult Fitness, and Exercise Testing.* 2nd ed. Philadelphia, Pa: Len & Febiger; 1981.

exercise tests are done under these circumstances, a physician should be present. Submaximal exercise tests are of little diagnostic use in this population, but if such tests are done it is not necessary to have a physician present if the patient is younger than 35 and has no symptoms of heart disease. Persons with symptoms suggestive of coronary, pulmonary, or metabolic disease should have a physician-supervised maximum exercise test prior to beginning a vigorous exercise program at any age.

Table 12.5
Medical History—Areas of Assessment

This is the most important part of the evaluation. Individuals should be questioned about a history of the following:

- Heart attack, coronary bypass, or other cardiac surgery
- Chest discomfort—especially with exertion
- High blood pressure
- Extra, skipped, or rapid heart beats/palpitations
- Heart murmurs, clicks, or unusual cardiac findings
- Rheumatic fever
- Ankle swelling
- Peripheral vascular disease
- Phlebitis, emboli
- Unusual shortness of breath
- Lightheadedness or fainting
- Pulmonary disease including asthma, emphysema, and bronchitis
- Abnormal blood lipids
- Diabetes
- Stroke
- Emotional disorders
- Medications of all types
- Recent illness, hospitalization, or surgical procedure
- Drug allergies
- Orthopedic problems, arthritis
- Family* history should be evaluated for the following:
    - Coronary disease—at what age
    - Sudden death—at what age
    - Congenital heart disease
- Other diet habits:
    - Caffeine including cola drinks
    - Alcohol
    - Tobacco
    - Other unusual habits or dieting
    - Exercise history with information on habitual level of activity:
        - type of exercise, frequency, duration, and intensity

*Family includes grandparents, parents, aunts, uncles, and siblings.
Reprinted with permission from American College of Sports Medicine. *Guidelines for Exercise Testing and Prescription.* 3rd ed. Philadelphia, Pa: Lea & Febiger; 1986.

People at any age with known cardiovascular pulmonary or metabolic disease should have an exercise test prior to beginning vigorous exercise. This is important not only to assess the safety of vigorous exercise, but to measure functional capacity so that progress can be monitored. Exercise testing in this group is valuable in establishing a prognosis and in making decisions about the need for further evaluation or intervention. A physician should be present.[3] *Table12.4* describes contraindications for entry into inpatient and outpatient programs.

The major components of the patient-selection evaluation process in a cardiac rehabilitation program are medical history (*Table 12.5*), physical examination (*Table 12.6*), and laboratory tests. Recommended laboratory tests include a plasma lipid and lipoprotein profile, complete blood count, submaximal treadmill test, and an ECG.

Table 12.6
Physical Examination—Areas of Assessment

A limited physical examination is useful to specifically assess:

- Presence of any acute illness
- Weight/body composition
- Orthopedic problems including arthritis

Most significant noncardiac problems which might influence exercise testing and prescription will be identified through the medical history. Areas of possible concern revealed by the history should be evaluated in the physical examination.

Cardiovascular evaluation: The following evaluation is recommended prior to exercise testing. If a physician is present, this evaluation can easily be completed in minutes. If the evaluation is being conducted without the presence of a physician, then as much of the evaluation that can be carried out competently should be performed.

- Pulse rate and regularity
- Blood pressure: supine, sitting, and standing
- Auscultation of the lungs with specific attention to rales, wheezes, rhonchi, and uniformity of breath sounds in all areas
- Palpation for carotid, femoral, and pedal pulses and for cardiac impulse and thrills
- Auscultation of the heart with specific attention to murmurs, gallops, clicks, and rubs
- Carotid, abdominal, or femoral bruits
- Edema
- Xanthoma and xanthelasma

Reprinted with permission from American College of Sports Medicine. *Guidelines for Exercise Testing and Prescription.* 3rd ed. Philadelphia, Pa: Lea & Febiger; 1986.

CARDIAC REHABILITATION COMMITTEE OR ADVISORY BOARD*

Personnel and rehabilitation activities are under the direction of a committee or advisory board that meets periodically to review objectives and services (*Table 12.7*). Emphasis is on an interdisciplinary approach, with team members contributing to daily care and weekly department conferences. Allied health personnel are given a strong role in direct patient care.

The number of team members as well as the role and function of each may vary from center to center. Some facilities may have one person performing more than one function. In all cases, primary patient care remains the responsibility of the referring physician. The team members identified here represent only a suggested model. The composition of the team will vary depending on organizational needs.

*By Patricia Peterson

Table 12.7 Cardiac Rehabilitation Committee or Advisory Board, Members and Duties

The membership shall include:

- At least three staff physicians who are cardiologists or internists with a special interest in rehabilitation and exercise physiology
- The medical director
- A representative from the institution's administration

The role of the committee or board shall be to establish policies and guidelines for the center. It must meet periodically to review the objectives, policies, and services of the center.

Medical director. Typically a cardiologist or internist with a special interest in exercise physiology, the medical director is in charge of the patient during the program. He or she prescribes successive steps in the rehabilitation process within the structure of the program, works with and uses the services of other team members, receives reports at successive stages of the program, and attends weekly ward rounds and monthly conferences.

Program director. This person has a degree in exercise physiology or physical therapy or is a registered nurse, is primarily responsible for the overall effectiveness and safety of the program, and is a member of the cardiac rehabilitation committee or advisory board. The program director should be skilled in personnel management, exercise techniques, arrhythmias, and cardiopulmonary resusitation. A person who is skilled in marketing and public speaking and involved with community programs will help insure the program's success.

The program director coordinates patients' admission to the program; oversees the inpatient and outpatient personnel and facilities; works with the medical director and committee and keeps them informed of progress and problems; instructs other team members in managing arrhythmias and giving CPR; monitors techniques; provides continuing-education programs; provides patient and family education; assists exercise technicians in monitoring cardiac patients when desirable for the safety of the patients; maintains accurate records of inpatient and outpatient services; and periodically reviews all active inpatient and outpatient records to assure that patients are receiving the prescribed program and have no complications.

Cardiovascular nurse coordinator. A registered nurse, the cardiovascular nurse coordinator is knowledgeable in exercise physiology, monitoring equipment, and arrhythmia recognition, as well as the intensive care of the inpatient. Primarily involved with coronary artery bypass graft patients from admission, the coordinator does presurgery teaching and coordinates patient care. By working closely with the referring physician, cardiologist, and surgeon, the coordinator insures that the patient receives maximum benefits from the program.[7]

Clinical psychologist. A professional skilled in behavioral evaluation and counseling techniques, the clinical psychologist is familiar with coping mechanisms, family interaction patterns, and available community resources. (For Medicare payments, Title XXII of the Social Security Act requires a graduate of an accredited master of social work program affiliated with the center.) The psychologist identifies psychosocial factors that may limit recovery; assesses the patient's and family's premorbid and present coping abilities; provides supportive counseling to the patient and his or her family in such areas as self-image, sexual functioning, and vocational goals; counsels patients in useful behavior changes; assists in vocational rehabilitation counseling; participates in team conferences; and keeps progress notes on each patient.

Registered dietitian. A professional knowledgeable in nutrition assessment and dietary counseling, planning, and modification, the registered dietitian works with the attending physician in providing the appropriate diet during hospitalization. He or she reviews the patient's chart and interviews the patient and interested family members for dietary history and factors affecting nutritional status; completes and implements a nutrition assessment and nutrition care plan for and with the patient; prepares appropriate nutrition-education talks to be given during the cardiac rehabilitation session; and works with all team members to promote good nutrition practices of the patients.

The registered dietitian in a cardiac rehabilitation program has many responsibilities. The most obvious is that of a nutrition educator. In this capacity, the registered dietitian becomes involved with each participant in the nutrition care process. Follow-up is scheduled on the basis of need; however, a four- or six-month follow-up should be part of the nutrition intervention to assure compliance and, more important, to provide feedback. Apart from the initial and follow-up nutrition assessment conducted with each cardiac rehabilitation participant, the registered dietitian provides nutrition education to the organization via small group sessions. These "minilectures" can be conducted before or after a participant's scheduled exercise sessions.

In addition to providing nutrition education, the registered dietitian must be skilled in marketing, psychology, sociology, and communications. Expertise in these areas is important when dietitians assume nutrition-counseling responsibilities. The goal of nutrition in a cardiac rehabilitation program should focus on the process of nutrition education. As such, the registered dietitian will recognize that compliance with new dietary recommendations does not occur immediately. Rather, compliance occurs over time and is dependent on each person's readiness to make changes.[8] Perhaps the most important issue in cardiac rehabilitation nutrition counseling is to encourage participants to make dietary changes gradually. In addition, participants should be encouraged to focus on only one nutrition behavior change at a time. Obviously, the most important dietary issues for individual patients should be addressed first. If the decision is to concentrate on reducing intake of dietary saturated fat, then the dietitian develops participant behavioral goals based solely around that larger goal. This approach gives the participant just one change to implement. One dietary change will be perceived to be reasonable and less threatening or disruptive than multiple changes and expectations.

It is the dietitian's responsibility to support the process of nutrition change and to provide guidance through nutrition education. The following ideas are a sample of some nutrition-education activities that could be offered in a cardiac rehabilitation program.

ACTIVITIES FOR A CARDIAC REHABILITATION PROGRAM*

Start a newsletter. This communication tool can provide a route for nutrition articles relevant to CHD. Recipes can be included, participants who are losing weight might have a support-group column, and community nutrition and exercise events (such as a local jogging or walking event or a restaurant that has added healthy entrees to its menu) could be publicized.

*By Kristine Clark

Establish set times for group nutrition presentations. These talks should be short, 10 to 15 minutes. One basic topic should be identified and discussed without the use of biochemical or other scientific jargon. The participants should have an objective for listening (a learner behavioral objective should be preestablished by the dietitian). A pretest or posttest is an important way of documenting participation in the activity as well as assessing the participants' acquisition of knowledge. Examples of topics that could be discussed include:

- Oat bran versus wheat bran
- Saturated fat
- Polyunsaturated fat
- Monounsaturated fat
- Use of dried beans
- Use of dried fruit
- Use of egg substitutes
- Use of soy products such as tofu
- Various frozen desserts
- Tropical oils
- Quick snacks
- How to pack a nutritious brown-bag lunch
- Low-calorie beverages
- Niacin
- Recipe modification
- Artificial fats
- Low-sodium products
- Alternative spices
- Caffeine
- Fads, such as garlic
- Fish oils and fish
- National Cholesterol Education Program
- What is cholesterol (HDL versus LDL)?
- What are triglycerides?
- Low-fat cheeses
- Label reading

Become familiar with new low-fat, low-cholesterol products. Obtain brochures on the products for educating participants. Write for samples and let participants taste new foods.

Provide recipes. Begin a recipe bulletin board for participants to exchange low-fat or low-cholesterol ideas. A participant could be delegated to keep it functioning and neat.

Schedule a guest speaker. Ask the assigned physician if he or she would discuss the use of niacin for cardiac patients.

Have a booth at community nutrition or exercise events. This is a prime opportunity to promote the dietitian's position within the cardiac rehabilitation program and to provide nutrition information to potential participants.

Other team members are occupational therapists, physical therapists, and exercise physiologists, professionals knowledgeable in exercise physiology, exercise techniques, activity levels, monitoring equipment, arrhythmia recognition, and CPR (including defibrillation).

These staff members are the core of the program, providing direct patient care thoughout all phases of the program. They perform and interpret physiologic assessments; monitor exercises and activities according to the patients' responses within prescribed levels; monitor and report patients' progress in the exercise program; provide evaluation and recommendations for patients' self-care activities; and instruct patients on how to take their pulse, monitor their symptoms, and adjust their activities.

ADMINISTRATIVE AND FINANCIAL STRATEGIES*

An organizational structure such as the one shown in *Figure 12.2* provides a clear delineation of financial and administrative responsibilities versus medical management and intervention responsibilities. This is an important concept, because many programs have definite medical as well as administrative needs and concerns.

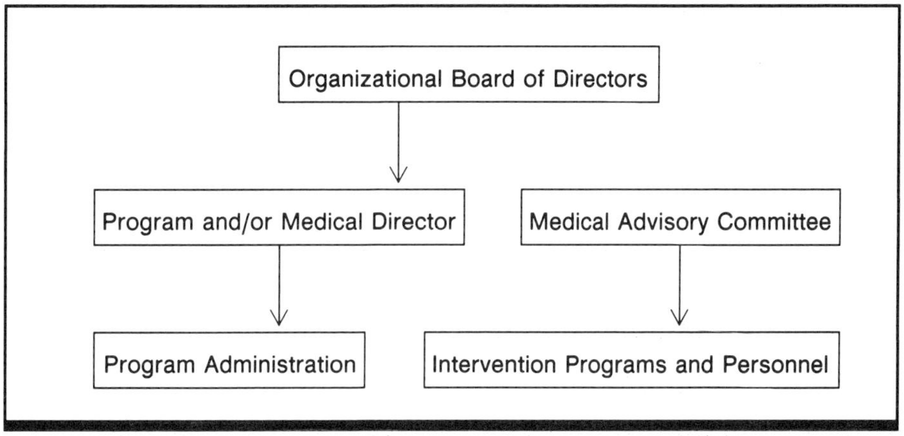

Fig. 12.2
Cardiac rehabilitation program organizational structure. Reprinted with permission from American Heart Association. **Guidelines for Cardiac Rehabilitation.** ***Los Angeles, Calif; 1978.***

An effective line of communication is necessary between the medical director and program director and the program administrator because of their contribution to the growth of the organization and the cardiac rehabilitation program. Many other organizational patterns are possible. It is important to have clear lines of accountability, an overall medical direction, and clearly delineated areas of responsibility.

Effective program administration is enhanced through well-defined organizational relationships that clearly identify specific personnel responsibilities and sources of authority. Ultimate accountability for the program should rest with a governing body or advisory committee comprising appropriate professionals who contribute their collective knowledge to the program. This governing body should include health educators, attorneys, insurance experts, business and accounting advisors, and local health agency representatives. The policies and procedures adopted by this body provide the guidelines for the development and operation of the exercise program and the delegation of responsibilities to appropriate administrators. Program guidelines should be reviewed and updated on an annual basis to integrate new techniques and delete apparently ineffective segments of the program. Five-year program goals and objectives should be written to prepare for future growth and program changes.[4]

The position of program director requires training and experience in leadership, planning, delegation of authority, and assumption of responsibility. The effective administrator has a broad academic understanding and insight into human relationships, practical intelligence, and a strong commitment to exercise program goals.

Financial Strategies

Income and expenditure accounting procedures are established within guidelines determined by the program governing board. A board member with

*By Patricia Peterson

accounting capabilities will facilitate a development of practical policies. Some financial planning is assured by a realistic and accurate appraisal of conditions affecting the program. Budget development should follow a reasonable sequence that includes inventory, staff input, analysis and review, submission and approval, revision, direct and indirect expense-revenue projection, and budget administration. Regular income sources must be managed carefully to ensure a consistent cash flow in balance with projected expenses.

Table 12.8
Sample Informed Consent Form

Informed Consent for Exercise Treatment

I desire to engage voluntarily in the Cardiac Rehabilitation Program in order to improve my cardiovascular function. This program has been recommended to me by my physician, Dr. ___________.

Before I enter this exercise program I will have a clinical evaluation. This evaluation will include a medical history, physical examination, resting ECG and graded exercise test. The purpose of this evaluation is to detect any condition which would indicate that I should not engage in this exercise program.

The program will follow an exercise prescription approved by the Medical Director and will be carefully followed by the supervisor of the exercise program. The amount of exercise will be regulated on the basis of my tolerance. I shall exercise only under the supervision of a qualified supervisor.

The activities are designed to place a gradually increasing workload on the circulation and thereby to improve its function. The reaction of the cardiovascular system to such activities cannot be predicted with complete accuracy. There is the risk of certain changes occurring during or following the exercise. These changes include abnormalities of blood pressure or heart rate, or ineffective "heart function," and in rare instances "heart attacks" or "cardiac arrest."

Before starting the program I will be instructed as to, and will understand, the signs and symptoms which I would report promptly to the supervisor of the exercises and which will alert me to modify my activities.

Every effort will be made to avoid such events by the preliminary examination and by observation during the exercise. Emergency equipment and trained personnel are available to deal with and minimize the dangers of untoward events should they occur.

I have read the foregoing and I understand it. Any questions that have arisen or occurred to me have been answered to my satisfaction.

Date ___________________

Patient Signature ___________________

Witness ___________________

Reprinted with permission from Wilson WK, Winga ER, Edgett JW, et al. *Policies and Procedures of a Cardiac Rehabilitation Program: Intermediate to Long-Term Care.* Philadelphia, Pa: Lea & Febiger; 1978.

The major source of income for preventive and rehabilitative exercise programs is through participant fees. These exercise programs should use written materials that explain the program fees to the participant, referring physician, and the insurance carriers prior to enrollment. Medicare, Medicaid, and vocational rehabilitation agencies should be considered as alternative income sources and developed and utilized. Such income may be reserved for research, capital expenditures, and contingencies. Line-item accountability is the most accurate method of bookkeeping and, with standard record-keeping practices, it provides reliable data for future financial planning.

Legal Considerations

It is essential that approved procedures are developed through a careful study of national and local practices with the guidance of medical and legal advisors to provide the best standards of reasonable and prudent care. Constant monitoring of personnel, activity selection, and environmental conditions, along with regular in-service staff training, should be provided within these standards. Specific policies for protection of the rights, confidentiality, and safety of patients must be developed and understood by all staff members. Such policies include, but are not limited to, obtaining informed consent (the basis of which provides documentation of the voluntary assumption of risk by the participant; *Tables 12.8* and *12.9*) and developing standing orders for emergency procedures. All such policies should be presented to those who enter the program in written form prior to their participation. Guidelines for safe exercise, exercise prescription, early warning signs of impending heart attack, and facility rules and regulations are a few items that can be covered in a participant handbook.

Table 12.9
Safety Equipment for Exercise Programs

Emergency equipment

- Defibrillation—portable Lifepak by Physiocontrol
- Emergency medications and means of parental administration
- Oxygen, airways, artificial respiration

Emergency procedure

- Availability of trained physician
- Immedicate application of AHA-approved CPR measures for cardiac assist.
- Facilities for direct hospitalization and follow-up cardiac monitor through critical periods

Reprinted with permission from American Heart Association. *Guidelines for Cardiac Rehabilitation.* Los Angeles, Calif; 1978.

Administrators must be aware that state statutes that govern the practice of medicine are generally restrictive, vary widely in scope and, if violated, can result in lawsuits. Self-protective procedures include: in-service training to be informed on current accepted procedures;[1] employing certified or licensed staff (all medical supervisory staff should be certified in advanced cardiac life support or the equivalent and nonmedical supervisory staff should be certified in basic life support as designated by the American Heart Association or the equivalent);[2] recertifying personnel periodically;[3] and securing satisfactory limits of liability insurance.[4] Written documentation of problems and staff recommendations are a necessary part of good medical management and legal coverage. All such documentations should be filed and kept per state requirement.

Careful screening and monitoring of participants and the written documentation of procedures provides for a safe and "legal" program (see Table 12.8).

Reimbursement and Documentation

Guidelines for obtaining reimbursement of payment for cardiac rehabilitation generally include[9]: the facility must meet certain requirements for location, space, safety, etc; the services to be covered are specifically outlined; certain procedures are followed for filing claims; medical necessity is documented and reviewed by a utilization committee.

Table 12.10
Cardiac Rehabilitation Progress Report

TO: ______________________________ MD   DATE: ______________________________

RE: ______________________________   STARTING DATE: ______________________________

This is a monthly progress report concerning the regular participation of this patient in the New England Center for Health Promotion. These sessions meet three times per week for 1 hour of exercise.

ATTENDANCE: From __________ To __________

- Total Number of Exercise Sessions __________
- Exercise Sessions Attended __________
- Reason(s) for Absence ______________________________
- Extracurricular Exercise Participation ______________________________

EXERCISE PRESCRIPTION:

- Prescribed Target Heart Rate __________
- Resting Heart Rate __________
- Average Exercise Heart Rate __________
- Resting Blood Pressure __________
- Average Exercise Blood Pressure __________

Mode/Duration: Calisthenics ______ Treadmill ______ Bicycle ______
Arm Ergometer ______ Rowing ______ Nautilus ______

Average Training MET Level __________ METs

WEIGHT MANAGEMENT/CONTROL:

- Initial Weight __________
- Desirable Weight __________
- Present Weight __________

COMMENTS:

Reprinted with permission from New England Center for Health Promotion—Cardiac Rehabilitation Program.

Program Coverage*

Currently most major medical insurances and health maintenance organizations (HMOs) cover cardiac rehabilitation for three visits per week for 12 weeks, with a maximum of 36 visits. However, coverage is constantly changing and is determined according to the patient's condition, diagnoses, and any new complications that occur during cardiac rehabilitation. The number of medical conditions that would qualify for cardiac rehabilitation are increasing, although there has been discussion of limiting phase II rhythm-monitored sessions to just six to eight weeks. Patients should investigate what their individual insurance will cover.

Medicare. As many as three cardiac rehabilitation visits are allowed per week over a 12-week period (procedure code W9007). Patients must begin rehabilitation within eight weeks of discharge. Coverage for continued participation in the cardiac exercise programs beyond 12 weeks is allowed only on a case-by-case basis, up to the maximum of 36 visits.

Claims should list the referring and supervising physicians and the date of the coronary event. The initial comprehensive office visit can be claimed at the beginning of the program if the evaluation has not already been completed by the referring physician. The ECG stress test can be claimed along with the initial evaluation. The claim should list the start and end date of the program. Documentation is made on forms such as the one in *Table12.10.*

References

1. Pollock ML, Peis AE. Exercise prescription for the cardiac patient. In: Franklin BA, Rubenfire M, eds. *Cardiac Rehabilitation.* Philadelphia, Pa: WB Saunders Co; 1984.
2. Wenger NK, Hellerstein HK. *Rehabilitation of the Coronary Patient.* New York, NY: John Wiley & Sons; 1978.
3. American Heart Association. *Guidelines for Cardiac Rehabilitation.* Los Angeles, Calif; 1978.
4. Wilson WK, Winga ER, Edgett JW, et al. *Policies and Procedures of a Cardiac Rehabilitation Program: Intermediate to Long-Term Care.* Philadelphia, Pa: Lea & Febiger; 1978.
5. Pollock M, Foster C, Ward A. Exercise prescription for rehabilitation of the cardiac patient. In: Pollock ML, Schmidt DH, eds. *Heart Disease and Rehabilitation.* New York, NY: Churchhill-Livingstone; 1986: 480.
6. McKay-Dee Hospital Cardiac Fitness Institute. *Cardiac Rehabilitation Program.* Ogden, Utah; 1987.
7. Froelicher VF, Pollock MI. Cardiac rehabilitation programs state of the art 1983. *J Cardiac Rehab.* 1982;2:429.
8. Hochbaum GM. Strategies and their rationale for changing people's eating habits. *J Nutr Educ.* 1981;13:S59.
9. Blue Cross, Blue Shield. *Physical Reimbursement for Cardiac Rehab Programs.* Prepared by the Professional Utilization Review Department, BC, BS of Rhode Island; June 1985.
10. American College of Sports Medicine. *Guidelines for Exercise Testing and Prescription.* 3rd ed. Philadelphia, Pa: Lea & Febiger; 1986.

*By Dottie Dolezal

PART 4
ADDITIONAL INFORMATION

13. RESOURCES*

BOOKS AND PUBLICATIONS

Beyond Cholesterol: The Johns Hopkins Complete Guide for Avoiding Heart Disease
P. Kwiterovich
Johns Hopkins University Press
701 W. 40th St
Baltimore,MD 21211

Building Nutrition Counseling Skills, vol 1:
Guidebook for Workshop Planning (1984)
NIH publication 84-2661
Information Services Section
Communications and Public Information Branch
National Heart, Lung and Blood Institute
Building 31, Room 4A21
Bethesda, MD 20892

Cholesterol: Current Concepts for Clinicians (1988)
Information Center
4733 Bethesda Ave, Suite 530
Bethesda, MD 20814

Current Status of Blood Cholesterol Measurement in Clinical Laboratories in the United States: A Report from the Laboratory Standardization Panel of the National Cholesterol Education Program (1988)
NIH publication 88-2928
(same address as *Cholesterol*)

Diet and Health: Implications for Reducing Chronic Disease Risk (1989)
Committee on Diet and Health, Food and Nutrition Board,
Commission on Life Sciences, National Research Council
National Academy Press
2101 Constitution Ave, NW
Washington, DC 20418

Diet and the Prevention of Coronary Heart Disease and Cancer (1986)
B. Halgren
Raven Press
1140 Avenue of the Americas
New York, NY 10036

Every Beat of Your Heart: An Idea Book for Community Health Programs (1987)
NIH publication 87-2641
(same address as *Building Nutrition Counseling Skills*)

A Guide to Healthy Eating: What You Need to Know About Fat, Cholesterol, Fiber and Salt (1985)
M. Franz
International Diabetes Center
Park Nicollet Medical Foundation
500 W 39th St
Minneapolis, MN 55416

*By Mary E. Russell, Janine M. Hughes, and Rita Johnson

Health Implications of Obesity
National Institutes of Health
Office of Medical Applications of Research
Building 1, Room 216
Bethesda, MD 20892

The Healthy Heart Book for Women (1987)
NIH publication 87-2720
(same address as *Building Nutrition Counseling Skills*)

Heart to Heart: A Manual in Nutrition Counseling for the Reduction in Cardiovascular Disease Risk Factors (1985)
NIH publication 85-1528
(same address as *Building Nutrition Counseling Skills*)

The LEARN Program for Weight Control (1989)
K.D. Brownell
LEARN Education Center
1555 W. Mockingbird Lane
Suite 203
Dallas, TX 75235

National Guidance for Hypertensives
L. Williams
Nutrition Consulting
15348 Sandridge Rd
Bowling Green, OH 43402

NHLBI Kit '90
Manual A: Information for Program Planners
Manual B: Information for Consumers
National Heart, Lung and Blood Institute
US Dept of Health and Human Services
Public Health Service
National Institutes of Health
Building 31, Room 4A21
Bethesda, MD 20892

Non-Pharmacologic Approaches to the Control of High Blood Pressure (1986)
(same address as *Cholesterol*)

Nutrition Counseling Skills: Assessment, Treatment and Evaluation (1989), 2nd ed
L. Snetselaar
Aspen Publishers, Inc.
1600 Research Blvd
Rockville, MD 20850

Public Screening for Measuring Blood Cholesterol: Issues for Special Attention (1988)
(same address as *Cholesterol*)

The Sodium Content of Your Food
USDA Home and Garden bulletin 233
Superintendent of Documents
US Government Printing Office
Washington, DC 20402

Sports Nutrition: A Guide for the Professional Working With Active People
The American Dietetic Association
216 W. Jackson Blvd
Suite 800
Chicago, IL 60606-6995

Surgeon General's Report on Nutrition and Health
US Dept of Health and Human Services
Public Health Service publication 88-50211
US Government Printing Office
Washington, DC 20402

Client education materials:
Cholesterol Countdown
Children, Cholesterol, and Diet: Answers to Questions Parents Often Ask
Pocket Supermarket Guide
Labels: The Buyer's Guide to Healthful Foods
Why Can't I Lose Weight?
Weighty Issues: Evaluating Fad Diets
Weight Expectations
Traveling Lite: A Traveler's Guide to Healthy Eating
The Dietary Guidelines
The American Dietetic Association
216 W. Jackson Blvd
Suite 800
Chicago, IL 60606-6995

Fact Sheets on Good Sources of Nutrients
(Vitamins A, E, C, B_6, B_{12}, folate, thiamin, riboflavin, niacin, calcium, iron, magnesium, copper, zinc, phosphorous, potassium, fiber)
Superintendent of Documents
US Government Printing Office
Washington, DC 20402
Stock No. 001-000-04548-2

COOKBOOKS

American Heart Association Cookbook (1984)
David McKay Co
750 Third Ave
New York, NY 10017

Cardiac Cuisine: A Guide to Healthy Living (1988)
G. Underbakke
University of Wisconsin Press
114 N. Murray St
Madison, WI 53715

Choices for a Healthy Heart (1987)
J. Piscatella
Workman Publishers
708 Broadway
New York, NY 10003

Cooking à la Heart (1990)
Mankato Heart Health Program Foundation, Inc
L. Hachfeld and B. Eykyn
Apple Tree Press, Inc
Good Counsel Dr, Suite 125
Mankato, MN 56001

Cooking Light Cookbooks (1988)
Oxmoor House Books
500 Office Park Dr
Birmingham, AL 35223

Deliciously Simple (1986)
H. Roth
New American Library, Inc
1633 Broadway
New York, NY 10019

Eater's Choice: A Food Lover's Guide to Lower Cholesterol (1987)
S. and N. Goor
Houghton Mifflin Co
52 Vanderbilt Ave
New York, NY 10017

Family Cookbook, vols 1–3 (1987)
American Diabetes Association/
The American Dietetic Association
Prentice-Hall Inc
General Publishing Division
Englewood Cliffs, NJ 07632

The Guiltless Gourmet (1987)
International Diabetes Center
5000 W. 39th St
Minneapolis, MN 55416

Jane Brody's Good Food Book: Living the High-Carbohydrate Way (1985)
J. Brody
W. W. Norton and Co
500 Fifth Ave
New York, NY 10110

The Living Heart Diet (1984)
M. DeBakey
Raven Press
630 Fifth Ave
New York, NY 10020

Low-Fat, Low-Cholesterol Cookbook (1989)
S.M. Grundy and M. Winston
American Heart Association
7320 Greenville Ave
Dallas, TX 75231

The New American Diet (1986)
S. and W. Connor
Simon and Schuster Publishers
1230 Avenue of the Americas
New York, NY 10020

Recipes for Your Heart's Delight: The Stanford Guide to Healthy Cooking (1983)
Health Policy and Research Building, Room 8
Stanford University
Stanford, CA 94305

Salute to a Healthy Heart (1990)
Shadyside Hospital Nutrition Services
5230 Centre Ave
Pittsburgh, PA 15232

NATIONAL RESOURCES

The American Dietetic Association
216 W. Jackson Blvd
Suite 800
Chicago, IL 60606-6995
312/899-0040

American Diabetes Association
1600 Duke St
Alexandria, VA 22314
703/549-1500

American Heart Association
7320 Greenville Ave
Dallas, TX 75231
800/527-6441

American Home Economics Association
2010 Massachusetts Ave, NW
Washington, DC 20036

American Medical Association
Nutrition Information Section
535 N. Dearborn St
Chicago, IL 60610

Dept of Community Health
1075 Ste-Foy Rd
7th Floor
Quebec City, Quebec
Canada G1S-2M1

Dept of Health and Human Services
Public Health Service
Food and Drug Administration
5600 Fishers Lane
Rockville, MD 20857

Home Economics Dictorate
2nd Floor
800 Portage Ave
Winnipeg, Manitoba
Canada R3G-OP1

National Cholesterol Education Program
National Heart, Lung and Blood Institute
National Institutes of Health
9000 Rockville Pike
Bethesda, MD 20892

National Heart, Lung and Blood Institute
National Institutes of Health
Building 31, Room 4A21
9000 Rockville Pike
Bethesda, MD 20892
301/496-4236

National High Blood Pressure Education Program
National Heart, Lung and Blood Institute
120/80 National Institutes of Health
Bethesda, MD 20892
301/496-1809

National Institute of Diabetes, Digestive, and Kidney Diseases
9000 Rockville Pike
Building 31, Room 9A04
Bethesda, MD 20892
301/496-3583

National Institutes of Health
9000 Rockville Pike
Bethesda, MD 20892
301/496-4000

Office of Disease Prevention and Health Promotion
Health Information Center
PO Box 1133
Washington, DC 20013
800/366-4797

Public Health Resource Service
15 Overlea Blvd
5th Floor
Toronto, Ontario
Canada M4H-1A9

INDUSTRY SOURCES

Abbott Laboratories
Abbott Park, IL 60064

American Egg Board/
United Egg Producers
Egg Nutrition Center
2501 M Street, NW, Room 410
Washington, DC 20037

American Soybean Association
PO Box 27300
St Louis, MO 63141
314/432-1600

Bertolli Olive Oil
1 Harmon Plaza
Secaucus, NJ 07096

Best Foods
CPC International
International Plaza
Englewood Cliffs, NJ 07623

Bristol-Myers
US Pharmaceutical and National Group
Evansville, IN 47721

Campbell's Soup Co
Home Economics Dept
375 Memorial Ave
Camden, NJ 08101
609/342-4825

Fleischmann's
PO Box 2695
Grand Central Station
New York, NY 10012

Frito-Lay, Inc
7701 Legacy Dr
Plano, TX 75024
214/353-2000

General Foods
Consumer Center
250 North St
White Plains, NY 10600

General Mills
Nutrition Dept
Dept 45
PO Box 1112
Minneapolis, MN 55440
612/540-2311

The Potato Board
1385 S. Colorado Blvd
Suite 512
Denver, CO 80222

McDonald's
McDonald's Plaza
Oakbrook, IL 60521
708/887-6198

National Sunflower Association
4023 N. State St
Bismarck, ND 58501

Procter and Gamble Co
Educational Materials Dept
301 E. 6th St
PO Box 599
Cincinnati, OH 45202
800/543-7276

Quaker Oats Consumer Affairs Center
PO Box 9001
Chicago, IL 60604-9001
312/222-8700

Safeway Stores, Inc
430 Jackson St
Oakland, CA 94660
415/891-3000

National Dairy Council
6300 N. River Rd
Rosemont, IL 60018-4233

Wheat Flour Institute
600 Maryland Ave
Washington, DC 20024

Kellogg Company
Dept of Home Economics
Battle Creek, MI 49016

NUTRITION RESOURCE CENTERS

Center for Science in the Public Interest
1501 16th St, NW
Washington, DC 20036-1499

Food and Nutrition Information Center
National Agricultural Library
10301 Baltimore Blvd
Room 304
Beltsville, MD 20705
301/334-3719

National Center for Nutrition and Dietetics, the Public Education Initiative of The American Dietetic Association and Its Foundation
Nutrition Resource Dept
216 W. Jackson Blvd
Chicago, IL 60606-6995
312/899-0040, ext 4854

Nutrition Information Service
University of Alabama at Birmingham
Webb Building
Room 101
Birmingham, AL 35294
205/934-3923

Nutrition Information Service
Ryerson Polytechnical Institute
50 Gould St
Room 2955
Toronto, Ontario, Canada M5B-1E8
416/595-5428

Penn State Nutrition Center
Penn State University
Benedict House
University Park, PA 16802
814/865-6323

Society for Nutrition Education
1736 Franklin St
9th Floor
Oakland, CA 94612
415/444-7133

Stanford University Hospital
Department of Dietetics
Room P1070
Stanford, CA 94305-5223
415/723-6904

SELECTED READINGS

The American Dietetic Association. Health implications of dietary fiber —technical support paper. *J Am Diet Assoc.* 1988;88:217.

American Heart Association Nutrition Committee and The Council on Arteriosclerosis. Recommendations for treatment of hyperlipidemia in adults. *Circulation.* 1984;69:1065A.

Grundy SM. Cholesterol and coronary heart disease, a new era. *JAMA.* 1986;256:2849-2858.

Kinsella JE. Food lipids and fatty acids: importance in food quality, nutrition and health. *Food Tech.* 1988;42:124-145.

Kris-Etherton PM, Krummel D, Russell M, et al. The effect of diet on plasma lipids, lipoproteins and coronary heart disease. *J Am Diet Assoc.* 1988;88:1373-1400.

National Cholesterol Education Program Expert Panel. Report on detection, evaluation and treatment of high blood cholesterol in adults. *Arch Intern Med.* 1988;148:36–69.

Rifai N. Lipoproteins and apolipoproteins. *Arch Pathol Lab Med.* 1986; 110:694-701.

Rock CL, Coulston AM. Weight-control approaches: a review by the California Dietetic Association. *J Am Diet Assoc.* 1988;88:44.

Steinberg D. Lipoproteins and the pathogenesis of artherosclerosis. *Circulation.* 1987;76:508-514.

EDUCATIONAL MATERIALS

Cholesterol Countdown
46 Stoneham Rd
Rochester, NY 14625

Cholesterol Counts—A Course to Promote Good Health with Good Food
Health Sciences Center for Educational Resources
Distribution Center, SB-56
University of Washington
Seattle, WA 98195

Cholesterol and Your Health (video)
Iowa State University
Media Resource Center
121 Pearson
Ames, IA 50011
515/294-8022

Cooking Without Your Salt Shaker, 1988
American Heart Association
7320 Greenville Ave
Dallas, TX 75231
800/527-6441

Dietary Treatment for Hypercholesterolemia: A Handbook for Counselors, 1988
American Heart Association
7320 Greenville Ave
Dallas, TX 75231
800/527-6441

Dietary Treatment for Hypercholesterolemia: A Manual for Patients, 1988
American Heart Association
7320 Greenville Ave
Dallas, TX 75231
800/527-6441

Eater's Choice
Cholesterol Treatment Program
Health Prospects
1801 Rockville Pike
Suite 550
Rockville, MD 20852

Healthy Dividends: A Do-It-Yourself Approach to Lowering Fat for Life
National Dairy Council
6300 N. River Rd
Rosemont, IL 60018-4233
708/696-1020

Healthy Dividends: Leader's Guide
National Dairy Council
6300 N. River Rd
Rosemont, IL 60018-4233

HeartCare Program Videos
Hall-Foushee Productions, Inc
1313 5th St SE
Suite 215A
Minneapolis, MN 55414
612/379-3829

Heart Healthy (video)
Penn State Audio-Visual Services
Special Services Building
University Park, PA 16802
800/826-0132

The Heart Wise Nutrition Program
463 Water St
Indiana, PA 15701

Lean Life Food Series and *The Lowdown on Cholesterol*
Nutrivisuals
PO Box 1367
Shingle Springs, CA 95682

Lofat Lifeline Publications
Dept 302
52 Condolea Ct
Lake Oswego, OR 97035

Lower Your Cholesterol Now! (video)
Family Experiences Productions, Inc
1509 Old W. 38th St
Suite 4
Austin, TX 78731

Patti's Plate Works
Sturgess PG
PO Box 20042
Englewood, CO 80110

Supermarket Savvy (video)
Family Experiences Productions, Inc
PO Box 5150805
Addison, TX 75251-5805
214/363-3996

Take Part for a Healthy Heart (video)
Penn State Nutrition Center
Ruth Building
University Park, PA 16802
814/865-6325

SOFTWARE REFERENCES

Annual Manual of Dietetic Software
Box 2565
Norman, OK 73070
405/360-5554

Nutrient Data Book Directory, 7th ed, 1988
L. Hoover, editor
University of Missouri-Columbia
Dept of Human Nutrition
Foods and Food Systems Management
College of Home Economics
217 Gwynn Hall
Columbia, MO 65211

SCAN's Software Resource Manual
SCAN
c/o Joanne Milkereit
7 Pitt St
Charleston, SC 29401
803/792-3100

NEWSLETTERS AND PERIODICALS

American Institute for Cancer Research Newsletter
American Institute for Cancer Research
500 N. Washington
Suite 100
Falls Church, VA 22046-3535

Ardell Wellness Report
D. Ardell, editor
University of Central Florida
Health Resource Center
Orlando, FL 32816

Contemporary Nutrition
G. Florey, editor
General Mills, Inc
PO Box 5588
Stacey, MN 55079

Cooking Light Magazine
PO Box 830549
Birmingham, AL 35282-9810

Current Diet Review
L.T. Harris, publisher
PO Box 1914
Rialto, CA 92376

Dairy Council Digest and
Dairy Council News and Views
National Dairy Council
6300 N. River Rd
Rosemont, IL 60018-4233

Dietetic Currents
J.D. Gussler, editor
Ross Laboratories
625 Cleveland Ave
Columbus, OH 43216

Environmental Nutrition
B. Goldblatt, publisher
2112 Broadway
Suite 200
New York, NY 10023

Food Facts for Dietitians
3535 Olentangy River Rd
Riverside Methodist Hospital
Columbus, OH 43214

Food Insight—Current Topics in Food Safety and Nutrition
International Food Information Council
1331 Pennsylvania Ave, NW
Suite 717
Washington, DC 20004

Food News for Consumers and
FDA Consumer
USDA
Superintendent of Documents
US Government Printing Office
Washington, DC 20402

Food and Nutrition News
E.M. Urenos, editor
National Live Stock and Meat Board
444 N. Michigan Ave
Chicago, IL 60611

Healthline
The C. V. Mosby Company
Attn: Circulation Dept
11830 Westline Industrial Dr
St Louis, MO 63146-9988

Health and Obesity (formerly the *International Obesity Newsletter*)
Rte 1, Box 6A
Hettinger, ND 58639

In Health (formerly *Hippocrates—The Magazine of Health and Medicine*)
PO Box 56963
Boulder, CO 80322-6863

Lowfat Lifeline
V. Parker, editor
52 Condolea Ct
Lake Oswego, OR 97033-1002

Nutrition Action Healthletter
Center for Science in the Public Interest
1501 16th St, NW
Washington, DC 20036-1499

Nutrition Clinics
George F. Stickley Co
210 W. Washington Sq
Philadelphia, PA 19106

Nutrition Forum
S. Barrett, editor
George F. Stickley Co
210 W. Washington Sq
Philadelphia, PA 19106

Nutrition and the MD
PO Box 2160
Van Nuys, CA 91405

Nutrition Today
H. Guthrie, editor
Williams & Wilkins
428 E. Preston St
Baltimore, MD 21202

Sports Medicine Digest
PO Box 2468
Van Nuys, CA 91404

Sports Nutrition News
J. Fishman, editor
PO Box 986
Evanston, IL 60204

Sports Science Exchange
Gatorade Sports Science Institute
PO Box 9005
Chicago, IL 60604-9005

Tufts University Diet and Nutrition Newsletter
PO Box 57957
Boulder, CO 80233-7857

University of California–Berkeley Wellness Letter
PO Box 10922
Des Moines, IA 50340

The University of Texas Lifetime Health Letter
PO Box 53819
Boulder, CO 80321

VNIS (Vitamin Nutrition Information Service)
Hoffman-LaRoche
340 Kingsland Ave
Nutley, NJ 07110

CHD- OR HYPERTENSION-RELATED CURRICULAR ACTIVITIES FOR CHILDREN AND ADOLESCENTS

A Dietary Alteration Program Trial (A.D.A.P.T.): Sodium Sense Curriculum Guide (1988)
Grades: 4–6
Louisiana State University
Medical Center
1542 Tulane Ave
New Orleans, LA 70112-2822

Eat, Think & Be Healthy! Creative Nutrition Activities for Children (1987)
Ages: 8–12 years
Center for Science in the Public Interest
1501 16th St, NW
Washington, DC 20036-1499

Food. . . Your Choice/Science (1981)
Grades: 7–10
National Dairy Council
6300 N. River Rd
Rosemont, IL 60018-4233

Heart Health Education of the Young (1983)
Grades: K–12
American Heart Association
7320 Greenville Ave
Dallas, TX 75231

The Heart Treasure Chest (1985)
Grades: Preschool, kindergarten
American Heart Association
7320 Greenville Ave
Dallas, TX 75231

Hearty Heart and Friends (1983)
Grades: Elementary
Minnesota Heart Health Project
Division of Epidemiology
University of Minnesota
Minneapolis, MN 55455

Know Your Body (1978)
Grades: Elementary; junior, senior high school
American Health Foundation
320 E. 43rd St
New York, NY 10019

New Horizons in Nutrition (1980)
Grades: Junior, senior high school
Luzerne Intermediate Unit 18
368 Tioga Ave
Kingston, PA 18704

Nutrition for Life (1987)
Grades: 7, 8
Division of Nutritional Sciences
Cornell University
Ithaca, NY 14853

Peanut Butter and Pickles (1981)
Grades: Elementary
California State Department of Education
Humboldt County
Office of Education/Nutrition Education Program
901 Myrtle Ave
Eureka, CA 95501

Putting Your Heart Into the Curriculum (1982)
Grades: K–12
American Heart Association
7320 Greenville Ave
Dallas, TX 75231

Your Heart and Its Future (1984)
Grades: High school
American Heart Association
7320 Greenville Ave
Dallas, TX 75231

14. APPENDIX

CONTENTS

Table 14.1
Plasma Total-Cholesterol (mg/dL) Population Distribution

	White Males							White Females						
	Percentile							Percentile						
Age yr	5	10	25	50	75	90	95	5	10	25	50	75	90	95
0–4	—	125	—	151	—	186	—	—	120	—	156	—	189	—
5–9	125	131	141	153	168	183	189	131	136	151	164	176	190	197
10–14	124	131	144	160	173	188	202	125	131	142	159	171	191	205
15–19	124	123	136	152	168	183	191	118	126	140	157	176	198	207
20–24	118	126	142	159	179	197	212	121	132	147	165	186	220	237
25–29	130	137	154	176	199	223	234	130	142	158	178	198	217	231
30–34	142	152	171	190	213	237	258	133	141	158	178	199	215	228
35–39	147	157	176	195	222	248	267	139	149	165	186	209	233	249
40–44	150	160	179	204	229	251	260	146	156	172	193	220	241	259
45–49	163	171	188	210	235	258	275	148	162	182	204	231	256	268
50–54	157	168	189	211	237	263	274	153	171	188	214	250	267	281
55–59	161	172	188	214	236	260	280	167	182	201	229	251	278	294
60–64	163	170	191	215	237	262	287	172	186	207	226	251	282	300
65–69	166	174	192	213	250	275	288	167	179	212	233	259	282	291
70+	155	160	185	214	236	253	265	173	181	196	226	249	268	280

Adapted from *The Lipid Research Clinics Population Studies Data Book*. 1980;1. US Dept of Health and Human Services publication NIH 80-1527.

Table 14.2
Plasma VLDL-Cholesterol (mg/dL) Population Distribution

	White Males							White Females						
	Percentile							Percentile						
Age yr	5	10	25	50	75	90	95	5	10	25	50	75	90	95
0–4	—	—	—	—	—	—	—	—	—	—	—	—	—	—
5–9	0	2	4	7	11	15	18	1	1	4	9	13	19	24
10–14	1	2	5	9	13	18	22	2	3	6	10	15	20	23
15–19	2	3	8	12	17	23	26	2	3	6	11	15	22	24
20–24	1	5	8	12	18	24	28	2	4	8	13	18	24	28
25–29	3	6	8	15	22	31	36	2	3	6	11	19	24	29
30–34	1	5	8	12	18	24	28	1	3	6	11	17	21	27
35–39	3	7	12	19	30	46	56	2	3	8	13	21	29	36
40–44	5	8	14	21	30	43	56	3	5	8	13	20	28	32
45–49	5	8	13	20	31	40	51	2	4	9	15	22	33	41
50–54	8	10	14	23	33	49	62	2	5	9	15	23	32	37
55–59	3	6	11	19	28	39	49	2	4	9	18	28	37	49
60–64	3	4	9	16	23	35	44	1	3	6	13	20	29	39
65–69	0	3	8	16	23	40	45	0	3	7	13	21	36	41
70+	0	3	7	15	23	31	38	0	1	6	13	19	32	48

Adapted from *The Lipid Research Clinics Population Studies Data Book*. 1980;1. US Dept of Health and Human Services publication NIH 80-1527.

Table 14.3
Plasma LDL-Cholesterol (mg/dL) Population Distribution

	White Males							White Females						
	Percentile							Percentile						
Age yr	5	10	25	50	75	90	95	5	10	25	50	75	90	95
0–4	—	—	—	—	—	—	—	—	—	—	—	—	—	—
5–9	63	69	80	90	103	117	129	68	73	88	98	115	125	140
10–14	64	72	81	94	109	122	132	68	73	81	94	110	126	136
15–19	62	68	80	93	109	123	130	59	65	78	93	111	129	137
20–24	66	73	85	101	118	138	147	57	65	82	102	118	141	159
25–29	70	75	96	116	138	157	165	71	77	90	108	126	148	164
30–34	78	88	107	124	144	166	185	70	77	91	109	128	147	156
35–39	81	92	110	131	154	176	189	75	81	96	116	139	161	172
40–44	87	98	115	135	157	173	186	74	84	104	122	146	165	174
45–49	98	106	120	141	163	186	202	79	89	105	127	150	173	186
50–54	89	102	118	143	162	185	197	88	94	111	134	160	186	201
55–59	88	103	123	145	168	191	203	89	97	120	145	168	199	210
60–64	83	106	121	143	165	188	210	100	105	126	149	168	191	224
65–69	98	104	125	146	170	199	210	92	99	125	151	184	205	221
70+	88	100	119	142	164	182	186	96	108	127	147	170	189	206

Adapted from *The Lipid Research Clinics Population Studies Data Book.* 1980;1. US Dept of Health and Human Services publication NIH 80-1527.

Table 14.4
Plasma HDL-Cholesterol (mg/dL) Population Distribution

	White Males							White Females						
	Percentile							Percentile						
Age yr	5	10	25	50	75	90	95	5	10	25	50	75	90	95
0–4	—	—	—	—	—	—	—	—	—	—	—	—	—	—
5–9	38	42	49	54	63	70	74	36	38	47	52	61	67	73
10–14	37	40	46	55	61	71	74	37	40	45	52	58	64	70
15–19	30	34	39	46	52	59	63	35	38	43	51	61	68	74
20–24	30	32	38	45	51	57	63	33	37	44	51	62	72	79
25–29	31	32	57	44	50	58	63	37	39	47	55	63	74	83
30–34	28	32	38	45	52	59	63	36	40	46	55	64	73	77
35–39	29	31	36	43	49	58	62	34	38	44	53	64	74	82
40–44	27	31	36	43	51	60	67	34	39	48	56	65	79	88
45–49	30	33	38	45	52	60	64	34	41	47	58	68	82	87
50–54	28	31	36	44	51	58	63	37	41	50	62	73	85	91
55–59	28	31	38	46	55	64	71	37	41	50	60	73	85	91
60–64	30	34	41	49	61	69	74	38	44	51	61	75	87	92
65–69	30	33	39	49	62	74	78	35	38	49	62	73	84	98
70+	31	33	40	48	56	70	75	33	38	48	60	71	82	92

Adapted from *The Lipid Research Clinics Population Studies Data Book.* 1980;1. US Dept of Health and Human Services publication NIH 80-1527.

Table 14.5
Plasma Triglycerides (mg/dL)
Population Distribution

	White Males							White Females						
	Percentile							Percentile						
Age yr	**5**	**10**	**25**	**50**	**75**	**90**	**95**	**5**	**10**	**25**	**50**	**75**	**90**	**95**
0–4	—	33	—	51	—	84	—	—	38	—	59	—	96	—
5–9	28	34	39	48	58	70	85	32	37	45	57	74	103	126
10–14	33	37	46	58	74	94	111	39	44	53	68	85	104	120
15–19	38	43	53	68	88	125	143	36	40	52	64	85	112	126
20–24	44	50	61	78	107	146	165	37	42	60	80	104	135	168
25–29	45	51	67	88	120	171	204	42	45	57	76	104	137	159
30–34	46	57	76	102	152	214	253	40	45	55	73	104	140	163
35–39	52	58	80	109	167	250	316	40	47	61	83	115	170	205
40–44	56	69	89	123	174	252	318	45	51	66	68	116	161	191
45–49	56	65	88	119	165	218	279	44	55	71	94	139	180	223
50–54	63	75	94	128	178	244	313	53	58	75	103	144	190	223
55–59	60	70	85	117	167	210	261	59	65	80	111	163	229	279
60–64	56	65	84	111	150	193	240	57	66	78	105	143	210	256
65–69	54	61	78	108	164	227	256	56	64	86	118	158	221	260
70+	63	71	87	115	152	202	239	60	68	83	110	141	189	289

Adapted from *The Lipid Research Clinics Population Studies Data Book.* 1980;1 US Dept of Health and Human Services publication NIH 80–1527.

Table 14.6
Desirable Weights for Men and Women, 1959

Height (With Shoes)	Weight (in Indoor Clothing), lb Small Frame	Medium Frame	Large Frame
Men			
5′ 2″	112–120	118–129	126–141
5′ 3″	115–123	121–133	129–144
5′ 4″	118–126	124–136	132–148
5′ 5″	121–129	127–139	135–152
5′ 6″	124–133	130–143	138–156
5′ 7″	128–137	134–147	142–161
5′ 8″	132–141	138–152	147–166
5′ 9″	136–145	142–156	151–170
5′10″	140–150	146–160	155–174
5′11″	144–154	150–165	159–179
6′ 0″	148–158	154–170	164–184
6′ 1″	152–162	158–175	168–189
6′ 2″	156–167	162–180	173–194
6′ 3″	160–171	167–185	178–199
6′ 4″	164–175	172–190	182–204
Women			
4′10″	92–98	96–107	104–119
4′11″	94–101	98–110	106–122
5′ 0″	96–104	101–113	109–125
5′ 1″	99–107	104–116	112–128
5′ 2″	102–110	107–119	115–131
5′ 3″	105–113	110–122	118–134
5′ 4″	108–116	113–126	121–138
5′ 5″	111–119	116–130	125–142
5′ 6″	114–123	120–135	129–146
5′ 7″	118–127	124–139	133–150
5′ 8″	122–131	128–143	137–154
5′ 9″	126–135	132–147	141–158
5′10″	130–140	136–151	145–163
5′11″	134–144	140–155	149–168
6′ 0″	138–148	144–159	153–173

Prepared by the Metropolitan Life Insurance Co in 1959. Derived primarily from data of the Build and Blood Pressure Study, 1959, Society of Actuaries.

Reprinted by permission.

Table 14.7
Desirable Weights for Men and Women, 1983

Height (With Shoes)	Weight (in Indoor Clothing), lb		
	Small Frame	**Medium Frame**	**Large Frame**
Men*			
5′ 2″	128–134	131–141	138–150
5′ 3″	130–136	133–143	140–153
5′ 4″	132–138	135–145	142–156
5′ 5″	134–140	137–148	144–160
5′ 6″	136–142	139–151	146–164
5′ 7″	138–145	142–154	149–168
5′ 8″	140–148	145–157	152–172
5′ 9″	142–151	148–160	155–176
5′10″	144–154	151–163	158–180
5′11″	146–157	154–166	161–184
6′ 0″	149–160	157–170	164–188
6′ 1″	152–164	160–174	168–192
6′ 2″	155–168	164–178	172–197
6′ 3″	158–172	167–182	176–202
6′ 4″	162–176	171–187	181–207
Women†			
4′10″	102–111	109–121	118–131
4′11″	103–113	111–123	120–134
5′ 0″	104–115	113–126	122–137
5′ 1″	106–118	115–129	125–140
5′ 2″	108–121	118–132	128–143
5′ 3″	111–124	121–135	131–147
5′ 4″	114–127	124–138	132–151
5′ 5″	117–130	127–141	137–155
5′ 6″	120–133	130–144	140–159
5′ 7″	123–136	133–147	143–163
5′ 8″	126–139	136–150	146–167
5′ 9″	129–142	139–153	149–170
5′10″	132–145	142–156	152–173
5′11″	135–148	145–159	155–176
6′ 0″	138–151	148–162	158–179

*Weights at ages 25–29 based on lowest mortality. Weight in pounds according to frame (in indoor clothing weighing 5 lb, shoes with 1″ heels).

†Weights at ages 25–29 based on lowest mortality. Weight in pounds according to frame (in indoor clothing weighing 3 lb, shoes with 1″ heels).

Prepared by the Metropolitan Life Insurance Co in 1983. Courtesy of Metropolitan Life Insurance Co.

Table 14.8
Probability of Developing Coronary Heart Disease in 6 Years. Men Aged 35–70

	Points										
	0	**1**	**2**	**3**	**4**	**5**	**6**	**7**	**8**	**9**	**10**
SBP	100	110	120	130	140	150	160	170	180	190	200
CIG	No				Yes						
LVH	No						Yes				
GLU	No		Yes								

	Age											
Chol	**36**	**38**	**40**	**42**	**44**	**46**	**48**	**50**	**55**	**60**	**65**	**70**
165	3	6	0	11	14	16	18	19	23	26	27	27
180	5	8	10	13	15	17	19	20	24	26	27	27
195	7	9	12	14	16	18	20	21	24	26	27	27
210	8	11	13	15	17	19	21	22	25	27	27	27
225	10	12	15	17	19	20	22	23	26	27	28	27
240	11	14	16	18	20	21	23	24	27	28	28	27
255	13	15	17	19	21	23	24	25	27	28	28	27
270	15	17	19	21	22	24	25	26	28	29	28	26
285	16	18	20	22	24	25	26	27	29	29	28	26
300	18	20	22	23	25	26	27	28	29	29	28	26
315	20	22	23	25	26	27	28	29	30	30	29	26

Calculation of Probability

Enter points for

_______ Systolic blood pressure (SBP)
\+ _______ Cigarette smoking (CIG)
\+ _______ Left ventricular hypertrophy (LVH)
\+ _______ Glucose intolerance (GLU)
\+ _______ Age/serum cholesterol
\=\=\=\=\=\=\= Total points (TP) → probability (prob)

TP	**Prob**	**TP**	**Prob**	**TP**	**Prob**
5	0.003	20	0.021	35	0.13
6	0.004	21	0.024	36	0.14
7	0.004	22	0.028	37	0.16
8	0.005	23	0.031	38	0.17
9	0.006	24	0.035	39	0.19
10	0.006	25	0.040	40	0.21
11	0.007	26	0.045	41	0.23
12	0.008	27	0.050	42	0.25
13	0.009	28	0.057	43	0.28
14	0.010	29	0.064	44	0.30
15	0.012	30	0.071	45	0.33
16	0.013	31	0.080	46	0.36
17	0.015	32	0.090	47	0.39
18	0.017	33	0.100	48	0.42
19	0.019	34	0.11	49	0.45

Reprinted with permission from Kannel WB, Shatzkin A. Risk factor analysis. *Prog Cardiovasc Dis.* 1984;26:309.

Table 14.9 Probability of Developing Coronary Heart Disease in 6 Years. Women Aged 35–70

	Points										
	0	**1**	**2**	**3**	**4**	**5**	**6**	**7**	**8**	**9**	**10**
SBP	100	110	120	130	140	150	160	170	180	190	200
LVH	No			Yes							
GLU	No			Yes							

Note: No points added for smoking

	Age											
Chol	**36**	**38**	**40**	**42**	**44**	**46**	**48**	**50**	**55**	**60**	**65**	**70**
165	0	2	4	5	7	9	10	12	15	18	20	21
180	1	3	4	6	8	9	11	12	16	18	20	22
195	2	3	5	7	9	10	13	13	16	19	21	22
210	3	4	6	8	10	11	13	14	17	19	21	22
225	4	5	7	9	10	12	13	15	17	20	21	22
240	4	6	8	10	11	13	14	15	18	20	22	23
255	5	7	9	11	12	13	15	16	19	21	22	23
270	6	8	10	11	13	14	16	17	19	21	23	24
285	7	9	11	12	14	15	16	17	20	22	23	24
300	8	10	12	13	15	16	17	18	21	22	24	24
315	9	11	13	14	15	17	18	19	21	23	24	25

Calculation of Probability

Enter points for

______ Systolic blood pressure (SBP)

\+ ______ Left ventricular hypertrophy (LVH)

\+ ______ Glucose intolerance (GLU)

\+ ______ Age/serum cholesterol

====== Total points (TP) → probability (prob)

TP	Prob	TP	Prob	TP	Prob
5	0.002	17	0.014	29	0.081
6	0.003	18	0.016	30	0.093
7	0.003	19	0.019	31	0.11
8	0.004	20	0.022	32	0.12
9	0.004	21	0.025	33	0.14
10	0.004	22	0.029	34	0.16
11	0.006	23	0.034	35	0.18
12	0.007	24	0.040	36	0.20
13	0.008	25	0.046	37	0.23
14	0.009	26	0.053	38	0.26
15	0.010	27	0.061	39	0.29
16	0.012	28	0.071	40	0.32

Reprinted with permission from Kannel WB, Shatzkin A. Risk factor analysis. *Prog Cardiovasc Dis.* 1984;26:309.

Table 14.10
Food-Intake Record

Directions:

1. Record date and day of the week for each day the diary is kept. Record all food and beverages ingested along with the time you eat or drink them. It is best to carry the diary with you and to record items immediately before or after consuming them.
2. Include an exact description of the item, the method of preparation when applicable, and your best estimate of portion size or amount. Be sure to include condiments, dressings, sauces, beverages, and snacks.
3. Evaluate your intake by listing in the Servings column the number of servings and food-group type. At the bottom of the page, tally servings from each group, compare it to your goal, and compute either a positive, negative, or neutral balance between your total daily intake and your goal.

Sample

Day 1 Date October 23 Day Mon.

Time	Item	Amount	Servings
8:15 AM	milk, 2%	1c	1 milk
	toast, wheat	2sl	2 grain
	margarine	1 tbsp	"other"
12:30 PM	ham, lunchmeat	2 oz	1 meat
	roll, kaiser	1	2 grain
	cheese, colby	1.5 oz	1 milk
	mayonnaise	1 tbsp	"other"
	apple	1	1 fruit

Food Group	Tally	Goal	Balance
Milk/dairy	||	2	0
Fruit/vegetable	|	4	–3
Cereal/grain	||||	4	0
Meat/protein	|	2	–1
Other	||	0	+2

Table 14.10
Food-Intake Record—(Cont.)

Day_____ Date ____________________________ Day ____

Time	**Item**	**Amount**	**Servings**

Food Group	**Tally**	**Goal**	**Balance**
Milk/dairy			+–
Fruit/vegetable			+–
Cereal/grain			+–
Meat/protein			+–
Other			+–

Table 14.11
Food Diary

Day of the week ______________ Name ______________

Time	Minutes Spent Eating	Activity While Eating	Location of Eating	Food Type	Quality	Eating With Whom	Food Cues
6:00							
11:00							
4:00							
9:00							

Table 14.12
Do-It-Yourself Caffeine Audit

The following exercise will help you to identify the sources of the caffeine you consume and to approximate your daily caffeine intake. To complete this audit, you need to recall your caffeine consumption during the past 24 hours. In column A, record the number of servings or doses for each of the items listed that you have consumed within the past 24 hours. Then multiply the column A value by its corresponding column B value and record the product in column C. Total the values in column C to arrive at your estimated daily intake of caffeine. Caffeine values have been rounded to the nearest 5 milligrams (mg) to make it easier to multiply.

Source of Caffeine	Column A Number of Servings per Day		Column B Amount of Caffeine per Serving (mg)		Column C Total Caffeine (mg)
Coffee (5-oz cup)					
Brewed, drip method	______	×	115	=	______
Brewed, percolator	______	×	80	=	______
Instant	______	×	65	=	______
Decaffeinated	______	×	3	=	______
Tea (5-oz cup)					
Brewed	______	×	50	=	______
Instant	______	×	30	=	______
Iced (12-oz glass)	______	×	70	=	______
Cocoa beverage (5-oz cup)	______	×	4	=	______
Chocolate milk beverage (8 oz)	______	×	5	=	______
Milk chocolate (1 oz)	______	×	6	=	______
Dark chocolate, semi-sweet	______	×	20	=	______
Chocolate flavored syrup	______	×	4	=	______
Soft drinks (12-oz serving)					
Jolt	______	×	71	=	______
Sugar-free Mr. Pibb	______	×	59	=	______
Mountain Dew	______	×	54	=	______
Mello Yello	______	×	54	=	______
TAB	______	×	53	=	______
Coca-Cola	______	×	46	=	______
Diet Coke	______	×	46	=	______
Shasta Cola	______	×	44	=	______
Mr. Pibb	______	×	41	=	______
Dr. Pepper	______	×	40	=	______
Sugar-free Dr. Pepper	______	×	40	=	______
Pepsi-Cola	______	×	39	=	______
Diet Pepsi	______	×	36	=	______

If your caffeine consumption is over 250 to 300 milligrams per day, you may be consuming too much. Some suggestions for reducing caffeine consumption include: (1) switching to decaffeinated coffee or soft drinks; (2) cutting down on caffeinated beverages; (3) mixing caffeinated and decaffeinated coffee grounds together before making coffee; or (4) limiting your consumption of caffeinated beverages to a preselected number and then switching to decaffeinated beverages.

Adapted with permission from Hale C, Davis RC. The do-it-yourself caffeine audit. *J Nutr Educ.* 1986;18:122A.

Table 14.13
Alcohol-Consumption Questionnaire

1. During the past three months, have you consumed any beer, wine, or hard liquor? *(Circle all that apply.)*
   Beer   Wine   Hard liquor   No alcohol

IF YOU DRANK BEER:

2. During the past three months, on average, how many days per week or per month did you drink *beer*?
   ____ per week or ____ per month
   days   days

3. About how many fluid ounces of *beer* did you usually drink on each day you drank?
   ____________ fluid ounces

4. Would you say your consumption of *beer* varies by season of the year?
   Yes   No

   (If no, go to question 6.)

5. In what season(s) of the year do you usually drink the most *beer*? *(Circle all that apply.)*
   Spring   Fall   Summer   Winter

IF YOU DRANK WINE:

6. During the past three months, on average, how many days per week or per month did you drink *wine*?
   ____ per week or ____ per month
   days   days

7. About how many fluid ounces of *wine* did you usually drink on each day you drank?
   ____________ fluid ounces

8. Would you say your consumption of *wine* varies by season of the year?
   Yes   No

   (If no, go to question 10.)

9. In what season(s) of the year do you usually drink the most *wine*? *(Circle all that apply.)*
   Spring   Fall   Summer   Winter

IF YOU DRANK HARD LIQUOR:

10. During the past three months, on average, how many days per week or per month did you drink *hard liquor*?
    ____ per week or ____ per month
    days   days

11. About how many fluid ounces of *hard liquor* did you usually drink on each day you drank?
    ____________ fluid ounces

12. Would you say your consumption of *hard liquor* varies by season of the year?
    Yes   No

    (If no, go to question 14.)

13. In what season(s) of the year do you usually drink the most *hard liquor*? *(Circle all that apply.)*
    Spring   Fall   Summer   Winter

IF YOU DRINK ANY ALCOHOLIC BEVERAGES:

14. On what days of the week do you usually consume alcoholic beverages? *(Circle all that apply.)*
    Monday   Tuesday   Wednesday   Thursday   Friday   Saturday   Sunday

Note to dietitians: More than two alcoholic drinks (24 oz beer, 8 oz wine, or 2 shots hard liquor) per day is not recommended.
Adapted from US Department of Agriculture. *Nationwide Food Consumption Survey.* 1987:16-17.

Table 14.14
Sodium-Assessment Questionnaire

Section I—This section measures food on a *daily* basis.

Food Groups	Serving Size	Circle One Box for Each Food Group Servings per Day	Servings per Day	Servings per Day	Servings per Day
Dairy foods: Milk (skim, 2%, whole, or chocolate) Yogurt Non-fat dry milk Evaporated milk	 1/2 cup 1/2 cup 2 tbsp (1/8 cup) 1/4 cup	5+ (15)	3–4 (11)	2 (6)	0–1 (2)
Meat items eaten at restaurant or at home: Beef, pork, lamb, or venison Chicken, turkey, or other poultry Fish (fresh or frozen) Crab, lobster, scallops, shrimp, clams, or oysters Eggs *(Processed meat and fast foods will be counted separately)*	 2 oz 2 oz 2 oz 2 oz 2	6+ (16)	4–5 (12)	2–3 (7)	0–1 (2)
Bread and cereals: Bread Dinner roll Bagel or kaiser roll Doughnut, muffin, biscuit, or pancake Tortilla or taco shell Dry cereal Cooked cereal (cooked with salt) Noodle, pasta, macaroni, or spaghetti (with salt)	 1 slice 1 small 1/2 1 small 2 shells 3/4 cup 1/2 cup 1/3 cup	7+ (61)	5–6 (48)	3–4 (30)	0–2 (9)
Grains, cereal, and pasta, cooked *without* salt: Cooked cereal (no salt added) Pasta (no salt added) Wheat germ White rice Brown rice	 1/2 cup 1/3 cup 1/2 tbsp 1/2 cup 1/4 cup	7+ (0)	5–6 (0)	3–4 (0)	0–2 (0)
Vegetables: Tossed salad Raw vegetables Cooked vegetables Tomato Low-sodium canned vegetables/tomato sauce *(Potato will be counted separately)*	 1 cup 1 cup 1/2 cup 1 small 1/2 cup	6+ (5)	4–5 (4)	2–3 (2)	0–1 (1)
Canned vegetables Tomato sauce or spaghetti sauce	1/2 cup 1/2 cup	6+ (46)	4–5 (34)	2–3 (19)	0–1 (4)
Fruits: Fresh fruits *(Whole grapefruit or banana will be counted as 2 servings)* Canned fruits Fruit juice Dried fruits (raisins, dates, figs, or prunes)	 1 small 1/2 cup 1/2 cup 2 tbsp (1/8 cup)	6+ (1)	4–5 (1)	2–3 (0)	0–1 (0)

Table 14.14
Sodium-Assessment Questionnaire—(Cont.)

Section I—This section measures food on a *daily* basis.

Food Groups	Serving Size	Circle One Box for Each Food Group			
		Servings per Day	**Servings per Day**	**Servings per Day**	**Servings per Day**
Fats and oils:					
Butter or margarine (salted)	1 tbsp				
Mayonnaise	1 tbsp				
Salad dressing (regular or low-calorie, salted)	1 tbsp	6+	4–5	2–3	0–1
(You do not have to count low-sodium butter or margarine or low-sodium salad dressings)		(33)	(30)	(14)	(3)
Beverages:					
Coffee or tea	1 cup (8 oz)				
Beer	12 oz	3	2	1	0
Wine	4 oz	(1)	(0)	(0)	(0)

Section II—This section measures food on a *weekly* basis.

Food Groups	Serving Size	Circle One Box for Each Food Group			
		Servings per Day	**Servings per Week**	**Servings per Week**	**Servings per Week**
Cheeses:					
Cheddar, colby, Swiss, provolone, mozzarella, or other natural cheeses	1 oz				
Cottage cheese	1/4 cup	1+	5–6	3–4	0–2
Cream cheese	2 oz (4 tbsp)				
Parmesan, grated	2 tbsp	(9)	(7)	(5)	(2)
Convenience foods:					
Soups (canned or prepared from powder mix)	1 cup				
Macaroni and cheese	1 cup				
Ready-to-serve products (eg, beef and vegetable stew, chili, ravioli or spaghetti with meat sauce)	1 cup	1+	5–6	3–4	0–2
Frozen dinners	1 dinner				
Ramen noodles (oriental noodles)	1 pkg	(43)	(34)	(22)	(6)
Fast foods:					
Hamburger or cheeseburger	1 burger				
Fish or chicken sandwich	1 sandwich				
Pizza	1/8 of large				
Hoagies	4 inches	1+	5–6	3–4	0–2
Fried chicken	1 thigh				
Chicken nuggets	6 nuggets				
Taco or burrito	1	(30)	(24)	(15)	(5)
Processed meat/processed cheese:					
Luncheon meat	1 oz				
Hot dog or sausage	1 (6 in)				
Bacon	1 slice				
Tuna or salmon (canned)	1 oz	1+	5–6	3–4	0–2
Sardines (canned)	2 med				
American or processed cheese	1 oz				
Cheese spread	1 oz (2 tbsp)	(15)	(12)	(8)	(3)

Table 14.14
Sodium-Assessment Questionnaire—(Cont.)

Section II—This section measures food on a *weekly* basis.

Food Groups	Serving Size	Circle One Box for Each Food Group: Servings per Day	Servings per Week	Servings per Week	Servings per Week
Snacks: Snack crackers Corn chips or Doritos Popcorn *(count only if salt is added)* Pretzels	 10 10 2 cups 1/2 oz (10 small)	1+ (7)	5–6 (5)	3–4 (3)	0–2 (1)
Milk-base desserts and drinks: Ice cream Ice milk Custard Pudding Milk shake or malted milk Eggnog Sorbet	 1 cup 1/2 cup 1/2 cup 1/2 cup 1/2 cup 1/2 cup 1 cup	1+ (4)	5–6 (3)	3–4 (2)	0–2 (1)
Potatoes: Baked potato Mashed potato (low-sodium) Hash browns (low-sodium) French fries (with no salt added)	 1/2 potato 1/2 cup 1/2 cup 10 fries	1+ (0)	5–6 (0)	3–4 (0)	0–2 (0)
Potato items with salt added: Mashed potato (with salt added) Hash browns (with salt added) French fries Potato chips Potato salad, potatoes au gratin, or scalloped potatoes	 1/2 cup 1/2 cup 10 fries 1 oz (10 chips) 1/2 cup	1+ (9)	5–6 (7)	3–4 (4)	0–2 (2)
Legumes, beans, nuts, and peanut butter: Lentils (cooked without salt) Beans, cooked without salt (ie, kidney beans, lima beans, pinto beans, navy beans) Split peas (cooked) Unsalted nuts (almonds, cashews, peanuts, macadamia nuts, walnuts, etc) Low-sodium peanut butter	 1/4 cup 1/4 cup 1/4 cup 1 oz (1/8 cup) 1 tbsp	1+ (0)	5–6 (0)	3–4 (0)	0–2 (0)
Salted beans, nuts, and peanut butter: Beans, cooked with salt or canned Nuts, salted Peanut butter	 1/4 cup 1 oz 1 tbsp	1+ (5)	5–6 (4)	3–4 (2)	0–2 (1)
Seasonings, spices, and sauces: Bacon bits Steak sauce, barbeque sauce, or catsup Chili sauce Seasonings with salt Soy sauce Gravy	 1/2 cup 1 tbsp 1 tbsp 1/8 tsp 1/2 tsp 2 tbsp	1+ (7)	5–6 (5)	3–4 (3)	0–2 (1)

Table 14.14
Sodium-Assessment Questionnaire—(Cont.)

Section II—This section measures food on a *weekly* basis.

Food Groups	Serving Size	Circle One Box for Each Food Group: Servings per Day	Servings per Week	Servings per Week	Servings per Week
Miscellaneous:					
Molasses	1 tsp				
Brown sugar	1 tbsp				
Apple butter	1 tbsp				
Chocolate candy	2 (1-in squares)	1+	5–6	3–4	0–2
Hershey kisses	3 pieces				
Pickle relish	1 tbsp				
Pickles	3 slices	(0)	(0)	(0)	(0)

How often do you or the person who prepares your food add salt during cooking?	always	sometimes	seldom	never	uncertain
How often do you use salt at the table?	always	sometimes	seldom	never	uncertain

Note to dietitians: Add up number in parentheses for each food group. If score is greater than 100 dietary modifications should be considered.
From Chan, Chi Yee (unpublished data).

Table 14.15
AHA-Recommended Fat Intakes

	Calorie Intake Level: 1600 (Adult Female)	2000 (Male/Female Age 9-11)	2400 (Adult Male)	2800 (Male Age 18)
Total fat,* g	53	67	80	93
Saturated fat,† g	18	22	27	31

*<30% of total calories.

†<10% of total calories, or one third of total fat.

Prepared by Frances Seligson.

Table 14.16
Effectiveness of Dietary Fat-Reduction Strategies

Strategy	Kcal Fat, %*	Chol, mg	SFA, %	MUFA, %	PUFA, %
1. Skim milk replaced higher-fat milk Medium-fat meat exchanges replaced higher-fat ones Use of fat-modified dressings, sauces, and spreads	27	402	9	10	6
2. Skim milk replaced higher-fat milk Lean-meat exchanges replaced higher-fat ones	28	264	9	10	7
3. Skim milk replaced higher-fat milk Lean-meat exchanges replaced higher-fat ones Use of fat-modified dressings, sauces, and spreads	24	247	8	9	5
4. Skim milk replaced higher-fat milk Use of fat-modified dressings, sauces, and spreads	30	422	11	12	5
5. Medium-fat meat exchanges replaced higher-fat ones Use of fat-modified dressings, sauces, and spreads	29	426	10	10	6
6. Lean-meat exchanges replaced higher-fat ones	30	288	10	11	7
7. Using all "OK" foods of the American Heart Association	23	293	6	7	9

*Kcal fat indicates kilocalories from fat; Chol, cholesterol; SFA, saturated fatty acids; MUFA, monounsaturated fatty acids; and PUFA, polyunsaturated fatty acids. Baseline diet was 37% of calories from fat, 13% of calories from saturated fatty acids and 465 mg of cholesterol.

Compiled by L. M. Smith, BS, M. Sigman, PhD, RD, and P. M. Kris-Etherton, PhD, RD, The Pennsylvania State University, University Park, PA, 1990.

Fig. 14.1
Fat in the US food supply. From* Nutrition Monitoring in the United States: An Update Report on Nutrition Monitoring. *US Dept of Health and Human Services; 1989. DHHS publication no. (PHS) 89-1225.

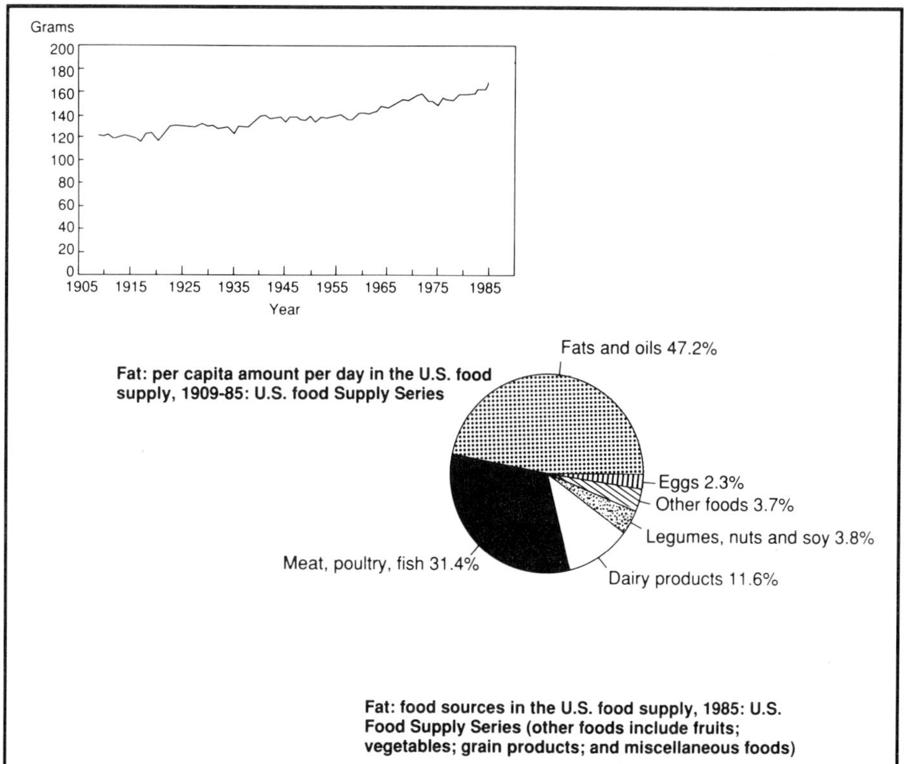

Fig. 14.2
Saturated fat in the US food supply. From* Nutrition Monitoring in the United States: An Update Report on Nutrition Monitoring. *US Dept of Health and Human Services; 1989. DHHS publication no. (PHS) 89-1225.

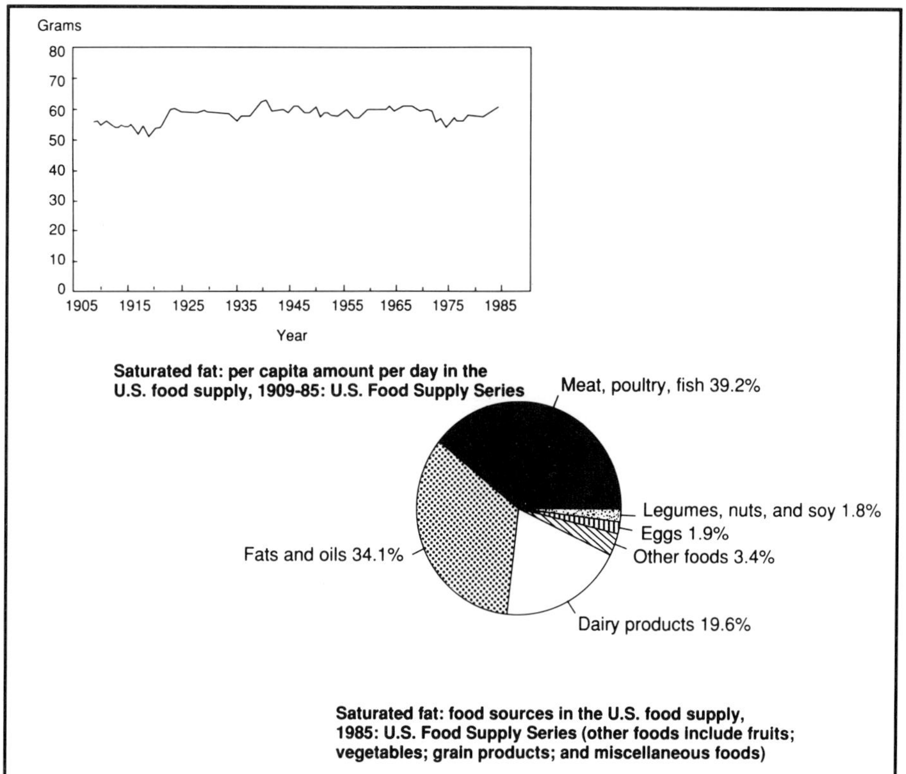

Table 14.17
Major Contributors of Total Fat in the US Diet

Item	Percentage of Total Fat
Hamburgers, cheeseburgers, meat loaf	7.02
Hot dogs, ham, lunch meats	6.39
Whole milk, whole-milk beverages	5.98
Doughnuts, cookies, cake	5.98
Beef steaks, roasts	5.45
White bread, rolls, crackers	4.88
Eggs	4.63
Cheeses, excluding cottage cheese	4.54
Margarine	4.50
Mayonnaise, salad dressings	4.30
Pork, including chops, roast	3.97
French fries, fried potatoes	2.70
Salad and cooking oils	2.59
Butter	2.39
Ice cream, frozen desserts	2.05
Salty snacks	2.02
Peanuts, peanut butter	1.86
Pies, excluding pumpkin	1.53
Bacon	1.38
2% milk	1.37
Spaghetti with tomato sauce	1.32
Sausage	1.26
Chicken or turkey, excluding fried	1.23
Fried fish	1.22
Gravy, other meat sauces	1.06
Candy (chocolate)	1.04
Chili	0.96
Potatoes, excluding fried	0.91
Fried chicken	0.86
Pizza	0.77
Pinto, navy, other dried beans	0.73
Tuna, tuna salad, tuna casserole	0.66
Cornbread, grits, tortillas	0.64
Mixed dishes with cheese	0.64
Beef stew, pot pie	0.62
Green salad	0.62
Soups other than vegetable, tomato	0.60
Cooking fat, lard	0.54
Mixed dishes with chicken	0.51
Nondairy coffee creamers	0.51
Whole-wheat, rye, other dark breads	0.47
Cream, half-and-half	0.44
Nuts (excluding peanuts)	0.43
Veal, lamb	0.39
Coleslaw, cabbage	0.38
Fish, broiled, baked, canned	0.35
Mixed dishes with beef	0.31
Bran and granola cereals	0.30
Pancakes, waffles, French toast	0.29
Vegetable, tomato, minestrone soups	0.27

Reprinted with permission from Block G, Dresser CM, Hartman A, et al. Nutrient sources in the American diet: data from the NHANES II survey. *Am J Epidemiol.* 1985;122:27.

Table 14.18
Major Contributors of Saturated Fatty Acids in the US Diet

Item	Percentage of Total Saturated Fat
Hamburgers, cheeseburgers, meat loaf	9.31
Whole milk, whole-milk beverages	9.11
Cheeses, excluding cottage cheese	7.28
Beef steaks, roasts	7.28
Hot dogs, ham, lunch meats	7.04
Doughnuts, cookies, cake	4.84
Eggs	4.52
Pork, including chops, roast	3.99
Butter	3.67
White bread, rolls, crackers	3.22
Ice cream, frozen desserts	3.11
Margarine	2.56
2% milk	2.48
Mayonnaise, salad dressings	2.41
French fries, fried potatoes	1.89
Salty snacks	1.53
Bacon	1.37
Nondairy coffee creamers	1.34
Sausage	1.28
Chili	1.25
Gravy, other meat sauces	1.16
Candy (chocolate)	1.13
Pies, excluding pumpkin	1.11
Chicken or turkey, excluding fried	1.10
Fried fish	1.04
Peanuts, peanut butter	1.02
Spaghetti with tomato sauce	0.98
Salad and cooking oils	0.82
Pinto, navy, other dried beans	0.78
Beef stew, pot pie	0.77
Fried chicken	0.70
Potatoes, excluding fried	0.70
Mixed dishes with cheese	0.69
Cream, half-and-half	0.68
Pizza	0.59
Cooking fat, lard	0.57
Veal, lamb	0.57
Green salad	0.50
Cornbread, grits, tortillas	0.46
Soups other than vegetable, tomato	0.46
Mixed dishes with chicken	0.35
Cottage cheese	0.33
Tuna, tuna salad, tuna casserole	0.33
Whole-wheat, rye, other dark breads	0.27
Sour cream, dips	0.25
Fish, broiled, baked, canned	0.23
Yogurt	0.22
Venison, gizzard, other unusual meats	0.21
Pancakes, waffles, French toast	0.20
Puddings	0.20

Reprinted with permission from Block G, Dresser CM, Hartman A, et al. Nutrient sources in the American diet: data from the NHANES II survey. *Am J Epidemiol.* 1985;122:27.

Table 14.19
Major Contributors of Monounsaturated Fatty Acids (Oleic Acid) in the US Diet

Item	Percentage of Total Oleic Acid
Hamburgers, cheeseburgers, meat loaf	8.26
Hot dogs, ham, lunch meats	7.38
Doughnuts, cookies, cake	6.71
Beef steaks, roasts	6.48
Margarine	5.56
White bread, rolls, crackers	5.45
Whole milk, whole-milk beverages	5.19
Eggs	5.08
Pork, including chops, roast	4.54
Cheeses, excluding cottage cheese	3.40
Salad and cooking oils	3.36
Mayonnaise, salad dressings	2.80
French fries, fried potatoes	2.35
Peanuts, peanut butter	2.29
Butter	2.14
Bacon	1.78
Ice cream, frozen desserts	1.74
Pies, excluding pumpkin	1.70
Spaghetti with tomato sauce	1.68
Salty snacks	1.55
Sausage	1.45
Candy (chocolate)	1.33
Chicken or turkey, excluding fried	1.24
Chili	1.13
Gravy, other meat sauces	1.03
Fried chicken	0.99
2% milk	0.93
Potatoes, excluding fried	0.84
Fried fish	0.81
Pizza	0.78
Beef stew, pot pie	0.72
Pinto, navy, other dried beans	0.70
Cooking fat, lard	0.67
Cornbread, grits, tortillas	0.64
Mixed dishes with cheese	0.58
Nuts (excluding peanuts)	0.55
Whole-wheat, rye, other dark breads	0.44
Veal, lamb	0.41
Cream, half-and-half	0.39
Soups other than vegetable, tomato	0.39
Mixed dishes with chicken	0.37
Green salad	0.34
Tuna, tuna salad, tuna casserole	0.30
Pancakes, waffles, French toast	0.29
Shellfish	0.27
Liver	0.26
Avocados	0.24
Coleslaw, cabbage	0.21
Venison, gizzard, other unusual meats	0.21
Pumpkin pie	0.20

Reprinted with permission from Block G, Dresser CM, Hartman A, et al. Nutrient sources in the American diet: data from the NHANES II survey. *Am J Epidemiol.* 1985;122:27.

Table 14.20
Major Contributors of Omega-6 Fatty Acids (Linoleic Acid) in the US Diet

Item	Percentage of Total Linoleic Acid
Mayonnaise, salad dressings	14.89
Margarine	10.16
French fries, fried potatoes	7.54
White bread, rolls, crackers	6.72
Salad and cooking oils	6.48
Doughnuts, cookies, cake	6.43
Salty snacks	5.42
Peanuts, peanut butter	3.55
Hot dogs, ham, lunch meats	2.83
Pork, including chops, roast	2.51
Fried fish	2.36
Eggs	2.18
Chicken or turkey, excluding fried	1.79
Potatoes, excluding fried	1.72
Pies, excluding pumpkin	1.61
Green salad	1.49
Hamburgers, cheeseburgers, meat loaf	1.39
Coleslaw, cabbage	1.31
Fried chicken	1.19
Tuna, tuna salad, tuna casserole	1.17
Gravy, other meat sauces	1.11
Bacon	1.04
Whole milk, whole-milk beverages	1.03
Nuts, excluding peanuts	0.92
Sausage	0.85
Spaghetti with tomato sauce	0.82
Cornbread, grits, tortillas	0.81
Beef steaks, roasts	0.77
Cheeses, excluding cottage cheese	0.76
Whole-wheat, rye, other dark breads	0.74
Mixed dishes with chicken	0.73
Candy (chocolate)	0.69
Soups other than vegetable, tomato	0.55
Pizza	0.53
Mixed dishes with cheese	0.52
Butter	0.51
2% milk	0.48
Pinto, navy, other dried beans	0.43
Ice cream, frozen desserts	0.40
Cooking fat, lard	0.39
Edible seeds	0.35
Cooked cereals	0.27
Pancakes, waffles, French toast	0.24
Avocados	0.18
Beef stew, pot pie	0.16
Fish, broiled, baked, canned	0.15
Vegetable, tomato, minestrone soup	0.14
Pumpkin pie	0.14
Candy (nonchocolate)	0.13
Liver	0.12

Reprinted with permission from Block G, Dresser CM, Hartman A, et al. Nutrient sources in the American diet: data from the NHANES II survey. *Am J Epidemiol.* 1985;122:27.

Table 14.21
Major Contributors of Cholesterol in the US Diet

Item	Percentage of Total Cholesterol
Eggs	35.88
Beef steaks, roasts	8.69
Hamburgers, cheeseburgers, meat loaf	7.28
Whole milk, whole-milk beverages	5.41
Hot dogs, ham, lunch meats	4.29
Pork, including chops, roast	3.61
Doughnuts, cookies, cake	3.61
Cheeses, excluding cottage cheese	3.05
Liver	2.70
Chicken or turkey, excluding fried	2.55
Fried chicken	1.75
Ice cream, frozen desserts	1.71
Butter	1.70
Spaghetti with tomato sauce	1.50
Cornbread, grits, tortillas	1.09
Shellfish	0.96
Fish, broiled, baked, canned	0.83
Beef stew, pot pie	0.80
Pies, excluding pumpkin	0.80
2% milk	0.79
Tuna, tuna salad, tuna casserole	0.73
White bread, rolls, crackers	0.72
Fried fish	0.65
Mayonnaise, salad dressings	0.63
Sausage	0.60
Potatoes, excluding fried	0.59
Veal, lamb	0.58
Chili	0.55
Bacon	0.50
Soups other than vegetable, tomato	0.48
Pancakes, waffles, French toast	0.48
Cream, half-and-half	0.37
Pizza	0.35
Mixed dishes with cheese	0.34
Vegetable, tomato, minestrone soups	0.33
Mixed dishes with chicken	0.33
Venison, gizzard, other unusual meats	0.32
Pumpkin pie	0.22
Skim milk, buttermilk	0.22
Liverwurst	0.21
Noodles, macaroni	0.21
Puddings	0.21
Cottage cheese	0.19
Salty snacks	0.18
Pinto, navy, other dried beans	0.16
Green salad	0.14
Dressings and stuffings	0.12
Cooking fat, lard	0.12
Mixed dishes with beef	0.08
Yogurt	0.08

Reprinted with permission from Block G, Dresser CM, Hartman A, et al. Nutrient sources in the American diet: data from the NHANES II survey. *Am J Epidemiol.* 1985;122:27.

Table 14.22
Composition of Dietary Fats

Dietary Fat	Saturated Fatty Acids, %	Polyunsaturated Fatty Acids, %	Monounsaturated Fatty Acids, %
Canola oil	6	32	62
Safflower oil	10	77	13
Sunflower oil	11	69	20
Corn oil	13	61	25
Olive oil	14	9	77
Soybean oil	15	61	24
Peanut oil	18	33	49
Margarine	19	32	49
Cottonseed oil	27	54	19
Vegetable shortening	28	28	44
Chicken fat	31	22	47
Lard	41	12	47
Butter	66	4	30
Beef fat	52	4	44
Sockeye-salmon oil	20	25	55
Palm oil	51	12	47
Palm kernel oil	86	2	12
Coconut oil	92	2	6

From Reeves JB III. *Composition of foods: Fats and Oils—Raw, Processed and Prepared.* 1979. USDA handbook 8-4.

Table 14.23
Foods High in Monounsaturates

Item	SFA, g*	MUFA, g	PUFA, g
Avocado (1/2)	4.5	19.0	3.5
Macadamia nuts (1 oz)	3.2	17.1	0.4
Olive oil (1 tbsp)	1.9	10.3	1.2
Pickled herring (3 oz)	2.0	10.0	1.4
Canola oil (1 tbsp)	1.0	9.0	4.0
Peanuts, roasted (1 oz)	1.9	6.9	4.4
Peanut oil (1 tbsp)	2.4	6.5	4.5
Butter (1 tbsp)	9.2	4.2	0.5
Scallops (6 breaded)	2.5	4.1	2.5
Peanut butter (1 tbsp)	1.4	4.0	2.5
Salmon (3 oz smoked)	2.6	3.9	0.7
Sardines (3 oz canned)	2.1	3.7	2.9
Corn oil (1 tbsp)	1.8	3.5	8.7
Soybean oil (1 tbsp)	2.1	3.4	8.5
Sunflower oil (1 tbsp)	1.5	2.8	9.7
Salmon (3 oz red)	1.2	2.4	1.4
Safflower oil (1 tbsp)	1.4	1.8	10.8

*SFA indicates saturated fatty acids; MUFA, monounsaturated fatty acids; PUFA, polyunsaturated fatty acids.

From Gebhardt SE, Matthews RH. *Nutritive Values of Foods.* Washington, DC: US Gov Printing Office and Proctor & Gamble Co; 1981. US Dept of Agriculture Home and Garden bulletin 72.

14.24
Fat, Omega-3 Fatty Acids, and Cholesterol Content of Selected Foods (100-g Raw Edible Portion)

	Fat, g	Omega-3 Fatty Acids, g*	Cholesterol, mg
Fish			
Anchovy, European	4.8	1.4	—†
Bass, striped	2.3	0.8	80
Bluefish	6.5	1.2	59
Carp	5.6	0.3	67
Catfish, channel	4.3	0.3	58
Cod, Atlantic	0.7	0.3	43
Cod, Pacific	0.6	0.2	37
Flounder, unspecified	1.0	0.2	46
Haddock	0.7	0.2	63
Halibut, Pacific	2.3	0.4	32
Herring, Atlantic	9.0	1.6	60
Herring, Pacific	13.9	1.7	77
Mackerel, Atlantic	13.9	2.5	80
Mullet, unspecified	4.4	1.1	34
Ocean perch	1.6	0.2	42
Pike, walleye	1.2	0.3	86
Pompano, Florida	9.5	0.6	50
Sablefish	15.3	1.4	49
Salmon, Atlantic	5.4	1.2	—
Salmon, chinook	10.4	1.4	—
Salmon, pink	3.4	1.0	—
Salmon, sockeye	8.6	1.2	—
Sardines, in sardine oil‡	15.5	21.1	—
Shark	1.9	0.5	44
Snapper, red	1.2	0.2	—
Sole	1.2	0.1	50
Sturgeon	3.3	0.3	—
Swordfish	2.1	0.2	39
Trout, brook	2.7	0.4	68
Trout, lake	9.7	1.6	48
Trout, rainbow	3.4	0.5	57
Tuna	2.5	0.5	54
Crustaceans			
Crab, Alaska king	0.8	0.3	—
Crab, Dungeness	1.0	0.3	59
Crayfish, unspecified	1.4	0.1	158
Lobster, northern	0.9	0.2	95
Shrimp, unspecified	1.1	0.3	147
Mollusks			
Abalone, New Zealand	1.0	Trace	—
Clam, hardshell	0.6	Trace	31
Clam, littleneck	0.8	Trace	—
Mussel, blue	2.2	0.5	38
Octopus, common	1.0	0.2	—
Oyster, Pacific	2.3	0.6	—
Scallop, unspecified	0.8	0.2	45
Squid, unspecified	1.1	0.3	—
Fish oils			
Cod liver oil	100.0	18.5	570
Herring oil	100.0	11.4	766
MaxEPA‡	100.0	29.4	600
Salmon oil	100.0	19.9	485

*20:5 plus 22:6.

†Dashes indicate a lack of reliable cholesterol data at the present time.

‡Hall Labs, Portland, OR 97219; Jones Medical Industries, St. Louis, MO 63146; Miller Pharmaceutical Group, West Chicago, IL 60185; Moore H.L. Drug Exchange, New Britain, CT 06050; Nature Made Vitamins, Los Angeles, CA 91331; The Rexall Group, Ft Lauderdale, FL 33334; Rugby Labs, Rockville Centre, NY 11570; Schein Pharmaceutical, Port Washington, NY 11050; and Sundown Vitamins, Ft Lauderdale, FL 33334.

From Hepburn FN, et al. Sources of omega-3 fatty acids in seafood. *J Am Diet Assoc.* 1986;86:788; and from USDA publication HNIS/PT-103.

For additional information the reader should see King I, Childs MT, Dorsett C, et al. Shellfish: proximate composition, minerals, fatty acids, and sterols. *J Am Diet Assoc.* 1990;90:677.

Table 14.25
Other Sources of Omega-3 Fatty Acids (100-g Raw Edible Portion)

	Fat, g	Omega-3 Fatty Acids, g	Cholesterol, mg
Broccoli	0.4	0.1	0
Butternuts, dried	57.0	8.7	0
Soybeans, green	21.3	3.2	0
Soybean oil	100.0	6.8	0
Strawberries	0.4	0.1	0
Beans, common, dry	1.5	0.6	0
Walnuts, black	56.5	3.3	0
Walnut oil	100.0	10.4	0
Beef, ground	27.0	0.2	85
Butter	81.1	1.2	219
Chicken, broiler fryers	14.8	0.1	90
Lamb, leg	17.6	0.3	71
Pork bacon	57.5	0.8	67

Adapted from Hepburn FN, et al. Sources of omega-3 fatty acids in seafood. *J Am Diet Assoc* 1986; 86:788.

Table 14.26
Leaner Meat Cuts—Less Than 200 Calories per 3-oz Cooked, Trimmed Serving

	Calories	Total Fat, g	Cholesterol, mg
Beef			
Eye round, roasted	155	5.5	59
Top round, broiled	162	5.3	72
Round tip, roasted	162	6.4	69
Top loin, broiled	172	7.6	65
Tenderloin, broiled	174	7.9	72
Sirloin, broiled	177	7.4	76
Brisket, point portion, braised	181	7.3	81
T-bone, broiled	182	7.4	68
Porterhouse, broiled	185	7.7	68
Rib, small end, broiled	188	9.6	68
Rib-eye, small end, broiled	191	8.8	68
Chuck arm, braised	196	8.5	85
Pork			
Boneless ham, canned, roasted	140	7.0	35
Tenderloin, roasted	141	4.1	79
Leg, shank portion, roasted	183	8.9	78
Leg, whole, roasted	187	9.4	80
Leg, rump portion, roasted	187	9.1	81
Shoulder, arm picnic, roasted	194	10.7	81
Loin, center, broiled	196	8.9	83
Lamb			
Leg, shank portion, roasted	153	5.7	74
Fore shank, braised	159	5.1	88
Leg, sirloin portion, roasted	174	7.8	78
Shoulder blade chop, broiled	181	9.5	77
Loin chop, broiled	183	8.2	80
Rack (rib), roasted	197	11.4	74
Veal			
Rib, roasted	151	6.3	97
Cutlet, pan-fried	156	3.9	91
Arm steak, braised	139	4.9	93
Blade steak, braised	168	5.5	135
Sirloin steak, braised	143	5.3	89

The USDA composition of foods is taken from: (1) USDA Human Nutrition Information Service. *Beef Products.* 1986. US Dept of Agriculture handbook 8-13. (2) *Pork Products.* 1983. US Dept of Agriculture handbook 8-10. (3) *Veal Products.* 1988. US Dept of Agriculture handbook 8-17. Preliminary data. (4) Ono K, Berry B, Johnson HK, et al. Nutrient composition of lamb of two age groups. *J Food Sci.* 1984; 49:1233.

Table 14.27
WIN (Willmar Involved in Nutrition) Against Cancer Program Meat, Poultry, and Fish Criteria for a High-Fiber, Low-Fat Diet

Message

- Trim fat from beef and pork
- Try low-fat cooking methods: bake, broil, roast, braise, stew, stir-fry
- Use 4 oz raw (3 oz cooked) per serving (about the size of a deck of cards)

Beef
All trimmed round cuts
- Round steak
- Bottom round roast
- Bottom round steak
- Cubed steak
- Eye of the round roast
- Eye of the round steak
- Heel of the round
- Rump roast
- Tip roast
- Tip steak
- Stew meat if trimmed and from round
- Specific round cuts may have a "local" name

Ground beef
- 85% extra-lean

Loin
All trimmed loin cuts
- Porterhouse steak
- T-bone steak
- Tenderloin roast
- Tenderloin steak
- Tenderloin tips
- Top loin steak
- Sirloin steak
- Sirloin roast

Chuck
- Chuck arm roast
- Chuck arm steak

Pork
- Canadian bacon
- Center loin chop
- Trimmed hams, cured
- Leg steak
- Tenderloin roast
- Tenderloin strips

Turkey and chicken
- All fresh or frozen turkey that is not breaded
- Remove skin before cooking

Fish and seafood
- All fresh or frozen fish and seafood that is not breaded

Reprinted with permission.

Table 14.28
Dietary Fiber Content (in g) of Selected Foods

Food	**Total Dietary Fiber**	**Water-Soluble Fiber**	**Percentage Soluble Fiber**
Oatmeal, dry, 1/3 cup	2.58	1.33	52
Oat bran, dry, 1/3 cup	4.03	2.01	50
All-bran, 1/3 cup	8.61	1.43	17
Corn flakes, 1 cup	0.36	0.11	29
Brown rice, 1/2 cup	2.4	0.5	20
Spaghetti, 1/2 cup	0.8	0.3	40
White bread, 1 slice	0.51	0.25	49
Whole-wheat bread, 1 slice	1.37	0.30	22
Carrots, raw, 1/2 cup	1.28	0.61	48
Broccoli, frozen, 1/2 cup	2.80	1.25	45
Kidney beans, canned, 1/2 cup	7.92	1.99	25
Pinto beans, canned, 1/2 cup	4.28	1.00	23
White beans, canned, 1/2 cup	4.98	1.49	30
Apple, raw, 1 small	2.74	0.97	35
Orange, 1 small	1.08	0.63	58
Purple plums, canned, 1/3 cup	2.89	0.95	33
Blueberries, 1/2 cup	2.5	0.29	40

Adapted with permission from Anderson JW, Bridges SA. Fiber. ©*Am J Clin Nutr.* 1988; 47:440, and from Anderson JW. *Plant Fiber in Foods.* HCF Nutrition Research Foundation, Inc, PO Box 22124, Lexington, KY 40522, 1986. A more extensive list can be purchased from Dr James Anderson, HCF Nutrition Research Foundation, Inc, PO Box 22124, Lexington, KY 40522.

Table 14.29
Some Commercial Cookies, Crackers, and Baked Goods Containing 30% or Less of Calories From Fat

Cookies

Archway
- Old Fashioned Molasses
- Date Oatmeal
- Apple Oatmeal
- Oatmeal Rounds

Sunshine
- Animal Crackers
- Golden Fruit Raisin Biscuit
- Lemon Coolers
- Gingersnaps
- Honey Grahams

Nabisco
- Honey Maid Grahams
- Fig, Apple, Blueberry, Cherry, and other Newtons

Nabisco (Cont)
- Gingersnaps
- Barnum's Animal Crackers
- Pantry Molasses
- Social Tea Biscuits
- Nilla Wafers
- Devils Food Cakes
- National Arrowroot Biscuit

Lance
- Fig Bar
- Choco-o-Lunch
- Van-o-Lunch
- Apple Cinnamon Cookie
- Strawberry Cookie
- Blueberry Cookie

FFV
- Devils Food Trolley Cake

Keebler
- Cinnamon Crisps

Health Valley
- Peanut Butter
- Oatmeal Jumbos

LU
- Les Petit-Beurre
- Milk Lunch Cookies

Rippin' Good
- Cookie Jar Assortment
- Lemon Crisp

Crackers

Sunshine
- Krispy Saltine
- Oyster Crackers

Lance
- Captains Wafers
- Rye Twins
- Sesame Twins
- Wheat Twins
- Wheatwafers
- Saltines
- Oyster Crackers

Melba toast: all flavors and brands

FFV
- Ocean Crisp
- Sesame Crisp
- Sesame Crisp Wafers

Hain
- Wheat Rye

Manischewitz
- All matzos except egg-type

OTC
- Oyster Chowder

Pepperidge Farms
- English Water Biscuits
- Sesame Crackers
- Goldfish, pretzel-type
- Snack Sticks: Rye and Pumpernickel

RyKrisp
- Original
- Seasoned

Stella D'Oro
- Dietetic Bread Sticks

Waldorf
- Low Sodium Crackers

Finn Crisp
- All Flavors

Kavli
- Thin Bread

Wasa
- Fiber

Nabisco
- Oysterettes
- Premium Saltines
- Triscuits
- Uneeda Biscuits
- Zwieback Toast
- Golden Rye
- Hearty Rye
- Light Rye

Rice cakes: all flavors and brands

Commercial Baked Goods

Snack Cakes
- Hostess: Lil' Angels

Frozen Muffins
- Pepperidge Farms
  - Carrot Walnut
  - Cinnamon Swirl

Frozen Cakes
- Weight Watchers
  - Strawberry Cheesecake
  - Pound Cake with Blueberries

Betty Crocker
- Applesauce Raisin Snackin' Cake

Reprinted with permission from Kwiterovich P. *Beyond Cholesterol.* Baltimore, Md: Johns Hopkins University Press; 1989.

Table 14.30
Low-fat Cheeses

Variety	Calories per 1 oz	Fat, g	Cholesterol, mg	Calcium, mg	Serving Suggestions
American flavor					Use for sandwiches, salads.
Pasteurized process					
Alpine Lace Fat Free	35	0	5	180	
Borden Light American Singles	70	5	15	200	
Cheese Smart (Gamay) Singles	35	0	0	200	
Harvest Moon	70	4	15	200	
Light'n Lively (Kraft)	70	4	15	200	
Lite-line (Borden)	50	2	10	200	
Lite-line Reduced Sodium Singles (Borden)	70	4	20	200	
Weight Watchers Dijon American	50	2	8	200	
Blue-cheese flavor					Sharp, distinctive flavor. Use for appetizers, salads, salad dressings.
Nauvoo Low Fat	76	4	15	88	
Cheddar flavor					Mild to sharp flavor. Use for snacks, sandwiches, casseroles, sauces, on pie.
Natural cheddar style					
Cabot Light Vitalait	70	5	15	250	
Heidi Ann Ched-Style	83	5	14	200	
Lake to Lake Cheddar Style	80	5	30	200	
Lifetime Mild Cheddar	65	3	9	400	
Kraft Light Naturals	84	5	18	215	
Olympia's Natural Low Fat	90	6	25	200	
Ryser	85	5	14	200	
Simon's Low Fat	89	6	17	NA*	
Swiss Valley	80	5	20	200	
Weight Watchers Natural, Shredded	80	5	28	200	
Pasteurized process					
Cheese Smart (Gamay) Bar, Shredded	35	0	0	200	
Light'n Lively (Kraft) Sharp Cheddar	70	4	15	150	
Lite-line (Borden) Mild, Sharp Cheddar	50	2	10	200	
Cheese food					Use for snacks, sandwiches, casseroles.
Maritime					
Sharp Cheddar, Vegetable Garden, Nacho Party Spreads	70	3.5	16	150	
Pine River					
Vegetable Garden Lite, French Onion Lite Party Spreads	70	3.5	16	150	
Rio Del Pino					
Nacho Lite Fiesta Spread	70	3.5	16	150	
Weight Watchers Cheese Cups					
Port Wine, Sharp Cheddar, Cheddar/Onion	70	4	10	200	
Cheese spread					
Cheese Smart (Gamay) Cheddar, nacho and jalapeno	25	0	0	150	
Cheez Whiz (Kraft)					
Pasteurized Process Mild Mexican, Hot Mexican, Jalapeno Peppers, Pimento, Jalapeno	80	6	20	100	
Cracker Barrel Brand					
Cheese Log, Cheese Ball	90	6	15	150	
Easy Cheese (Nabisco)					
All flavors	80	6	15	100	
Heritage House American Singles					
Pasteurized Process	80	6	16	150	
Hickory Farms					
Light Choice					
Sharp Cheddar, Creamy Swiss	70	4	15	200	
Port Wine	80	4	10	200	
Premium Sharp Cheese Ball	80	4	13	150	

Table 14.30
Low-fat Cheeses—(Cont.)

Variety	Calories per 1 oz	Fat, g	Cholesterol, mg	Calcium, mg	Serving Suggestions
Hernke Lite Spread, all flavors	70	3.5	15	150	
Kraft Flavored Spreads					
Jalapeno Pepper	70	5	15	150	
Olive & Pimento	60	5	15	40	
Pimento	70	5	15	40	
Pineapple	70	5	15	40	
Relish	70	5	15	20	
Kraft Pasteurized Process Spreads					
American	80	6	20	150	
Cheese Spread with Garlic	80	6	15	150	
Laughing Cow Pasteurized Process Wedges	72	6	18	140	
Reduced Calorie Wedges	47	3	7	160	
Mohawk Valley Limburger	70	6	20	100	
Old Fashioned Non Fat Spreads	40	1	1	200	
Roka Blue Spread	70	6	20	60	
Velveeta Pasteurized Process Spread					
All flavors	80	6	20	150	
Velveeta Cheese Slices	90	6	20	150	
Colby flavor					Mild to mellow flavor. Use for sandwiches, salads, snacks.
Natural					
Alpine Lace Colby	85	5	20	200	
Kraft Light Natural	84	5	18	224	
Lake to Lake Colby Style	80	5	25	200	
Swiss Valley Farms	80	5	20	200	
Pasteurized process					
Lite-line (Borden)	50	2	10	200	
Cottage cheese (4-oz serving, ½ cup)†					Mild table cheese. Use for salads, dips, baking.
Dry curd, 0.5% milkfat‡	96	0.5	8	36	
Low-fat, 1% milkfat‡	82	1	5	69	
Low-fat, 2% milkfat‡	101	2	9	77	
Creamed, 4% milkfat‡	117	5	17	68	
Cream cheese					Mild flavor. Use for sandwiches, dips, spreads.
Light Philadelphia	60	5	15	40	
Farmer cheese					Clean, mild flavor. Use for salads, snacks, cooking.
Natural					
Holland Farm	81	5	18	217	
Simon's	80	5	21	200	
Ryser Part Skim	85	5	14	200	
White Clover Dairy	81	5	18	217	
Koch kaese or cook cheese					Use for snacks, spreads.
Tupper, Plain or Caraway	25	0	0.015	100	
Monterey jack flavor					Mild to mellow flavor. Use for salads, sandwiches, Mexican cooking.
Natural					
Alpine Lace	80	4	14	195	
Lake to Lake	80	5	20	200	
Lifetime Natural	65	3	9	400	
Kraft Light Natural	84	5.5	19	217	
Ryser Part Skim	80	4	14	200	
Swiss Valley	80	5	20	200	
Pasteurized process					
Lite-line (Borden)	50	2	10	200	
Mozzarella					Mild flavor. Use for Italian cooking, pizza, lasagna, grilled sandwiches.
Alpine Lace Fat Free	35	0	5	180	
Natural (part-skim)‡	72	5	16	183	
Natural (low-moisture, part-skim)‡	79	5	15	207	

Table 14.30
Low-fat Cheeses—(Cont.)

Variety	Calories per 1 oz	Fat, g	Cholesterol, mg	Calcium, mg	Serving Suggestions
Mozzarella flavor					
Natural					
Lifetime Natural	60	2	7	350	
Polly-O-Lite	70	4	15	200	
Weight Watchers					
Natural, Shredded	70	4	28	250	
Pasteurized process					
Cheese Smart (Gamay)	35	0	0	200	
Muenster flavor					A semisoft cheese, with a mild to mellow flavor. Use for sandwiches, snacks.
Natural					
Ryser Part Skim	85	5	14	200	
Pasteurized process					
Heidi Ann Thinline	85	5	15	200	
Lite-line (Borden)	50	2	10	200	
Pot cheese					Use for snacks, sandwich spread.
Sargento	25	0.2	NA	80	
Tupper Cheese					
Cajun Style, Italian Style, Mexican Style, Natural Flavor	25	0	0.015	100	
Ricotta					Semisweet flavor. Use for cooked dishes, salads, dips, fillings, desserts.
Natural (part-skim)					
Frigo	45	3	10	60	
Sargento	30	2	10	60	
Natural (whole-milk)					
Frigo	50	4	15	60	
Sargento	50	4	15	80	
Frigo Low-Fat	20	1	5	60	
Polly-O-Lite	40	2	7	100	
Sargento Lite	23	1	14	34	
Scamorza					Mild flavor. Use for cooking Italian dishes.
Natural (part-skim)‡	70	5	16	180	
Natural (low-moisture, part-skim)‡	79	5	15	207	
Semisoft part-skim cheese/skim-milk cheese					Creamy yellow or white. Mild to robust flavors. Use for snacks, sandwiches, cheese trays.
Dairy Lean (Zimmerman)	72	4.5	17	200	
Fromage Blanc	19	0	5	NA	
Laughing Cow					
Mini-BonBel Reduced Calorie	60	4	11	200	
Cheesebits Reduced Calorie					
Pasteurized Process	48	2	18	150	
String/strip					Mild flavor. Use for snacks.
Natural					
Arpin	85	6	15	200	
Baker	80	5	15	200	
Dorman Light Strip	85	6	12	200	
Dorman Strip Low Sodium	70	4	12	200	
Kraft with Jalapeno Peppers	80	5	20	200	
Falbo	90	6	NA	200	
Sargento	80	5	15	200	
Sargento Smoked	80	5	15	200	
Tolibia	72	5	16	200	

Table 14.30
Low-fat Cheeses—(Cont.)

Variety	Calories per 1 oz	Fat, g	Cholesterol, mg	Calcium, mg	Serving Suggestions
Swiss flavor					Mild, nutty, sweet flavor. Use for sandwiches, salads, fondue, casseroles.
Natural					
Heidi Ann Swiss Style	97	6	19	274	
Kraft Light Natural	86	5	21	326	
Lifetime	60	3	9	350	
Swiss Valley Farms	80	6	20	400	
Weight Watchers	50	2	8	200	
Pasteurized processed					
Light'n Lively (Kraft)	70	4	15	200	
Lite-line (Borden)	50	2	10	200	
Whey cheese					Slightly sweet, caramel colored. Use as wafer-thin slices on crackers.
Northern Light Primost	84	0.9	5	120	

*NA indicates information not available.

†Calories per ½-cup, 4-oz serving.

‡Nutrient values for cheeses with a standard of identity are from *Composition of Foods: Dairy and Egg Products, Raw, Processed, Prepared.* US Dept of Agriculture handbook 8-1, 1976. For cheese varieties with no standard of identity, brand names have been given with the nutrient values provided by the manufacturers.

Adapted and reprinted with permission from "A Cheese Lover's Guide to Low Fat Cheeses." ©April 1989. Dairy Council of Wisconsin, Inc. Westmont, IL 60559. All rights reserved. "A Cheese Lover's Guide to Low Fat Cheeses" may be ordered from Dairy Council of Wisconsin, Inc., 999 Oakmont Plaza Drive, Suite 510, Westmont, IL 60559.

Table 14.31
Bruce Protocol for Treadmill Testing*

Time, min	Stage	Speed, mph	Elevation, %	Approximate METs
0–3	I	1.7	10	5
3–6	II	2.5	12	7
6–9	III	3.4	14	9
9–12	IV	4.2	16	13
12–15	V	5.0	18	17
15–18	VI	5.5	20	20

*This protocol may be too strenuous for cardiac patients. Modified protocols are listed in Tables 14.32 and 14.33. Note that all protocols will get the patients to the maximum end point; however, some test protocols will get them there faster than others.

$$\dagger\text{MET} = \frac{\text{Oxygen Required for Exercise}}{\text{Oxygen Required at Rest (3.5 mL/kg/min)}}$$

Reprinted with permission from Bruce RA. Exercise testing of patients with coronary heart disease. *Ann Clin Res.* 1971;3:323.

Table 14.32
Balke Protocol for Treadmill Testing

Time, min	Speed, mph	Elevation, %	Approximate METs
0–2	3.0	2.5	4
3–4	3.0	5.0	5
5–6	3.0	7.5	6
7–8	3.0	10.0	7
9–10	3.0	12.5	8
11–12	3.0	15.0	9
13–14	3.0	17.5	11
15–16	3.0	20.0	12
17–18	3.0	22.5	13
19–20	3.0	25.0	14

From Balke B, Ware RW. An experimental study of physical fitness of Air Force personnel. *US Armed Forces Med J.* 1959;10:675.

Table 14.33
Low-Level Treadmill Test

Time, min	Stage	Speed, mph	Grade, %	METs
3	1	1.5	0	2.8
3	2	1.5	4	3.2
3	3	1.5	8	3.7
3	4	1.7	10	4.0
3	5	2.0	12	5.0

Reprinted with permission from Ellestad M. *Stress Testing Principals and Practice*. Philadelphia, Pa: F. A. Davis Co; 1980.

Table 14.34
Taking Your Pulse

For you fitness program to provide a good conditioning effect, you must exercise your heart within its target heart-rate zone. To monitor your heart rate, you must learn how to count your pulse. Two pulse points are felt most easily during or after exercise:

Radial Pulse

The radial pulse point is located in the wrist at the base of the thumb; it is best felt with the pads of two fingers of the opposite hand. Pressing the artery too hard will obliterate the pulse.

Carotid Pulse

The carotid pulse point is located in the neck on either side of the windpipe at the jaw angle. With the thumb on the chin, the fingers can easily feel the pulse just inside the vertical strip of muscles in the neck.

Measure your exercise heart rate by performing your prescribed exercise for 3 minutes; then stop and immediately count your pulse for 10 seconds. Multiply this number by 6 to obtain your pulse rate per minute. Modify your exercise intensity to keep your pulse rate within the recommended range established by the program.

Pulse rate is not the only indicator of your exercise continuation. Modify the intensity when you feel that your level of exertion has become too intense.

Table 14.35
Average Work Intensities for Activities Suitable for Exercise Prescription

Activity	Average Work Intensity	
	METs	kcal/hr (75 kg)
Walking, 0% grade		
2.5 mph	3.0	225
3.0	3.3	240
3.5	3.5	262
4.0	4.6	345
Jogging-running		
4.5 mph	5–7*	375-490
5.0	8.4	630
6.0	10.0	750
7.0	11.4	855
8.0	12.8	960
Cycling (ergometer)		
300 kpm	3.7	278
450	5.0	375
600	6.0	450
750	7.0	525
900	8.5	630
1,050	10.0	750
1,200	11.0	825
1,500	13.5	1,010
Swimming, crawl†		
20 yd/min	6.0	420
30	9.0	675
40	12.0	900
Games (average intensity)		
basketball	7-15	525-1,125
volleyball	5-12	375-900
soccer	7-15	525-1,125
handball	8-12	600-900
tennis	6-10	450-750

*The metabolic cost of jogging at 4 to 5 mph is variable owing to the transition between a fast walk and slow jog.

†The metabolic cost of swimming is highly variable owing to efficiency, buoyancy, and technique; values may vary by 25%.

Reprinted with permission from Acierno LJ. *Comprehensive Cardiac Rehabilitation and Prevention: A Model Program.* New York, NY: Immergut Siolek Pub; 1985.

Table 14.36
Suggested Exercise-Equipment Suppliers

Exercise Bicycles

Allegheny International Exercise Co
Vitamaster
PO Box 778
Lincolnton, NC 28092
704/735-6582

Amerec Corp
1776 136th Pl, NE
Bellevue, WA 98009
800/426-0858

AMF
American Athletic Equipment Div
200 American Ave
Jefferson, IA 50129
800/247-3978

Bally Fitness Products Corp
10 Thomas Rd
Irvine, CA 92714

Bodyguard, Inc
245 W. Roosevelt Rd
Bldg 15, Suite 6
West Chicago, IL 60185
800/553-1186

Eclipse, Inc
Box 3701
Ann Arbor, MI 48106
800/521-3092

Engineering Dynamics Corp
120 Stedman St
Lowell, MA 01851-2797

Excel
9935 Beverly Blvd
Pico Rivera, CA 90660

Excelsior Fitness Equipment Co
615 Landwehr Rd
Northbrook, IL 60062

Exxersource
14940 Clavert St
Van Nuys, CA 91411
800/241-4593 (in Calif)
800/421-6758

Feumex, Inc
Cybex Div
2100 Smithtown Ave
Ronkonkoma, NY 11779

Fitness Products Corp
9601 Jeronimo Rd
PO Box 19704
Irvine, CA 92718

Heart Mate
260 W. Beach Ave
Inglewood, CA 90302
213/677-8131

Hooker Performance
1024 W. Brooks St
Ontario, CA 91761
714/983-5871

Kreitler Custom Rollers, Inc
5102 Bannister Rd
Kansas City, MO 64137
816/765-0635

Marcy
2801 W. Mission Rd
Alhambra, CA 91803
818/570-1222

M&R Industries
7140 180th Ave, NE
Redmond, WA 98052
800/222-9995
206/885-1010 (in Wash)

Monark Ergometers and Exercise Cycles
(Universal Fitness Products)
50 Commercial St
Plainview, NY 11803
800/645-7554
516/349-8600 (in NY)

J. Oglaend, Inc
40 Radio Cir
Mt Kisco, NY 10549
800/828-1186
914/666-2272 (in NY)

Precor Co
9449 151st Ave, NE
Redmond, WA 98052
206/881-8982

Racer Mate, Inc
3016 NE Blakely
Seattle, WA 98105
206/524-7392

Schwinn Air-Dyne
Excelsior Fitness Equipment Co
615 Landwehr Rd
Northbrook, IL 60062
or
Schwinn Bicycle Co
Air-Dyne Division
217 N. Jefferson
Chicago, IL 60606

Tunturi, Inc
Box 3825
Bellevue, WA 98009

Universal Gym Equipment, Inc
PO Box 1270
Cedar Rapids, IA 52406
800/553-7901

Wimbledon Industries
260 W. Beach Ave
Inglewood, CA 90302

Table 14.36
Suggested Exercise-Equipment Suppliers—(Cont.)

Treadmills

Amerec Corp
1776 136th Pl, NE
Bellevue, WA 98009
800/426-0858

Allegheny International Exercise Co
Vitamaster
PO Box 778
Lincolnton, NC 28092
704/735-6582

Eaton Medical Corp
854 Phoenix Dr
Ann Arbor, MI 48104-7502

Landice Products
269 E. Blackwell St
Dover, NJ 07801
201/328-6560

M&R Industries
9215 151st Ave, NE
Redmond, WA 98052
800/222-9995

Pacer Industries
8201 Sovereign Row
Dallas, TX 75247
800/874-9090

Precor Co
9449 151st Ave, NE
Redmond, WA 98052
206/881-8982

Quinton Instrument Co
2121 Terry Ave
Seattle, WA 98121-2791
800/426-0337

Roadmaster
Radio Tower Rd
Olney, IL 62450
618/393-2991

Sportech
Box 99101
Cleveland, OH 44199
800/221-1258
216/566-7873

Trotter Treadmills, Inc
24 Hopedale St
Hopedale, MA 01747
617/473-0600

Universal Gym Equipment, Inc
PO Box 1270
Cedar Rapids, IA 52406
800/553-7901

Rowing Machines

Allegheny International Exercise Co
Vitamaster
PO Box 778
Lincolnton, NC 28092
704/735-6582

Amerec Corp
1776 136th Place, NE
Bellevue, WA 98009
800/426-0858

AMF
American Athletic Equipment Div
200 American Ave
Jefferson, IA 50129
800/247-3978

Concept II, Inc
RR1, Box 1100
Morrisville, VT 05661-9727

Diversified Products
PO Box 100
Opelika, AL 36803
205/749-9001

Excel
9935 Beverly Blvd
Pico Rivera, CA 90660
213/699-0311

Excelsior Fitness Equipment Co
615 Landwehr Rd
Northbrook, IL 60062
800/228-3737

Fitness Products Corp
9601 Jeronimo Rd
PO Box 19704
Irvine, CA 92718

G.E. Miller, Inc.
484 S. Broadway
Yonkers, NY 10705

Universal Fitness Products
50 Commercial St
Plainview, NY 11803

Stair Machines

Stair Master Sports/Medical Products
259 Rt 17K
Newburgh, NY 12550
800/772-0089

Heart-Rate Monitors

Amerec Pulse Meter
Amerec Corp
1776 136th Pl, NE
Bellevue, WA 98009
800/426-0858

Other

NordicTrack
(Cross-country ski simulator)
141C Jonathan Blvd N
Chaska, MN 55318
800/328-5888

Universal Gym Equipment, Inc
Box 1270
Cedar Rapids, IA 52406

INDEX

NOTES